Differential Diagnoses in Surgical Pathology
Non-Neoplastic Dermatopathology

Differential Diagnoses in Surgical Pathology: Non-Neoplastic Dermatopathology

Deborah L. Cook, MD

Professor, Department of Pathology
Robert Larner, MD College of Medicine at The University of Vermont Medical Center
Dermatopathologist
Department of Pathology and Laboratory Medicine
University of Vermont Medical Center
Burlington, Vermont

SERIES EDITOR

Jonathan I. Epstein, MD

Professor of Pathology, Urology, and Oncology
The Reinhard Professor of Urological Pathology
Director of Surgical Pathology
The Johns Hopkins Medical Institutions
Baltimore, Maryland

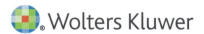

Philadelphia • Baltimore • New York • London
Buenos Aires • Hong Kong • Sydney • Tokyo

Acquisitions Editor: Nicole Dernoski
Development Editor: Ariel S. Winter
Editorial Coordinator: Sunmerrilika Baskar
Marketing Manager: Kirsten Watrud
Production Project Manager: Bridgett Dougherty
Manager, Graphic Arts & Design: Stephen Druding
Manufacturing Coordinator: Lisa Bowling
Prepress Vendor: TNQ Technologies

Copyright © 2024 Wolters Kluwer.

All rights reserved. This book is protected by copyright. No part of this book may be reproduced or transmitted in any form or by any means, including as photocopies or scanned-in or other electronic copies, or utilized by any information storage and retrieval system without written permission from the copyright owner, except for brief quotations embodied in critical articles and reviews. Materials appearing in this book prepared by individuals as part of their official duties as U.S. government employees are not covered by the above-mentioned copyright. To request permission, please contact Wolters Kluwer at Two Commerce Square, 2001 Market Street, Philadelphia, PA 19103, via email at permissions@lww.com, or via our website at shop.lww.com (products and services).

9 8 7 6 5 4 3 2 1

Printed in Mexico

Library of Congress Cataloging-in-Publication Data

ISBN-13: 978-1-975184-65-0

Cataloging in Publication data available on request from publisher.

This work is provided "as is," and the publisher disclaims any and all warranties, express or implied, including any warranties as to accuracy, comprehensiveness, or currency of the content of this work.

This work is no substitute for individual patient assessment based upon healthcare professionals' examination of each patient and consideration of, among other things, age, weight, gender, current or prior medical conditions, medication history, laboratory data and other factors unique to the patient. The publisher does not provide medical advice or guidance and this work is merely a reference tool. Healthcare professionals, and not the publisher, are solely responsible for the use of this work including all medical judgments and for any resulting diagnosis and treatments.

Given continuous, rapid advances in medical science and health information, independent professional verification of medical diagnoses, indications, appropriate pharmaceutical selections and dosages, and treatment options should be made and healthcare professionals should consult a variety of sources. When prescribing medication, healthcare professionals are advised to consult the product information sheet (the manufacturer's package insert) accompanying each drug to verify, among other things, conditions of use, warnings and side effects and identify any changes in dosage schedule or contraindications, particularly if the medication to be administered is new, infrequently used or has a narrow therapeutic range. To the maximum extent permitted under applicable law, no responsibility is assumed by the publisher for any injury and/or damage to persons or property, as a matter of products liability, negligence law or otherwise, or from any reference to or use by any person of this work.

shop.lww.com

PREFACE

We work with differential diagnoses in our everyday practice of medicine. In the arena of dermatopathology, we are charged with utilizing microscopic features to distinguish between skin diseases that are similar histopathologically but different clinically and in biologic behavior. Perhaps no other organ in the body has as many diseases that look alike histologically than does the skin. Because of this, nonneoplastic dermatopathology is one of the more difficult areas of surgical pathology for trainees, general pathologists, and dermatopathologists. Distinction between two entities often relies on very subtle histologic features and, ultimately, correlation with the clinical presentation.

This book provides an approach to inflammatory dermatopathology, with each chapter focusing on pathology of a specific anatomic component of the skin or disease category. Each section within a chapter examines two entities that histologically simulate one another. The apparent similarities for each differential diagnosis are compared and contrasted in outline form and illustrated with microscopic images. Essential ancillary studies, including histochemical and immunohistochemical stains, direct immunofluorescence, and molecular analyses, are incorporated into the differential diagnosis. Importantly, the clinical presentation of each entity is discussed for clinicopathologic correlation.

The scope of nonneoplastic dermatopathology is exceptionally broad, and this book does not attempt to address every possible differential diagnosis. Emphasis is on the more common diseases that one could encounter in their daily sign-out. The objective is to dispel some of the confusion and trepidation concerning inflammatory dermatoses.

We hope that trainees and practicing pathologists will enjoy this volume in the *Differential Diagnoses in Surgical Pathology* series and find it useful in their study of dermatopathology and diagnosis of dermatologic specimens.

ACKNOWLEDGMENTS

I would like to thank my teachers and mentors at the University of Vermont and the Medical University of South Carolina who instilled in me the love of surgical pathology and dermatopathology. It is a pleasure to work in an academic environment with energetic residents, inquisitive fellows, and supportive colleagues in both pathology and dermatology. I would also like to acknowledge the administrative staff at the University of Vermont Medical Center who assisted in collecting cases for this book. I am indebted to the patients who challenge my knowledge and inspire me to continue learning every day. Last, and most importantly, I would like to thank and dedicate this book to my loving and supportive husband, Joe, and daughter, Grace.

CONTENTS

Preface v
Acknowledgments vii

Chapter 1	**INFLAMMATORY DISEASES OF THE EPIDERMIS**	1
Chapter 2	**INFLAMMATORY DISEASES OF THE DERMIS**	80
Chapter 3	**VESICULOBULLOUS DISEASES**	154
Chapter 4	**DISORDERS OF THE ADNEXAE**	210
Chapter 5	**DISORDERS OF THE SUBCUTIS**	244
Chapter 6	**ALTERATIONS OF THE EPIDERMIS AND DERMIS**	283
Chapter 7	**INFECTIOUS DISEASES AND INFESTATIONS OF THE SKIN**	344

Index 417

1 Inflammatory Diseases of the Epidermis

1.1 Allergic Contact Dermatitis vs Irritant Contact Dermatitis
1.2 Photoallergic Dermatitis vs Phototoxic Dermatitis
1.3 Dyshidrotic Dermatitis vs Palmoplantar Pustular Psoriasis
1.4 Atopic Dermatitis (Eczema) vs Mycosis Fungoides
1.5 Pityriasis Rosea vs Erythema Annulare Centrifugum
1.6 Pityriasis Rosea vs Guttate Psoriasis
1.7 Nummular Dermatitis vs Dermatophytosis
1.8 Nummular Dermatitis vs Psoriasis (Plaque Type)
1.9 Psoriasis (Plaque Type) vs Seborrheic Dermatitis
1.10 Pityriasis Rubra Pilaris vs Psoriasis (Plaque Type)
1.11 Psoriasis vs Lichen Simplex Chronicus
1.12 Acute Generalized Exanthematous Pustulosis vs Psoriasis (Pustular Type)
1.13 Lichen Planus vs Lupus Erythematosus
1.14 Lichen Planus vs Lichen Planus–Like Keratosis
1.15 Lichenoid Drug Eruption vs Lichen Planus
1.16 Lichen Planus vs Lichen Sclerosus
1.17 Hypertrophic Lichen Planus vs Squamous Cell Carcinoma
1.18 Lichen Nitidus vs Lichen Striatus
1.19 Lichen Nitidus vs Langerhans Cell Histiocytosis
1.20 Pityriasis Lichenoides et Varioliformis Acuta vs Pityriasis Lichenoides Chronica
1.21 Pityriasis Lichenoides et Varioliformis Acuta vs Lymphomatoid Papulosis
1.22 Erythema Multiforme vs Pityriasis Lichenoides et Varioliformis Acuta
1.23 Graft-Versus-Host Disease, Acute vs Erythema Multiforme
1.24 Fixed Drug Eruption vs Erythema Multiforme
1.25 Erythema Multiforme vs Morbilliform Drug Eruption
1.26 Toxic Epidermal Necrolysis vs Staphylococcal Scalded Skin Syndrome
1.27 Radiation Dermatitis, Chronic vs Lichen Sclerosus
1.28 Dermatomyositis vs Lupus Erythematosus (Discoid)
1.29 Lupus Erythematosus (Subacute Cutaneous) vs Polymorphous Light Eruption

1.1 ALLERGIC CONTACT DERMATITIS VS IRRITANT CONTACT DERMATITIS

	Allergic Contact Dermatitis	Irritant Contact Dermatitis
Age	Any age.	Any age.
Location	Hands and face, especially eyelids, most common sites of involvement although any area of body may be affected. Distribution aids in diagnosis and identification of allergen. May also present in a generalized fashion.	Any location but face and hands predominately in adults. Diaper area in infants and perioral area in children.
Etiology	Type IV delayed hypersensitivity reaction that occurs as a result of activation of a specific population of T cells by an allergen. Sensitization is the first phase when the individual is exposed to the allergen causing an immune response. This is followed by the elicitation phase during which reexposure to the allergen causes a release of cytokines and inflammation that mediate the cutaneous symptoms.	Caused by direct toxic effect of an irritant on keratinocytes of the epidermis. An irritant may cause direct death of keratinocytes or facilitate disruption of the epithelial barrier, leading to increased permeability. Repetitive injury triggers an innate immune response with release of cytokines. There is activation of Langerhans cells and dermal dendritic cells with subsequent recruitment of lymphocytes, histiocytes, neutrophils, and mast cells to the skin.
Presentation	Pruritic scaly, erythematous papules and vesicles. Chronic lesions have lichenification and fissuring.	Acute phase characterized by bright erythema and burning sensation. Subacute and chronic forms present with scaly, erythematous plaques with fissuring. Severe cases may have vesiculation and necrosis.
Histology	1. A basket-weave stratum corneum in acute stage *(Fig. 1.1.1)*. Parakeratosis and a serum crust in subacute and chronic lesions. 2. Epidermal hyperplasia with spongiosis and microvesicle formation *(Figs. 1.1.1 and 1.1.2)*. 3. Lymphocytic and eosinophilic exocytosis with aggregates of Langerhans cells within the epidermis *(Fig. 1.1.2)*. 4. A superficial perivascular infiltrate of lymphocytes and eosinophils *(Fig. 1.1.3)*.	1. Focal parakeratosis and mild epidermal hyperplasia *(Fig. 1.1.4)*. 2. Epidermal necrosis with neutrophil exocytosis *(Figs. 1.1.5 and 1.1.6)*. Individual necrotic keratinocytes within the superficial epidermis with mild irritants and confluent superficial necrosis with harsh irritants. 3. Mild epidermal spongiosis *(Fig. 1.1.5)*. 4. A superficial dermal lymphocytic infiltrate *(Fig. 1.1.4)*; eosinophils are not prominent.
Special studies	Patch testing to clinically identify the allergen.	None.
Treatment	Avoidance of the offending allergen. Topical steroids are first-line treatment and topical calcineurin inhibitors are second-line. Antihistamines for itch and emollients to decrease dryness.	Avoidance of the irritant. Emollients to enhance barrier function of skin. Corticosteroids, topical or systemic, or other immunomodulators.
Prognosis	Good prognosis if the individual is able to avoid the allergen.	Isolated lesions generally resolve if the offending irritant is strictly avoided. The condition has a chronic course with relapses if unable to discontinue contact with the irritant.

1.1 Allergic Contact Dermatitis vs Irritant Contact Dermatitis

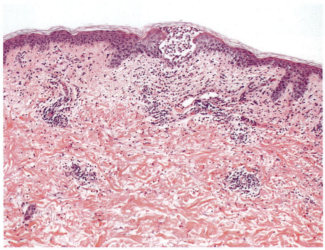

Figure 1.1.1 Allergic contact dermatitis, acute phase. A superficial perivascular and interstitial infiltrate with papillary dermal edema and epidermal spongiosis.

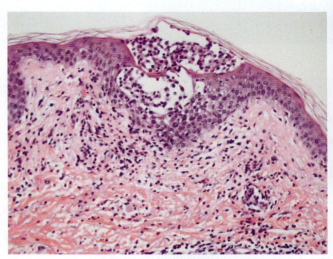

Figure 1.1.2 Allergic contact dermatitis, acute phase. An epidermal spongiotic vesicle with exocytosis of lymphocytes and eosinophils. Aggregates of Langerhans cells within spongiotic focus.

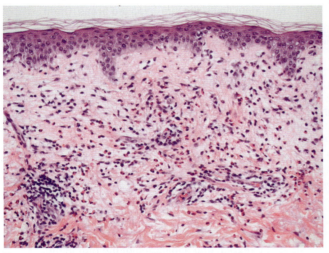

Figure 1.1.3 Allergic contact dermatitis, acute phase. Papillary dermal edema with a moderately dense infiltrate of lymphocytes and eosinophils.

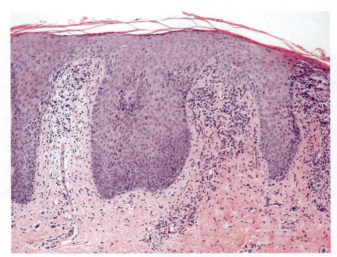

Figure 1.1.4 Irritant contact dermatitis. Epidermal hyperplasia with parakeratosis and lymphocytic exocytosis. A superficial dermal infiltrate of lymphocytes.

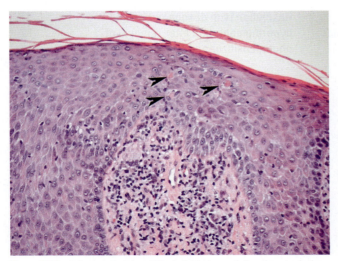

Figure 1.1.5 Irritant contact dermatitis. Individual necrotic keratinocytes in the mid and upper levels of the epidermis (arrowheads).

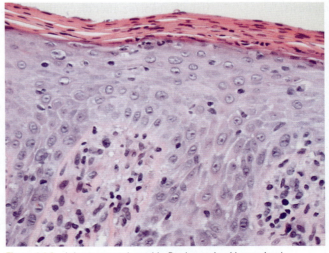

Figure 1.1.6 Irritant contact dermatitis. Parakeratosis with occasional neutrophils within the superficial epidermis and stratum corneum.

1.2 PHOTOALLERGIC DERMATITIS VS PHOTOTOXIC DERMATITIS

	Photoallergic Dermatitis	**Phototoxic Dermatitis**
Age	Any age.	Any age.
Location	Sun-exposed regions but may extend beyond exposed areas.	Sun-exposed regions; face, neck and chest, extensor forearms and hands.
Etiology	Immunologically mediated process in which a photoproduct generates a type IV hypersensitivity reaction. Requires prior sensitization and minimal exposure to the offending agent. Less common than phototoxic reactions.	Direct tissue or cellular injury by a photoproduct after exposure to phototoxic agent and appropriate UVR. It is dose dependent and does not require prior sensitization. More common than photoallergic reactions.
Presentation	Develops 24 h or more after exposure. Presents as an eczematous eruption with pruritic, erythematous, scaly plaques that may extend beyond areas of sun exposure.	Occurs minutes to hours after exposure to sunlight. Presents as an exaggerated sunburn with erythema, edema, and vesicle formation limited to sun-exposed areas. Often resolves with hyperpigmentation. There may be associated burning, stinging, and mild pruritus.
Histology	1. Mild epidermal hyperplasia with focal parakeratosis *(Fig. 1.2.1)*. 2. Epidermal spongiosis with exocytosis of lymphocytes and vesiculation *(Figs. 1.2.2 and 1.2.3)*. May have eosinophils within the epidermis. 3. A superficial and deep perivascular lymphocytic infiltrate with eosinophils *(Fig. 1.2.1)*.	1. Epidermal keratinocyte necrosis ("sunburn cells") *(Fig. 1.2.6)*. 2. May have confluent epidermal necrosis with strong phototoxic agents *(Figs. 1.2.4 and 1.2.5)*. 3. A dermal infiltrate of lymphocytes and neutrophils *(Fig. 1.2.4)*.
Special studies	Photopatch testing.	None.
Treatment	Sun avoidance and discontinuation of the offending agent, generally a medication. Topical steroids and sun-protective measures to minimize symptoms.	Identification and avoidance of the offending agent. Strict photoprotection (UVA and UVB) necessary. Analgesics for any pain and topical steroids for severe episodes.
Prognosis	Usually resolves after discontinuation of the offending agent. Rarely, can persist and evolves into chronic actinic dermatitis.	Resolution with desquamation and hyperpigmentation after removal of photosensitizer and UVR source.

1.2 Photoallergic Dermatitis vs Phototoxic Dermatitis

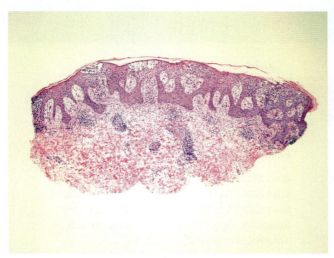

Figure 1.2.1 Photoallergic dermatitis. A superficial and deep perivascular infiltrate with epidermal spongiosis and papillary dermal edema.

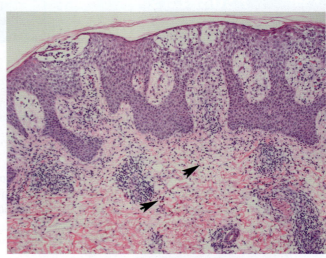

Figure 1.2.2 Photoallergic dermatitis. Mild epidermal hyperplasia with vesiculation, papillary dermal edema, and a dermal lymphocytic infiltrate with eosinophils (arrows).

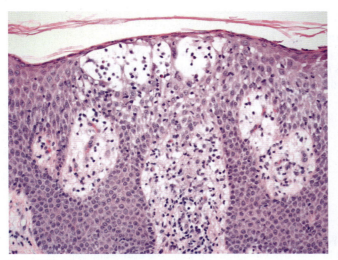

Figure 1.2.3 Photoallergic dermatitis. Epidermal spongiosis with vesiculation and exocytosis of lymphocytes and occasional eosinophils.

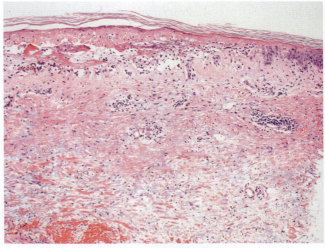

Figure 1.2.4 Phototoxic dermatitis. A superficial to mid-dermal lymphocytic infiltrate with neutrophils and overlying epidermal necrosis.

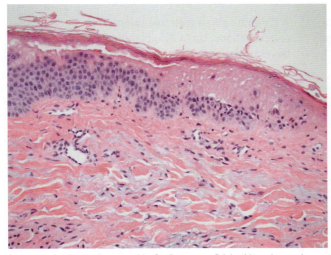

Figure 1.2.5 Phototoxic dermatitis. Confluent superficial epidermal necrosis (seen in severe photosensitizing reactions).

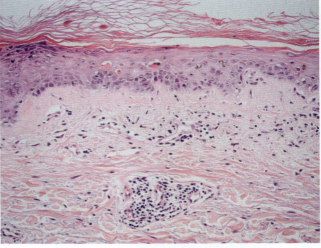

Figure 1.2.6 Phototoxic dermatitis. Other areas of individual necrotic keratinocytes ("sunburn cells") at all levels of the epidermis.

1.3 DYSHIDROTIC DERMATITIS VS PALMOPLANTAR PUSTULAR PSORIASIS

	Dyshidrotic Dermatitis	**Palmoplantar Pustular Psoriasis**
Age	Any age with peak incidence in middle-aged individuals.	Middle-aged adults, between 30 and 50 y of age. Predilection for women.
Location	Palms and soles.	Palms and soles.
Etiology	Unknown but close association with atopy. May be triggered by metal (nickel, cobalt) exposure, warm weather, fungal infection, and psychological stress.	A combination of genetic factors and environmental triggers. Possible association to variations in the genes in the IL-19 family. Antigenic triggers include smoking, stress, irritants, and repetitive trauma.
Presentation	Symmetric, intensely pruritic deep-seated vesicles ("tapioca-like") on lateral aspects of fingers and toes. May progress to bullae.	Pustules that develop a yellow scale or crust and resolve with brown macules. May have hyperkeratosis and fissuring. Symptoms include pruritus and pain with fissuring.
Histology	1. Prominent epidermal spongiosis with formation of large, discrete intraepidermal vesicles *(Figs. 1.3.1-1.3.3)*. 2. Exocytosis of lymphocytes; neutrophils not present unless eroded or superinfected *(Fig. 1.3.2)*. 3. A superficial perivascular lymphohistiocytic infiltrate with occasional eosinophils.	1. Focal parakeratosis with entrapped neutrophils *(Figs. 1.3.5* and *1.3.6)*. 2. Mild epidermal hyperplasia with diminished granular layer and spongiform neutrophilic microabscesses *(Figs. 1.3.5* and *1.3.6)*. 3. A superficial perivascular infiltrate of lymphocytes and occasional neutrophils; eosinophils generally not present *(Fig. 1.3.4)*.
Special studies	PAS stain to exclude fungal infection.	PAS and tissue Gram stains to exclude superficial fungal and bacterial infection.
Treatment	High-potency topical steroids with soaks and cold compresses are first-line therapy. Calcineurin inhibitors may be used in mild to moderate cases. Systemic corticosteroids may be necessary in severe disease. Avoidance of triggers.	Topical treatments include corticosteroids, tar, salicylic acid, calcipotriol, and anthralin. Systemic therapies include oral retinoids, methotrexate, and cyclosporine. A number of biologics are approved for treatment of psoriasis, including the palmopustular variant.
Prognosis	Although episodes typically resolve within a month, it is a chronic condition with frequent recurrences.	A chronic course with remissions and exacerbations. Up to 20% of patients may develop plaque-type psoriasis.

1.3 Dyshidrotic Dermatitis vs Palmoplantar Pustular Psoriasis

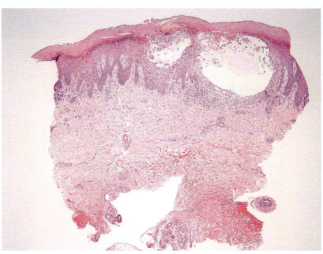

Figure 1.3.1 Dyshidrotic dermatitis. Acral skin with mild epidermal hyperplasia and large, discrete spongiotic vesicles.

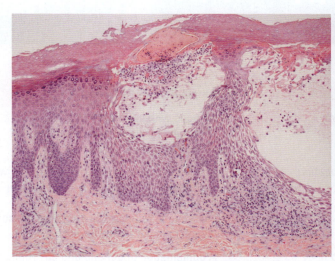

Figure 1.3.2 Dyshidrotic dermatitis. A serum crust with a preserved granular layer and large, discrete spongiotic vesicles with lymphocytic exocytosis. Neutrophils present only in area of erosion.

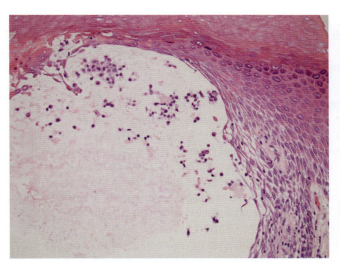

Figure 1.3.3 Dyshidrotic dermatitis. A spongiotic vesicle with lymphocytic exocytosis.

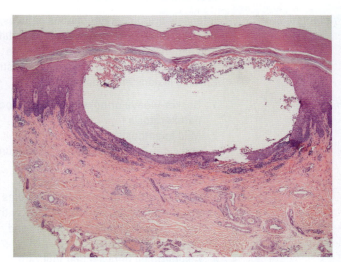

Figure 1.3.4 Palmoplantar pustular psoriasis. Acral skin with discrete spongiform neutrophilic microabscess.

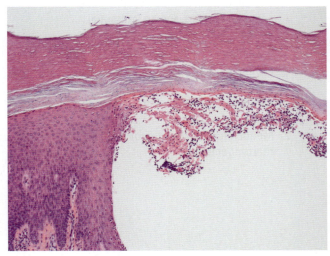

Figure 1.3.5 Palmoplantar pustular psoriasis. Parakeratosis with spongiform microabscess containing neutrophils and degenerated keratinocytes. A diminished granular layer.

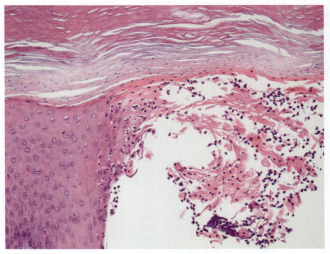

Figure 1.3.6 Palmoplantar pustular psoriasis. Parakeratosis with a diminished granular layer and an edge of spongiform neutrophilic microabscess.

1.4 ATOPIC DERMATITIS (ECZEMA) VS MYCOSIS FUNGOIDES

	Atopic Dermatitis (Eczema)	**Mycosis Fungoides**
Age	All ages with infantile, childhood, and adulthood forms. Approximately 85% of cases begin before 5 y of age.	Any age but primarily adults with highest incidence in those greater than 70 y of age.
Location	May be limited to hands or generalized with erythroderma. Face, neck, and extensor surfaces in infants. Flexural surfaces, including antecubital and popliteal fossae, typical in children and adults.	Sun-protected regions typically, including lower trunk and buttocks.
Etiology	A combination of genetic and environmental factors with a loss of epidermal barrier function and IgE-mediated sensitization to food and environmental allergens.	Chronic antigen stimulation leading to monoclonal proliferation of skin tropic malignant memory T-cell lymphocytes.
Presentation	Intensely pruritic, erythematous papules, plaques, and vesicles with serous exudate and excoriations. Lesions often become superinfected with more extensive crusting. Chronic lesions are lichenified.	Progressive, erythematous, serpiginous patches or thin plaques with variable scale. Lesions progress, at a variable rate, to thicker plaques and tumors.
Histology	1. Basket-weave orthokeratosis with focal parakeratosis *(Fig. 1.4.1)*. 2. Mild acanthosis of epidermis *(Figs. 1.4.1 and 1.4.2)*. Acanthosis is more pronounced in subacute and chronic forms. 3. Variable spongiosis with spongiotic vesicle formation; spongiotic vesicles are "urn-shaped" and associated with exocytosis of small lymphocytes and Langerhans cells *(Figs. 1.4.1-1.4.3)*. 4. A superficial perivascular infiltrate of small lymphocytes and occasional eosinophils *(Figs. 1.4.1 and 1.4.2)*.	1. Slight parakeratosis *(Fig. 1.4.4)*. 2. Epidermotropism of lymphocytes that are larger than lymphocytes in the superficial dermis. Lymphocytes are not associated with appreciable spongiosis. Lymphocytes are aligned along the basal zone and form round aggregates (Pautrier microabscesses) within the epidermis *(Figs. 1.4.5 and 1.4.6)*. 3. Lymphocytes have irregular, hyperchromatic, cerebriform nuclei and are surrounded by a pale cytoplasmic halo *(Fig. 1.4.6)*. 4. The superficial dermis has thickened collagen bundles and an interstitial infiltrate of small lymphocytes with occasional eosinophils and plasma cells.
Special studies	None.	1. Intraepidermal lymphocytes typically show CD3+, CD4+, CD8- phenotype with decreased expression of CD5 and CD7 *(Figs. 1.4.7-1.4.9)*. 2. Monoclonal T-cell receptor gene rearrangement.

1.4 Atopic Dermatitis (Eczema) vs Mycosis Fungoides

	Atopic Dermatitis (Eczema)	**Mycosis Fungoides**
Treatment	Therapy is aimed at controlling symptoms and preventing flares. Hydration of skin with emollients. Topical corticosteroids and topical immunomodulators. Avoidance of irritants and potential allergens.	Treatment is dependent on stage and includes watchful waiting, skin-directed remedies, and systemic therapies. Skin-directed therapies including topical corticosteroids, mechlorethamine, and bexarotene; UV phototherapy, total skin electron beam therapy, extracorporeal phototherapy, and localized radiotherapy. Systemic therapies include retinoids, interferon, and chemotherapy, and targeted immunotherapy.
Prognosis	A chronic, relapsing course. Childhood form shows remission by adolescence in majority of cases.	A chronic condition with a highly variable time course. Age greater than 60 y, generalized skin involvement, large cell transformation, extracutaneous disease, and increased lactate dehydrogenase level are associated with worse prognosis.

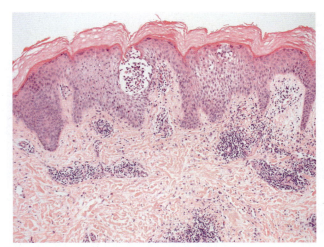

Figure 1.4.1 Atopic dermatitis (eczema). Acute phase with a superficial perivascular infiltrate and epidermal spongiosis.

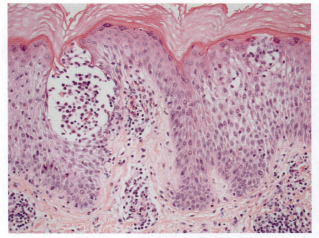

Figure 1.4.2 Atopic dermatitis (eczema). Epidermal spongiosis with "urn-shaped" microvesicle formation. Lymphocytes are small and without nuclear atypia.

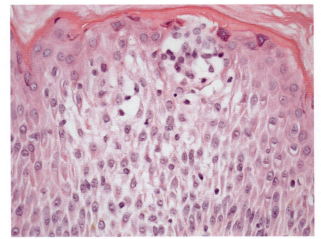

Figure 1.4.3 Atopic dermatitis (eczema). Lymphocytic exocytosis is in proportion to the degree of spongiosis. Intraepidermal lymphocytes are small with round nuclear contours.

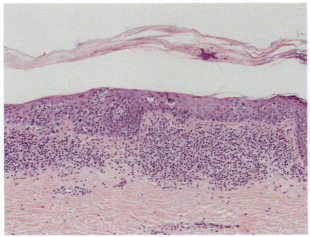

Figure 1.4.4 Mycosis fungoides. A moderately dense superficial interstitial infiltrate with lymphocytic epidermotropism and focal parakeratosis.

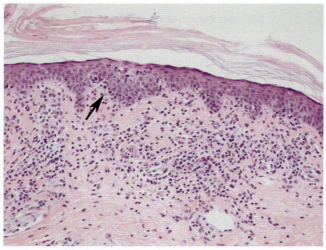

Figure 1.4.5 Mycosis fungoides. Epidermotropism of atypical lymphocytes out of proportion with spongiosis. Atypical lymphocytes focally aligned along the basal zone (arrow).

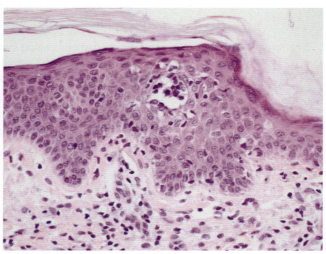

Figure 1.4.6 Mycosis fungoides. Pautrier microabscess (round aggregate vs urn-shaped) containing large, atypical lymphocytes with convoluted nuclei.

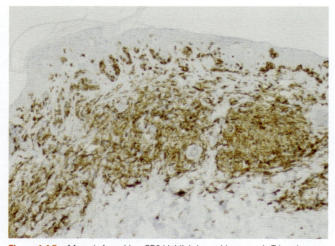

Figure 1.4.7 Mycosis fungoides. CD3 highlighting epidermotropic T lymphocytes within the epidermis, many aligned along the basal zone.

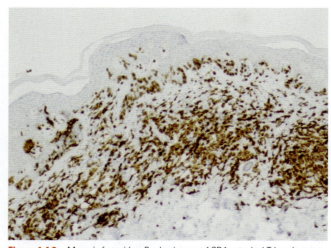

Figure 1.4.8 Mycosis fungoides. Predominance of CD4+ atypical T lymphocytes within the epidermis.

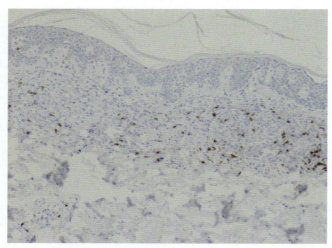

Figure 1.4.9 Mycosis fungoides. Lack of CD8+ atypical T lymphocytes within the epidermis.

1.5 PITYRIASIS ROSEA VS ERYTHEMA ANNULARE CENTRIFUGUM

	Pityriasis Rosea	**Erythema Annulare Centrifugum**
Age	Adolescents and young adults, between 15 and 30 y of age.	Any age.
Location	Chest, back, abdomen, and proximal extremities.	Trunk and proximal extremities.
Etiology	Uncertain; human herpesvirus 6 and 7 implicated.	Unknown but hypersensitivity reaction to medication, underlying infection, chronic disease, and malignancy is postulated.
Presentation	Begins as solitary red and scaly "herald patch" followed days to weeks later by multiple, symmetric, salmon-pink, oval papules with delicate scale; papules follow skin tension lines imparting a "Christmas tree" pattern on the trunk.	Asymptomatic, often multiple, gradually expanding plaques that become annular with central clearing. Often with delicate "trailing scale" along the inner portion of the advancing edge.
Histology	1. Delicate mounds of parakeratosis *(Fig. 1.5.1)*. 2. Minimal epidermal hyperplasia *(Figs. 1.5.1 and 1.5.2)*. 3. Slight epidermal spongiosis *(Figs. 1.5.1 and 1.5.2)*. 4. A sparse superficial perivascular lymphomononuclear infiltrate that extends into interstitium *(Fig. 1.5.3)*. 5. Erythrocyte extravasation *(Fig. 1.5.3)*.	1. Delicate mounds of parakeratosis *(Fig. 1.5.5)*. 2. No or slight spongiosis *(Fig. 1.5.4)*. 3. Tight cuffing ("coat sleeve") of the superficial vascular plexus by a lymphohistiocytic infiltrate *(Figs. 1.5.4 and 1.5.6)*. 4. No appreciable erythrocyte extravasation.
Special studies	None.	None.
Treatment	No treatment necessary but emollients, antihistamines, and topical corticosteroids may be used for symptomatic cases.	Typically resolves spontaneously and requires no treatment.
Prognosis	Excellent. Self-limiting disease.	Excellent. Cases may persist or recur over months to years but eventually resolve spontaneously.

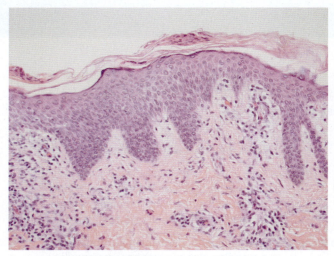

Figure 1.5.1 Pityriasis rosea. Slight epidermal hyperplasia with delicate mounds of parakeratosis. A sparse superficial perivascular and interstitial lymphocytic infiltrate.

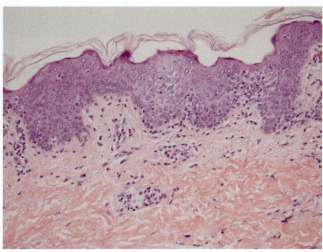

Figure 1.5.2 Pityriasis rosea. Much of the stratum corneum is thin and composed of basket-weave orthokeratin. The epidermis has slight spongiosis and lymphocytic exocytosis.

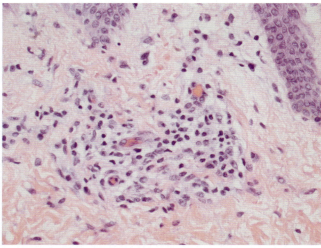

Figure 1.5.3 Pityriasis rosea. A sparse superficial perivascular and interstitial infiltrate of small lymphocytes. There is erythrocyte extravasation within the papillae.

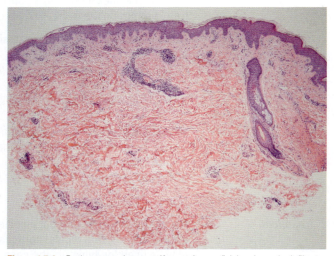

Figure 1.5.4 Erythema annulare centrifugum. A superficial perivascular infiltrate with mild epidermal hyperplasia and slight spongiosis.

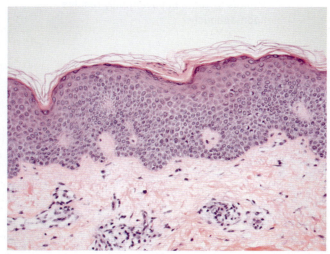

Figure 1.5.5 Erythema annulare centrifugum. Subtle mounds of parakeratosis correlating with "trailing scale" seen clinically.

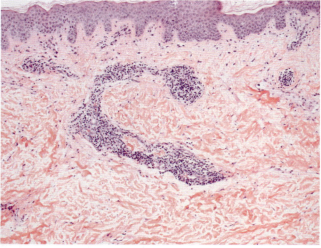

Figure 1.5.6 Erythema annulare centrifugum. A dermal lymphocytic infiltrate tightly cuffs the vascular plexus in a "coat sleeve" fashion. No appreciable erythrocyte extravasation within the papillary dermis.

1.6 PITYRIASIS ROSEA VS GUTTATE PSORIASIS

	Pityriasis Rosea	**Guttate Psoriasis**
Age	Adolescents and young adults, between 15 and 30 y of age.	Children and young adults.
Location	Chest, back, abdomen, and proximal extremities.	Trunk, upper extremities, and thighs.
Etiology	Uncertain; human herpesvirus 6 and 7 implicated.	Genetic predisposition with HLA-Cw6. Often follows streptococcal pharyngitis or viral upper respiratory infection. May also be drug-induced.
Presentation	Begins as solitary red and scaly "herald patch" followed days to weeks later by multiple, symmetric, salmon-pink, oval papules with delicate scale; papules follow skin tension lines imparting a "Christmas tree" pattern on the trunk.	Acute onset of 1-10 mm, salmon-pink papules with overlying fine scale.
Histology	1. Delicate mounds of parakeratosis without neutrophils *(Figs. 1.6.1 and 1.6.2)*. 2. Minimal epidermal hyperplasia *(Figs. 1.6.1 and 1.6.2)*. 3. Slight epidermal spongiosis *(Figs. 1.6.1 and 1.6.2)*. 4. A sparse superficial perivascular and interstitial lymphomononuclear infiltrate *(Fig. 1.6.3)*. 5. Erythrocyte extravasation *(Fig. 1.6.3)*.	1. Mounded parakeratosis with entrapped neutrophils *(Figs. 1.6.4-1.6.6)*. 2. Mild epidermal hyperplasia with reactive changes *(Figs. 1.6.4 and 1.6.5)*. 3. Minute superficial neutrophilic collections *(Fig. 1.6.5)*. 4. Dilated capillaries within papillae associated with a relatively sparse superficial perivascular lymphomononuclear infiltrate *(Figs. 1.6.4 and 1.6.6)*.
Special studies	None.	PAS to exclude superficial fungal infection.
Treatment	No treatment necessary but emollients, antihistamines, and topical corticosteroids may be used for symptomatic cases.	Given the propensity for spontaneous resolution, individuals may opt for no therapy. If treatment is preferred, phototherapy and topical corticosteroids or vitamin D analogues are first-line therapies. Systemic immunomodulatory agents may be utilized for refractory disease.
Prognosis	Excellent. Self-limiting disease.	Generally self-limiting but may recur with repeated streptococcal infections. There is risk of later development of plaque psoriasis.

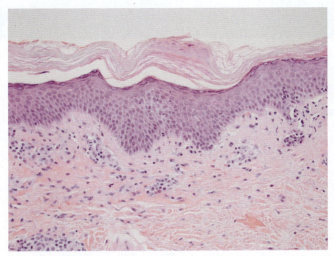

Figure 1.6.1 Pityriasis rosea. Delicate mounds of parakeratosis (without neutrophils), mild epidermal hyperplasia, and slight spongiosis.

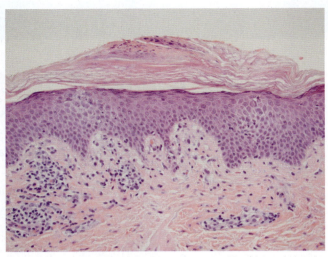

Figure 1.6.2 Pityriasis rosea. Mounded parakeratosis with mild spongiosis and a sparse superficial perivascular lymphocytic infiltrate. No neutrophils associated with the parakeratosis.

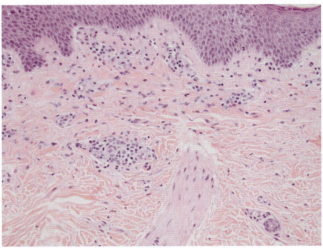

Figure 1.6.3 Pityriasis rosea. A sparse superficial perivascular and interstitial lymphocytic infiltrate with erythrocyte extravasation. Note absence of dilated papillary dermal capillaries.

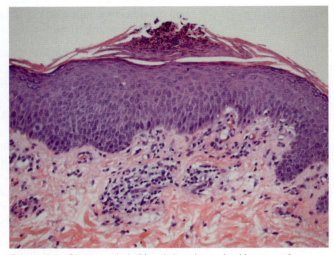

Figure 1.6.4 Guttate psoriasis. Mounded parakeratosis with entrapped neutrophils. Dilated capillaries within papillae.

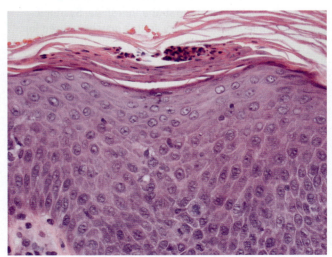

Figure 1.6.5 Guttate psoriasis. Mild epidermal hyperplasia with reactive changes, focally diminished granular layer, and overlying parakeratotic mound with neutrophils.

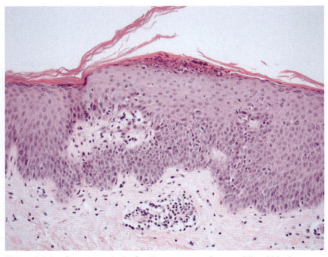

Figure 1.6.6 Guttate psoriasis. Small aggregates of neutrophils within the superficial epidermis and mounds of parakeratosis. Often need to perform multiple levels to illustrate the neutrophils.

1.7 NUMMULAR DERMATITIS VS DERMATOPHYTOSIS

	Nummular Dermatitis	**Dermatophytosis**
Age	Bimodal distribution, women 15–25 y of age and men 50–65 y of age.	Any age. Most forms occur in postpubertal individuals except tinea capitis, which occurs primarily in children.
Location	Lower extremities > upper extremities, trunk	Any area of body; tinea corporis (glabrous skin), tinea cruris (groin), tinea capitis (scalp), tinea faciei (face), tinea barbae (beard area), tinea pedis (foot).
Etiology	Compromise of the epidermal lipid barrier followed by release of cytokines with recruitment of T-cell lymphocytes, dendritic cells, and Langerhans cells.	Infection of the keratinized tissues of skin, nails, and hair by fungi of the *Trichophyton*, *Microsporum*, and *Epidermophyton* genera.
Presentation	Symmetrically distributed, well-circumscribed, round or coin-shaped, erythematous plaques with overlying scale. Associated with mild to intense pruritus.	Expanding annular, arcuate, or circinate, red-pink scaly plaques with a raised border. May have vesicles or pustules in the advancing edge. Symptoms may include mild burning or pruritus.
Histology	1. Confluent parakeratosis *(Figs. 1.7.1 and 1.7.2)*. 2. Epidermal hyperplasia with variable spongiosis and exocytosis of lymphocytes *(Figs. 1.7.2 and 1.7.3)*. 3. A superficial perivascular infiltrate of lymphocytes and eosinophils *(Fig. 1.7.3)*. 4. Widening of the dermal papillae by thickened collagen bundles *(Fig. 1.7.3)*.	1. Parakeratosis with entrapped neutrophils *(Fig. 1.7.5)*. 2. Mild epidermal spongiosis with exocytosis of lymphocytes and neutrophils *(Fig. 1.7.4)*. 3. A superficial dermal infiltrate of lymphocytes and neutrophils *(Fig. 1.7.4)*. 4. Septate, branching hyphae within stratum corneum; may be evident on H&E stain but fungal stain may be required to detect *(Figs. 1.7.6 and 1.7.7)*.
Special studies	PAS stain to exclude superficial fungal infection.	PAS or GMS stain. Microbiologic culture if confirmation and speciation of fungi is necessary for treatment.
Treatment	Moisturization with thick emollients and use of mid- to high-potency topical corticosteroids. Topical calcineurin inhibitors as steroid-sparing agents. Narrowband UVB phototherapy or dupilumab for widespread disease.	Topical azoles and allylamines for localized infection. Systemic antifungal therapy for extensive infection, immunosuppression, or infections recalcitrant to topical therapy.
Prognosis	A chronic course with flares and remissions over months to years.	Excellent. Resolution with treatment in 70%-100% of cases. Recurrence higher in tinea cruris and tinea pedis.

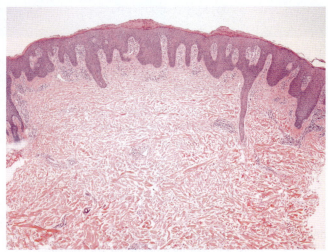

Figure 1.7.1 Nummular dermatitis. Irregular psoriasiform epidermal hyperplasia with confluent parakeratosis and a superficial perivascular infiltrate.

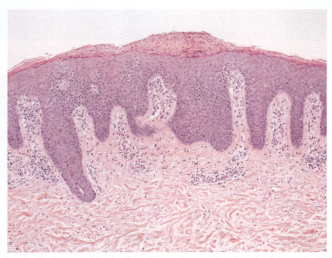

Figure 1.7.2 Nummular dermatitis. Hyperplastic epidermis with mild spongiosis, lymphocytic exocytosis, and scale crust.

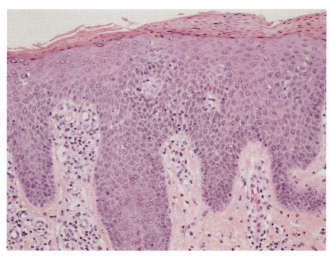

Figure 1.7.3 Nummular dermatitis. Confluent parakeratosis without evidence of fungal hyphae on H&E (or PAS stain, not illustrated). The epidermis has mild spongiosis and lymphocytic exocytosis.

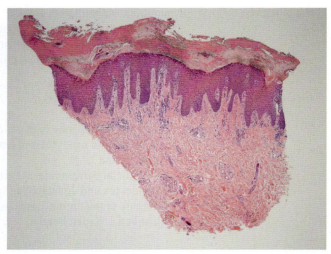

Figure 1.7.4 Dermatophytosis. Ragged, irregular parakeratosis and scale crust with underlying epidermal hyperplasia and superficial dermal inflammation.

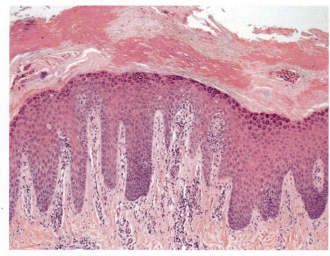

Figure 1.7.5 Dermatophytosis. Irregular psoriasiform epidermal hyperplasia with parakeratosis, scale crust, and entrapped neutrophils.

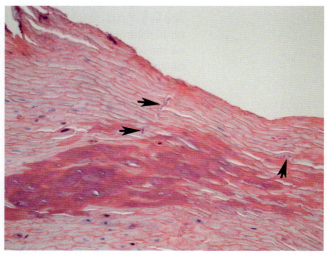

Figure 1.7.6 Dermatophytosis. Hyaline fungal hyphae (arrows) within stratum corneum evident on H&E stain.

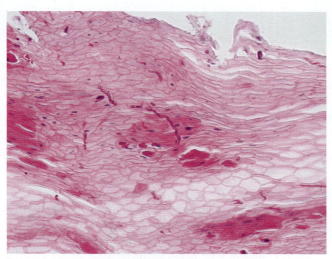

Figure 1.7.7 Dermatophytosis. PAS stain often necessary to confirm presence of fungal hyphae.

1.8 NUMMULAR DERMATITIS VS PSORIASIS (PLAQUE TYPE)

	Nummular Dermatitis	**Psoriasis (Plaque Type)**
Age	Bimodal distribution; women 15-25 y, men 50-65 y.	Any age, peak onset in young adulthood.
Location	Lower extremities > upper extremities, trunk.	Bilateral and symmetric; elbows, knees, buttock, scalp.
Etiology	Exact etiology unknown; xerosis, venous stasis, and autoeczematization may contribute.	A complex, multifactorial disease resulting from a combination of genetic, environmental, and immunologic factors. There is a genetic predisposition associated with certain HLA alleles, with HLA-Cw6 being most strongly associated. Environmental triggers are many and include infection, trauma, alcohol ingestion, medications, and cold weather. The triggers evoke excess T-cell activity that causes stimulation of epidermal keratinocytes with an increase in keratinocyte turnover rate.
Presentation	Well-demarcated, coin-shaped, erythematous, scaly plaques; 1-10 cm; associated with pruritus.	Monomorphic, sharply demarcated erythematous plaques covered by silvery scale.
Histology	1. Irregular psoriasiform epidermal hyperplasia with parakeratosis and a scale crust *(Figs. 1.8.1* and *1.8.2)*. 2. Thickened suprapapillary plate with hypergranulosis *(Figs. 1.8.3* and *1.8.4)*. 3. Mild epidermal spongiosis with lymphocytic exocytosis *(Figs. 1.8.3* and *1.8.4)*. 4. A superficial perivascular lymphohistiocytic infiltrate with occasional eosinophils *(Fig. 1.8.5)*. 5. Widening of the papillae with slightly thickened collagen bundles in chronic forms *(Fig. 1.8.5)*.	1. Regular psoriasiform epidermal hyperplasia with thinning of suprapapillary plate *(Figs. 1.8.6* and *1.8.7)*. 2. Confluent parakeratosis with entrapped neutrophils *(Figs. 1.8.7* and *1.8.8)*. 3. Neutrophilic microabscesses in the superficial epidermis and stratum corneum *(Fig. 1.8.8)*. 4. Dilated, tortuous thin-walled vessels in papillae *(Fig. 1.8.9)*.
Special studies	None.	PAS to exclude superficial fungal infection.
Treatment	Moisturization and topical corticosteroids; narrowband UVB for widespread disease; dupilumab for moderate to severe cases.	Treatment is based upon the extent and severity of the disease along with comorbidities. Limited disease is treated with topical corticosteroids and emollients. Phototherapy may be added for moderate to severe disease. Alternatively, systemic agents including retinoids, methotrexate, cyclosporine, and a variety of biologic immune-modifying agents.

1.8 Nummular Dermatitis vs Psoriasis (Plaque Type)

	Nummular Dermatitis	**Psoriasis (Plaque Type)**
Prognosis	A chronic course with relapses and remissions over months to years.	A chronic disease characterized by exacerbations and remissions. Individuals with cutaneous psoriasis are at risk for development of psoriatic arthritis.

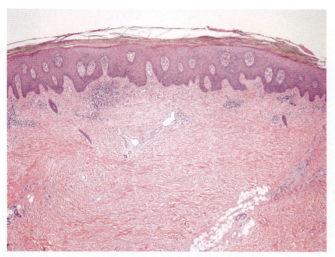

Figure 1.8.1 Nummular dermatitis. Confluent parakeratosis with irregular psoriasiform epidermal hyperplasia and a superficial dermal inflammatory infiltrate.

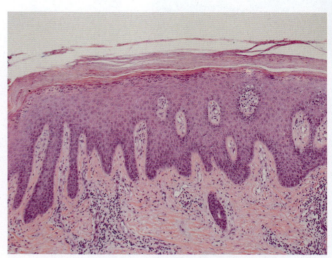

Figure 1.8.2 Nummular dermatitis. Irregular psoriasiform hyperplasia with retained granular layer and confluent parakeratosis.

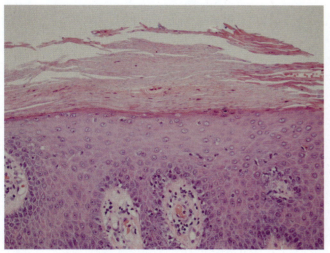

Figure 1.8.3 Nummular dermatitis. Ragged parakeratosis with entrapped serum. Epidermal hyperplasia with lymphocytic exocytosis.

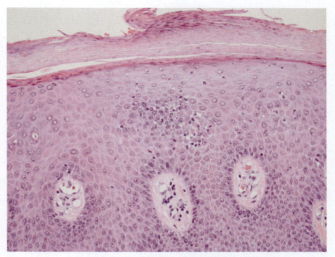

Figure 1.8.4 Nummular dermatitis. Mild spongiosis and lymphocytic exocytosis.

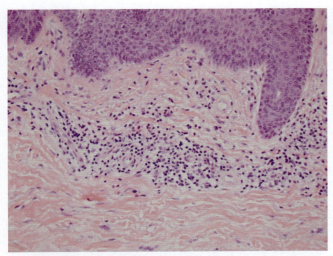

Figure 1.8.5 Nummular dermatitis. A superficial perivascular lymphocytic infiltrate with eosinophils. Mild thickening of papillary dermal collagen bundles.

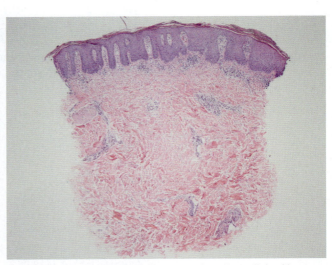

Figure 1.8.6 Psoriasis. Regular psoriasiform epidermal hyperplasia with confluent parakeratosis and a superficial dermal inflammatory infiltrate.

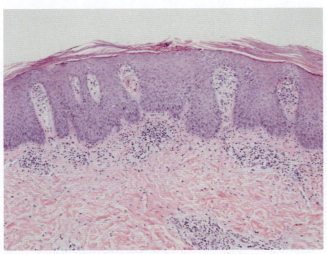

Figure 1.8.7 Psoriasis. Regular psoriasiform epidermal hyperplasia with confluent parakeratosis, diminished granular layer, and thinned suprapapillary plate.

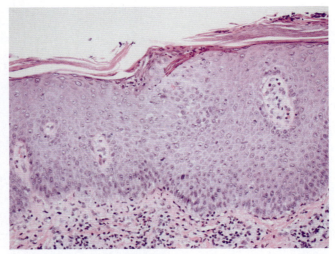

Figure 1.8.8 Psoriasis. Neutrophilic aggregates within the epidermis and the stratum corneum.

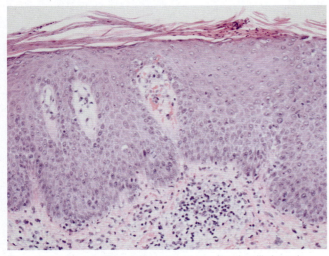

Figure 1.8.9 Psoriasis. Thin papillae with tortuous, dilated capillaries and erythrocyte extravasation. A superficial lymphocytic infiltrate without appreciable eosinophils.

1.9 PSORIASIS (PLAQUE TYPE) VS SEBORRHEIC DERMATITIS

	Psoriasis (Plaque Type)	Seborrheic Dermatitis
Age	Any age, peak onset in young adulthood.	Infants; adolescents and adults with peak at middle age.
Location	Bilateral and symmetric; elbows, knees, buttock, scalp.	Nasolabial folds, brows, ears, scalp, and chest.
Etiology	Complex, multifactorial disease resulting from a combination of genetic, environmental, and immunologic factors. There is a genetic predisposition associated with certain HLA alleles, with HLA-Cw6 being most strongly associated. Environmental triggers are many and include infection, trauma, alcohol ingestion, medications, and cold weather. The triggers evoke excess T-cell activity that causes stimulation of epidermal keratinocytes with an increase in keratinocyte turnover rate.	Not fully known but believed to be associated with overproduction of sebum and *Malassezia* (*Pityrosporum ovale*). More common in immunosuppressed individuals, suggesting dysregulation of immune system may play a role.
Presentation	Monomorphic, sharply demarcated erythematous plaques covered by silvery scale.	Well-demarcated, pink-yellow to red-brown, thin plaques with "greasy" scale.
Histology	1. Confluent parakeratosis, not restricted to follicular ostia *(Fig. 1.9.1)*. 2. Neutrophils in the stratum corneum and the superficial epidermis forming microabscesses *(Figs. 1.9.2* and *1.9.3)*. 3. Regular psoriasiform hyperplasia *(Figs. 1.9.1* and *1.9.2)*. 4. Diminished granular layer *(Fig. 1.9.2)*. 5. Dilated, tortuous vessels in dermal papillae *(Fig. 1.9.3)*.	1. Mounds of parakeratosis and scale crust at follicular ostia *(Figs. 1.9.4* and *1.9.5)*. No appreciable interfollicular parakeratosis. 2. Neutrophils present in the scale crust *(Fig. 1.9.5)*. 3. Variable degree of irregular psoriasiform epidermal hyperplasia with preserved granular layer *(Fig. 1.9.6)*. 4. Mild spongiosis in epidermis and follicular epithelium *(Fig. 1.9.6)*.
Special studies	PAS stain to exclude superficial fungal infection.	PAS stain to exclude superficial fungal infection.
Treatment	Treatment is based upon the extent and severity of the disease along with comorbidities. Limited disease is treated with topical corticosteroids and emollients. Phototherapy may be added for moderate to severe disease. Alternatively, systemic agents including retinoids, methotrexate, cyclosporine, and a variety of biologic immune-modifying agents.	Topical antifungal agents to reduce *Malassezia*. Topical corticosteroids or calcineurin inhibitors to decrease inflammation. Shampoos containing selenium sulfide, zinc pyrithione, and salicylic acid for scalp disease.
Prognosis	A chronic disease characterized by exacerbations and remissions. Individuals with cutaneous psoriasis are at risk for development of psoriatic arthritis.	A chronic, relapsing disease.

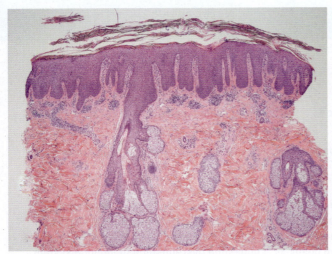

Figure 1.9.1 Psoriasis. Confluent, loose, laminated parakeratosis with underlying regular psoriasiform epidermal hyperplasia.

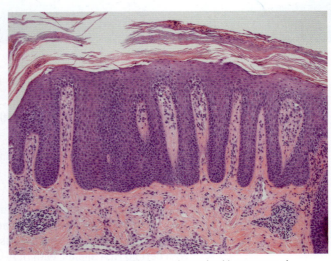

Figure 1.9.2 Psoriasis. Interfollicular parakeratosis with aggregates of neutrophils alternating with orthokeratosis. The epidermis has regular psoriasiform hyperplasia, reactive changes, and an absent granular layer.

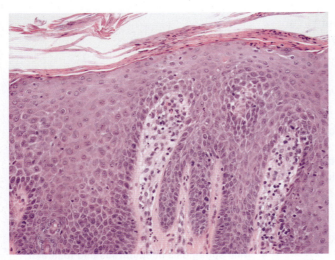

Figure 1.9.3 Psoriasis. Thin suprapapillary plate with exocytosis of neutrophils. The papillae are thin and have tortuous capillaries.

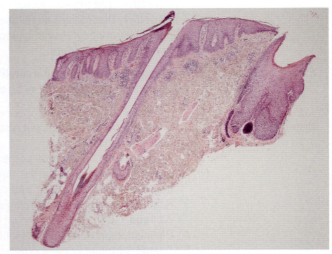

Figure 1.9.4 Seborrheic dermatitis. Psoriasiform epidermal hyperplasia with mounds of parakeratosis at the ostia of follicular units.

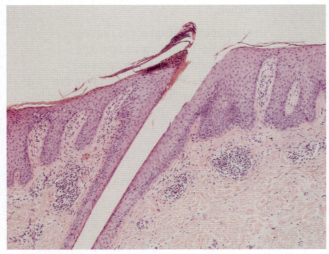

Figure 1.9.5 Seborrheic dermatitis. Mound of parakeratosis with entrapped neutrophils at the ostium of a follicular infundibulum.

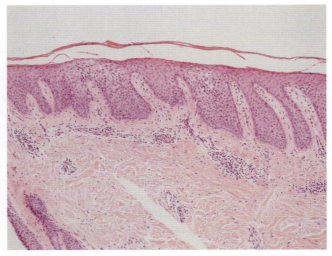

Figure 1.9.6 Seborrheic dermatitis. Psoriasiform epidermal hyperplasia with mild spongiosis. Note the lack of significant interfollicular parakeratosis and absence of neutrophilic exocytosis.

1.10 PITYRIASIS RUBRA PILARIS VS PSORIASIS (PLAQUE TYPE)

	Pityriasis Rubra Pilaris	**Psoriasis (Plaque Type)**
Age	Bimodal age distribution; peaking in first and second decades; six subtypes based on age of onset, presentation, course, and prognosis.	Any age, peak onset in young adulthood.
Location	Type I: Classic Adult: face and neck progressing to trunk and extremities. Type II: Atypical Adult: lower extremities with palmoplantar keratoderma. Type III: Classic Juvenile: face and neck progressing to trunk and extremities. Type IV: Circumscribed Juvenile: elbows and knees. Type V: Atypical Juvenile: similar to type II. Type VI: HIV-associated: similar to type I with concomitant features of follicular occlusion.	Bilateral and symmetric; elbows, knees, buttock, and scalp.
Etiology	Unknown. Clinical and histologic similarities to vitamin A deficiency disorder suggest possible vitamin A metabolism abnormalities. Genetic predisposition in autosomal dominant type V with mutations in the caspase recruitment domain family, member 14 gene (*CARD14*).	Complex, multifactorial disease resulting from a combination of genetic, environmental, and immunologic factors. There is a genetic predisposition associated with certain HLA alleles, with HLA-Cw6 being most strongly associated. Environmental triggers are many and include infection, trauma, alcohol ingestion, medications, and cold weather. The triggers evoke excess T-cell activity that causes stimulation of epidermal keratinocytes with an increase in keratinocyte turnover rate.
Presentation	Red-orange keratotic follicular papules coalescing into plaques with islands of sparing. Orange waxy palmoplantar keratoderma. Nail changes include subungual hyperkeratosis, nail plate thickening, and splinter hemorrhages.	Sharply demarcated salmon pink plaques with thick silvery scale. Oil-drop changes, pits, and marginal onycholysis of nails.
Histology	1. Alternating orthokeratosis and parakeratosis in both vertical and horizontal directions creating a "checkerboard" pattern; no neutrophils within parakeratosis *(Figs. 1.10.3* and *1.10.4)*. 2. Focal or confluent hypergranulosis *(Fig. 1.10.3)*. 3. Psoriasiform epidermal hyperplasia with short and broad rete ridges *(Figs. 1.10.1* and *1.10.2)*. 4. Thick suprapapillary plates *(Fig. 1.10.3)*. 5. Follicular plugging *(Figs. 1.10.1* and *1.10.2)*. 6. A sparse superficial perivascular dermal lymphohistiocytic infiltrate.	1. Alternating orthokeratosis and parakeratosis in vertical fashion (early lesions) or confluent parakeratosis (older lesions); neutrophils present within parakeratosis *(Fig. 1.10.5)*. 2. Regular psoriasiform hyperplasia with hypogranulosis *(Fig. 1.10.6)*. 3. Neutrophilic exocytosis with microabscess formation *(Figs. 1.10.6* and *1.10.7)*. 4. Dilated, tortuous thin-walled vessels in papillae *(Fig. 1.10.6)*.

(continued)

	Pityriasis Rubra Pilaris	**Psoriasis (Plaque Type)**
Special studies	None.	PAS stain to exclude superficial fungal infection.
Treatment	Systemic retinoids and methotrexate, either alone or in combination. Biologics in recalcitrant cases.	Treatment is based upon the extent and severity of the disease along with comorbidities. Limited disease is treated with topical corticosteroids and emollients. Phototherapy may be added for moderate to severe disease. Alternatively, systemic agents including retinoids, methotrexate, cyclosporine, and a variety of biologic immune-modifying agents.
Prognosis	Classic types typically resolve within 3-5 y. Other types have a more chronic course.	A chronic disease characterized by exacerbations and remissions. Individuals with cutaneous psoriasis are at risk for development of psoriatic arthritis.

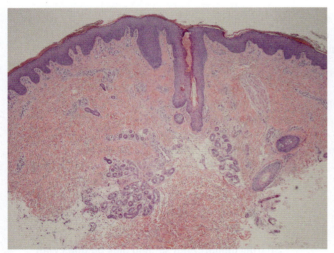

Figure 1.10.1 Pityriasis rubra pilaris. Irregular psoriasiform epidermal hyperplasia with short and broad rete ridges.

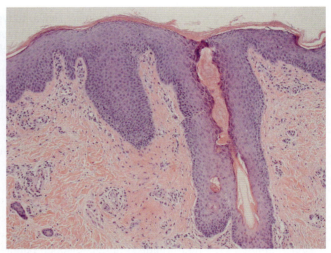

Figure 1.10.2 Pityriasis rubra pilaris. Irregular psoriasiform epidermal hyperplasia with hyperkeratosis, parakeratosis, and follicular plugging.

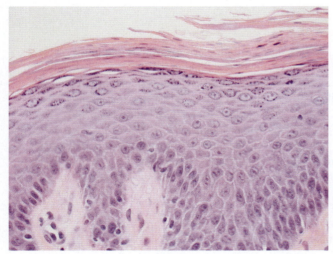

Figure 1.10.3 Pityriasis rubra pilaris. Preserved granular layer with alternating orthokeratosis and parakeratosis creating a "checkerboard" pattern.

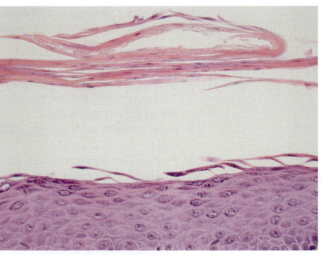

Figure 1.10.4 Pityriasis rubra pilaris. Laminated stratum corneum with "checkerboard" pattern of parakeratotic nuclei.

1.10 Pityriasis Rubra Pilaris vs Psoriasis (Plaque Type)

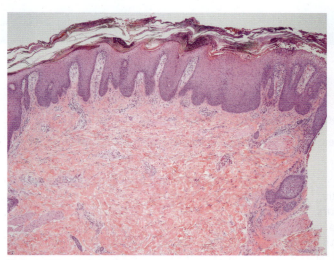

Figure 1.10.5 Psoriasis. Relatively regular psoriasiform epidermal hyperplasia with confluent parakeratosis.

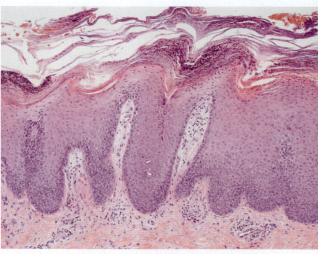

Figure 1.10.6 Psoriasis. Parakeratosis with aggregates of neutrophils (Munro microabscesses). Psoriasiform epidermal with diminished granular layer, thinning of the suprapapillary plate, and dilated papillary dermal capillaries.

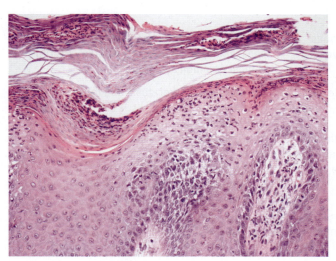

Figure 1.10.7 Psoriasis. Neutrophilic exocytosis with microabscess formation (Kogoj microabscess). Pallor of the superficial epidermis.

1.11 PSORIASIS VS LICHEN SIMPLEX CHRONICUS

	Psoriasis (Plaque Type)	Lichen Simplex Chronicus
Age	Any age, peak onset in young adulthood.	Middle to late adulthood.
Location	Bilateral and symmetric; elbows, knees, buttock, scalp.	Self-accessible areas including posterior neck, scalp, extremities, genitals.
Etiology	Complex, multifactorial disease resulting from a combination of genetic, environmental, and immunologic factors. There is a genetic predisposition associated with certain HLA alleles, with HLA-Cw6 being most strongly associated. Environmental triggers are many and include infection, trauma, alcohol ingestion, medications, and cold weather. The triggers evoke excess T-cell activity that causes stimulation of epidermal keratinocytes with an increase in keratinocyte turnover rate.	Thickening of the skin from chronic, habitual rubbing or scratching.
Presentation	Sharply delineated erythematous plaques with thick, micaceous scale. May have mild pruritus or be asymptomatic.	Discrete dry plaques with exaggerated skin lines, scale, and hyperpigmentation. Pruritus is most common symptom.
Histology	1. Mounded and confluent parakeratosis with entrapped neutrophils *(Figs. 1.11.1* and *1.11.2)*. 2. Regular epidermal hyperplasia with rete ridges of relatively equal length and thinning of the suprapapillary plate *(Figs. 1.11.1* and *1.11.2)*. 3. Hypogranulosis *(Fig. 1.11.2)*. 4. Neutrophil exocytosis with formation of microabscesses within the epidermis and the stratum corneum *(Figs. 1.11.2* and *1.11.3)*. 5. Tortuous and dilated capillaries within dermal papillae *(Fig. 1.11.3)*. 6. A superficial perivascular infiltrate of lymphocytes and occasional neutrophils *(Fig. 1.11.3)*.	1. Marked hyperkeratosis and focal parakeratosis *(Figs. 1.11.4* and *1.11.5)*. 2. Epidermal acanthosis with irregular elongation of rete ridges *(Figs. 1.11.4* and *1.11.5)*. 3. Hypergranulosis *(Fig. 1.11.5)*. 4. Vertically oriented thick collagen bundles in the papillary dermis and a sparse superficial perivascular lymphohistiocytic infiltrate *(Figs. 1.11.5* and *1.11.6)*.
Special studies	PAS to exclude superficial fungal infection.	None.
Treatment	Treatment is based upon the extent and severity of the disease along with comorbidities. Limited disease is treated with topical corticosteroids and emollients. Phototherapy may be added for moderate to severe disease. Alternatively, systemic agents including retinoids, methotrexate, cyclosporine, and a variety of biologic immune-modifying agents.	Topical corticosteroids, with or without occlusion. Antihistamines or topical antipruritics as well as treatment of any underlying cause of pruritus and interruption of itch-scratch cycle.

	Psoriasis (Plaque Type)	**Lichen Simplex Chronicus**
Prognosis	A chronic disease characterized by exacerbations and remissions. Individuals with cutaneous psoriasis are at risk for development of psoriatic arthritis.	A chronic course and often recalcitrant to therapy.

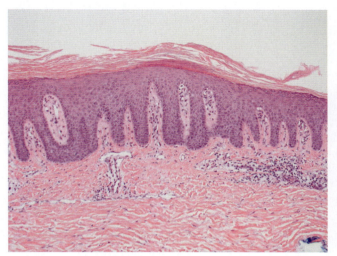

Figure 1.11.1 Psoriasis. Regular psoriasiform epidermal hyperplasia with orthohyperkeratosis and mounds of parakeratosis. Papillae are elongated and thin.

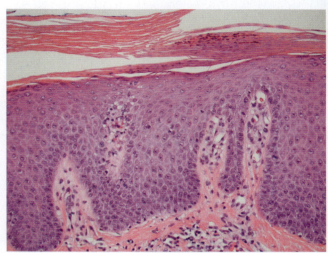

Figure 1.11.2 Psoriasis. Foci of parakeratosis with entrapped neutrophils overlying psoriasiform epidermal hyperplasia with a diminished granular layer. Papillae are thin and have tortuous and dilated capillaries.

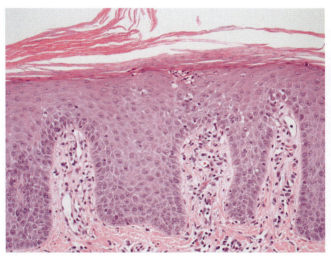

Figure 1.11.3 Psoriasis. Small neutrophilic microabscess in the superficial epidermis with slight spongiosis. Dilated and tortuous capillaries within thin papillae.

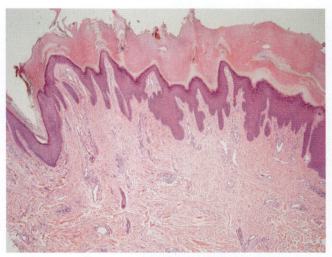

Figure 1.11.4 Lichen simplex chronicus. Prominent compact hyperkeratosis and focal parakeratosis with focal entrapped serum and blood. Markedly irregular epidermal hyperplasia with sparse superficial perivascular inflammation.

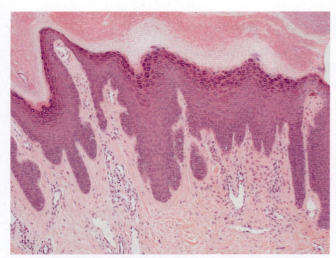

Figure 1.11.5 Lichen simplex chronicus. Irregular epidermal hyperplasia with hypergranulosis. Widened dermal papillae with reactive vessels and thick bundles of collagen.

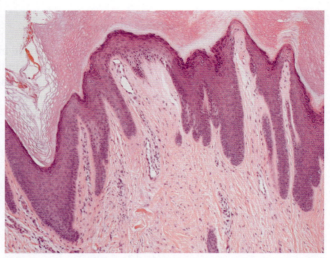

Figure 1.11.6 Lichen simplex chronicus. Widening of dermal papillae by thick collagen bundles in a vertical array. A minimal inflammatory infiltrate.

1.12 ACUTE GENERALIZED EXANTHEMATOUS PUSTULOSIS VS PSORIASIS (PUSTULAR TYPE)

	Acute Generalized Exanthematous Pustulosis	**Psoriasis (Pustular Type)**
Age	Adults.	Children, especially infants; adults, ages 40–50 y.
Location	Trunk and intertriginous areas are favored. Mucous membranes rarely involved.	Generalized and localized forms; localized forms primarily involving extremities.
Etiology	Adverse drug reaction most frequently associated with antibiotics, antifungal agents, and antimalarials.	Abnormal immune response, in genetically susceptible individuals (*IL36RN* mutations), triggered by a number of factors including medications, sudden withdrawal of systemic steroids, infection, and pregnancy.
Presentation	Acute onset of numerous, small, pruritic, nonfollicular pustules on erythematous base. Often associated with fever and neutrophilia. Onset is within 48 hours of exposure to medication. May have systemic involvement of lungs, liver, and kidneys.	Tender red papules or plaques that evolve into superficial pustules on background of erythema. Pustules may coalesce into lakes of pus. The diffuse variant may be associated with systemic symptoms including arthralgias, fever, malaise, and leukocytosis.
Histology	1. A normal basket-weave orthokeratotic stratum corneum; may have thin, delicate mounds of parakeratosis *(Figs. 1.12.1 and 1.12.2)*. 2. Exocytosis of neutrophils with formation of intracorneal, subcorneal, or intraepidermal pustules *(Figs. 1.12.1-1.12.3)*. 3. No increase in mitotic figures within the epidermis. 4. A sparse superficial perivascular infiltrate of lymphocytes with occasional neutrophils and eosinophils *(Fig. 1.12.3)*. 5. Blood vessels within papillae are not dilated or tortuous *(Fig. 1.12.3)*.	1. Discrete mounds of parakeratosis *(Fig. 1.12.4)*. 2. Mild psoriasiform epidermal hyperplasia *(Fig. 1.12.4)*. 3. Spongiform pustules within the superficial epidermis and stratum corneum; may have associated necrotic keratinocytes *(Figs. 1.12.4 and 1.12.5)*. 4. A superficial perivascular lymphocytic infiltrate; eosinophils not present *(Fig. 1.12.6)*. 5. Dilated and tortuous capillaries within dermal papillae *(Fig. 1.12.6)*.
Special studies	PAS to exclude superficial fungal infection.	PAS and tissue gram stain to exclude superficial fungal and bacterial infection.
Treatment	Discontinuation of the offending medication. Moist dressings and topical steroids may be appropriate to reduce symptoms.	Generalized forms require systemic therapy. First-line treatments include acitretin, methotrexate, infliximab, and cyclosporine. Biologics may also be efficacious. Localized variants are treated with topical and systemic therapies depending upon severity. Topical treatments include corticosteroids, calcipotriol, mechlorethamine hydrochloride, and fluorouracil.

(continued)

	Acute Generalized Exanthematous Pustulosis	Psoriasis (Pustular Type)
Prognosis	Typically resolves, with desquamation, within 2 w after withdrawal of the offending agent. Greater degree of morbidity and mortality with systemic involvement.	A chronic disease characterized by flares and remissions. The diffuse variant has higher risk of mortality particularly in individuals with preexisting conditions. Complications include hypocalcemia, hyperthermia, secondary infection, as well as liver and renal failure.

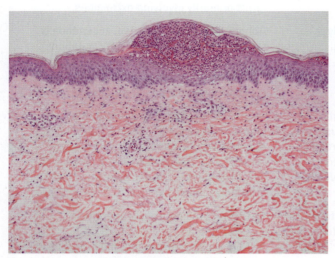

Figure 1.12.1 Acute generalized exanthematous pustulosis. Exocytosis of neutrophils with subcorneal pustule formation.

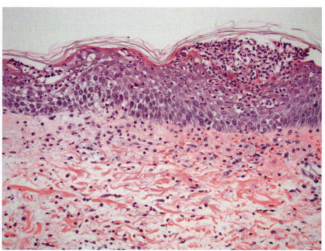

Figure 1.12.2 Acute generalized exanthematous pustulosis. An epidermis of normal thickness with a basket-weave stratum corneum, superficial pustule formation, and a background of spongiosis.

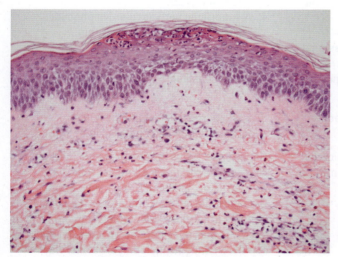

Figure 1.12.3 Acute generalized exanthematous pustulosis. Basket-weave orthokeratosis, without parakeratosis, and a delicate superficial epidermal pustule. Dermal edema with a mixed infiltrate that includes eosinophils. No tortuous capillaries within papillae.

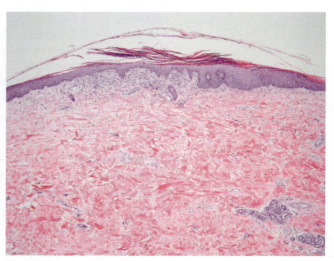

Figure 1.12.4 Pustular psoriasis. Mounded parakeratosis with epidermal hyperplasia and a sparse superficial perivascular infiltrate.

1.12 Acute Generalized Exanthematous Pustulosis vs Psoriasis (Pustular Type)

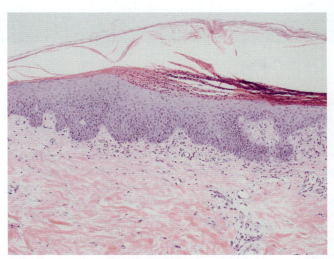

Figure 1.12.5 Pustular psoriasis. Parakeratosis with entrapped neutrophils. Epidermal hyperplasia with reactive nuclear changes and diminished granular layer.

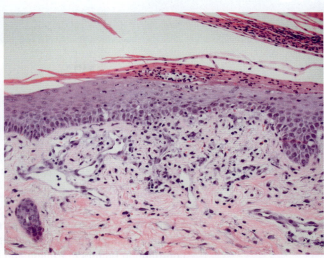

Figure 1.12.6 Pustular psoriasis. A superficial epidermal pustule with rare degenerated keratinocytes. Dilated and tortuous thin-walled vessels in papillae with erythrocyte extravasation.

1.13 LICHEN PLANUS VS LUPUS ERYTHEMATOSUS

	Lichen Planus	**Lupus Erythematosus**
Age	Any age, most commonly between 30 and 60 y of age.	Fourth to fifth decades; women more frequently than men.
Location	Predilection for flexor surfaces, wrists, forearms, legs. Oral and genital mucosal involvement common.	Sun-exposed areas favored. Localized forms most commonly on head and neck, especially scalp and ears. Generalized forms also involving extensor forearms and hands.
Etiology	T-cell–mediated autoimmune disorder with underlying genetic predisposition and contributing factors of trauma and infection.	Autoimmune disease with contributions from genetic (HLA) and environmental (UV exposure and smoking) factors.
Presentation	Pruritic, flat-topped, polygonal, violaceous papules and plaques. Surface has reticular, lacy white lines (Wickham striae). May show koebnerization. Oral lesions often erosive.	Well-demarcated, erythematous macules or papules with adherent scale. Late-stage lesions with peripheral hyperpigmentation surrounding central hypopigmentation and atrophy.
Histology	1. Compact orthohyperkeratosis. No parakeratosis *(Figs. 1.13.1* and *1.13.2)*. 2. Epidermal hyperplasia with tapered ("saw-tooth") rete ridges *(Figs. 1.13.2* and *1.13.3)*. 3. Keratinocytes have eosinophilic, glassy cytoplasm with wedge-shaped hypergranulosis *(Fig. 1.13.2)*. 4. Lichenoid lymphocytic inflammation with interface vacuolar alteration of the basal layer and necrotic keratinocytes ("Civatte", "colloid", "cytoid" bodies). No significant deeper perivascular infiltrates *(Figs. 1.13.2* and *1.13.3)*.	1. Epidermal atrophy with interface vacuolar change and occasional necrotic basal keratinocytes *(Figs. 1.13.5* and *1.13.6)*. 2. Follicular plugging *(Fig. 1.13.5)*. 3. A superficial and deep perivascular and periadnexal lymphocytic infiltrate *(Fig. 1.13.4)*. 4. Mucin deposition within the reticular dermis with colloidal iron or Alcian Blue stain *(Fig. 1.13.7)*.
Special studies	Direct immunofluorescence (DIF) may be performed and shows shaggy deposition of fibrin and globular deposition of multiple immunoglobulins at the dermal-epidermal junction (corresponding to cytoid bodies).	Colloidal iron or Alcian Blue stain to detect extracellular mucin. DIF (lesional lupus band test) sometimes utilized in unclear cases to detect granular deposits of IgG, IgM, and sometimes IgA at the dermal-epidermal junction.
Treatment	Medium- to high-potency topical corticosteroids are first-line therapy. Systemic corticosteroids or phototherapy for severe or widespread disease. Systemic retinoids may also be used for steroid resistant cases. Antihistamines for pruritus.	Strict sun avoidance and protection. Localized disease treated with topical corticosteroids or calcineurin inhibitors. Widespread or scarring disease treated with antimalarials drugs or other systemic immunosuppressants if refractory to antimalarials.
Prognosis	Classic lesions tend to resolve within 6–12 months. May recur. Generalized cases resolve in less time but have a higher likelihood of recurrence.	An unpredictable course with exacerbations and remissions. May cause considerable morbidity even when limited to the skin. Approximately 10%-20% may progress to systemic lupus erythematosus.

1.13 Lichen Planus vs Lupus Erythematosus

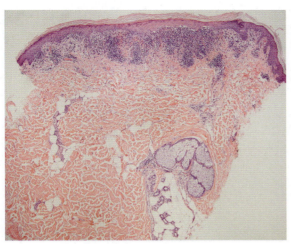

Figure 1.13.1 Lichen planus. Compact orthohyperkeratosis with epidermal acanthosis and a lichenoid inflammatory infiltrate.

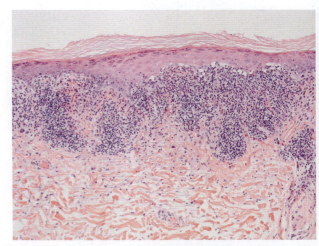

Figure 1.13.2 Lichen planus. Epidermal acanthosis with tapered ("sawtooth") rete ridges, wedge-shaped hypergranulosis, and lichenoid inflammation.

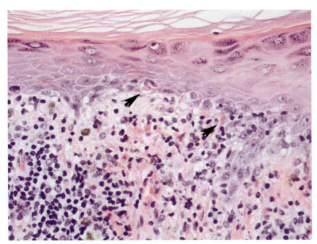

Figure 1.13.3 Lichen planus. Lichenoid lymphomononuclear inflammation with vacuolar interface change and necrotic basal keratinocytes ("Civatte bodies") (arrows).

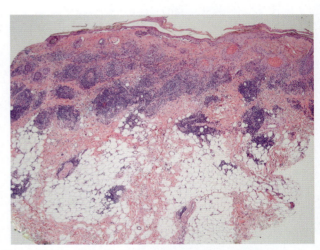

Figure 1.13.4 Lupus erythematosus. Parakeratosis and epidermal atrophy. A superficial and deep perivascular and periadnexal lymphocytic infiltrate.

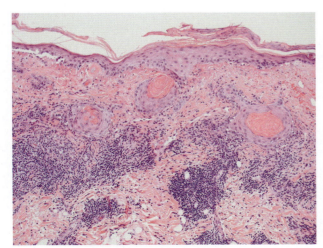

Figure 1.13.5 Lupus erythematosus. Parakeratosis with epidermal atrophy and effacement of the rete ridges. Interface vacuolar change with areas of squamatization of the basal zone. Follicular units are dilated and plugged with keratin.

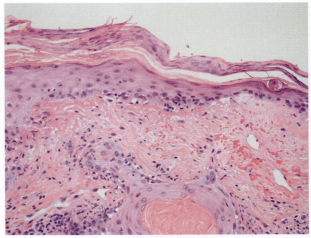

Figure 1.13.6 Lupus erythematosus. Interface vacuolar change with occasional degenerated keratinocytes and thickened basement membrane.

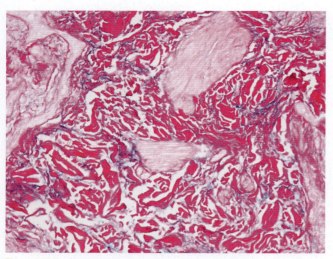

Figure 1.13.7 Lupus erythematosus. Mucin accumulation between the collagen bundles of the reticular dermis on colloid iron stain.

1.14 LICHEN PLANUS VS LICHEN PLANUS–LIKE KERATOSIS

	Lichen Planus	**Lichen Planus–Like Keratosis**
Age	Middle-aged adults.	Middle aged adults, fifth to sixth decades of life; women > men.
Location	Flexor surfaces of extremities primarily; other sites less frequently. Oral and genital mucosa often involved, with or without cutaneous lesions.	Sun-exposed areas of skin, most commonly chest and proximal aspects of upper extremities; less frequently on face and other sites.
Etiology	Unknown, theorized to be due to a combination of immune, genetic, and environmental factors.	Cell-mediated immune involution of benign entities such as seborrheic keratosis, solar lentigo, and actinic keratosis.
Presentation	Polygonal, pruritic, violaceous, flat-topped papules and plaques with overlying white, lacy, reticular lines (Wickham striae).	Abrupt onset of a solitary, pink to violaceous, shiny, plaque with overlying scale or crust. Older lesions may be hyperpigmented. May have burning or pruritic symptoms. A solitary lesion, vs multiple lesions of an eruption, aids in distinguishing it from lichen planus.
Histology	1. Compact orthohyperkeratosis *(Figs. 1.14.1 and 1.14.2)*. Absence of parakeratosis, unless irritated or excoriated. 2. Mild epidermal hyperplasia with tapered ("sawtooth") rete ridges and wedge-shaped hypergranulosis *(Fig. 1.14.2)*. 3. Lichenoid band of lymphocytes that obscures the dermal-epidermal junction *(Figs. 1.14.1 and 1.14.2)*. 4. Vacuolar change of the basal zone with necrotic/apoptotic keratinocytes ("Civatte", "cytoid", or "colloid" bodies) *(Fig. 1.14.3)*.	1. Parakeratosis and crust *(Fig. 1.14.4)*. 2. Epidermal hyperplasia with low papillomatosis representing residual seborrheic keratosis or adjacent clubbed-shaped rete ridges with basal hyperpigmentation representing residual solar lentigo *(Figs. 1.14.5 and 1.14.6)*. 3. A dense lichenoid infiltrate of lymphocytes and occasional eosinophils *(Figs. 1.14.5 and 1.14.6)*. 4. Interface vacuolar change with necrotic keratinocytes along the dermal-epidermal junction, in upper levels of epidermis, and clustering in the papillary dermis *(Fig. 1.14.5)*. Variable number of dermal melanophages *(Fig. 1.14.6)*.
Special studies	DIF reveals staining of colloid bodies with IgM, IgG, or IgA and a shaggy band with fibrinogen along the dermal-epidermal junction.	None.
Treatment	High-potency topical or intralesional corticosteroids are first-line therapy. Topical calcineurin inhibitors for mucosal disease. Systemic glucocorticoids, phototherapy, and oral retinoids for severe, widespread disease.	No treatment necessary, lesions generally resolve within weeks. If desired, can be removed by cryosurgery, electrosurgery, or curettage
Prognosis	Resolution of lesions generally within 1-2 y. Mucosal lesions may be more persistent and recalcitrant to treatment.	Excellent. Benign lesions with no reports of malignant transformation.

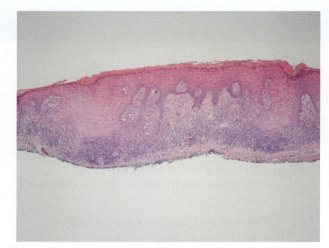

Figure 1.14.1 Lichen planus. Compact hyperkeratosis, irregular epidermal hyperplasia, and a band-like lichenoid inflammatory infiltrate.

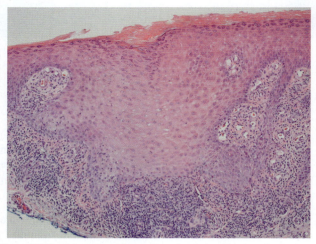

Figure 1.14.2 Lichen planus. Compact hyperkeratosis, without parakeratosis, tapered rete ridges, and hypergranulosis. Epidermal keratinocytes have reactive "glassy" eosinophilic cytoplasm.

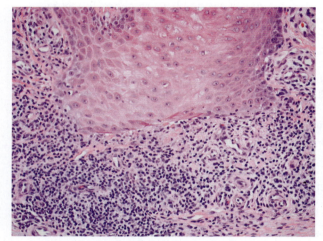

Figure 1.14.3 Lichen planus. A lichenoid lymphomononuclear infiltrate with interface vacuolar change and necrotic keratinocytes ("Civatte bodies").

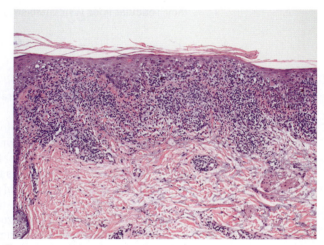

Figure 1.14.4 Lichen planus–like keratosis. Shaggy parakeratosis overlying epidermis of variable thickness and dense lichenoid inflammation. Elastosis in the reticular dermis.

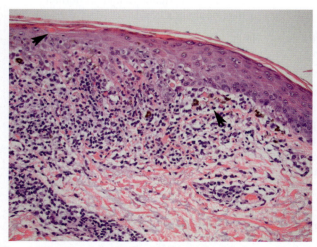

Figure 1.14.5 Lichen planus–like keratosis. Lichenoid interface change with necrotic keratinocytes at all levels of the epidermis and clustered at the junction with the dermis (arrows). Lichenoid lymphomononuclear inflammation with pigment dropout.

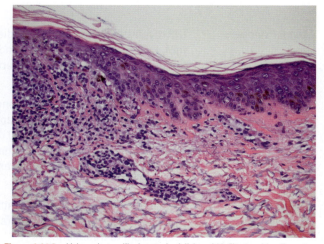

Figure 1.14.6 Lichen planus–like keratosis. A lichenoid infiltrate with adjacent clubbed rete ridges and basal hyperpigmentation representing residual solar lentigo.

1.15 LICHENOID DRUG ERUPTION VS LICHEN PLANUS

	Lichenoid Drug Eruption	**Lichen Planus**
Age	Adults.	Middle-aged adults.
Location	Trunk and extensor surfaces of extremities. Less likely involving flexural surfaces, genitalia, and mucosa.	Flexor surfaces of extremities primarily, other sites less frequently. Oral and genital mucosa often involved, with or without cutaneous lesions.
Etiology	Not completely known. Theorized that medications act as haptens causing production of T helper cell cytokine response that then recruits CD8+ T cells to the skin. The CD8+ T cells then react against keratinocytes.	Unknown, theorized to be due to a combination of immune, genetic, and environmental factors.
Presentation	Symmetric, pruritic, scaly papules or plaques. Usually develops months to years after medication is started. Hyperpigmentation in older lesions. No Wickham striae.	Polygonal, pruritic, violaceous, flat-topped papules and plaques with overlying white, lacy, reticular lines (Wickham striae).
Histology	1. Hyperkeratosis and focal parakeratosis *(Figs. 1.15.1* and *1.15.2).* 2. Interface vacuolar change with necrotic keratinocytes in upper levels of the epidermis, in addition to those in the basal zone *(Fig. 1.15.2).* 3. A lichenoid infiltrate that extends deeper in the dermis around the vascular plexus *(Fig. 1.15.1).* 4. A dermal infiltrate includes eosinophils and/or plasma cells in addition to lymphocytes *(Fig. 1.15.3).*	1. Compact orthohyperkeratosis *(Figs. 1.15.4* and *1.15.5).* 2. Mild epidermal hyperplasia with tapered ("sawtooth") rete ridges and wedge-shaped hypergranulosis *(Figs. 1.15.4* and *1.15.5).* 3. A lichenoid band of lymphocytes that obscures the dermal-epidermal junction *(Figs. 1.15.5* and *1.15.6).* 4. Vacuolar change of the basal zone with necrotic/apoptotic keratinocytes ("Civatte," "cytoid," or "colloid" bodies) *(Fig. 1.15.6).*
Special studies	None.	DIF reveals staining of colloid bodies with IgM, IgG, or IgA and a shaggy band with fibrinogen along the dermal-epidermal junction.
Treatment	Removal of the offending medication. Topical or systemic corticosteroids in cases with slow resolution, extensive lesions, or inability to remove the causal medication.	High-potency topical or intralesional corticosteroids are first-line therapy. Topical calcineurin inhibitors for mucosal disease. Systemic glucocorticoids, phototherapy, and oral retinoids for severe, widespread disease.
Prognosis	Good; in majority of cases resolution occurs after discontinuation of the medication, although it may take weeks to months to fully resolve.	Resolution of lesions generally within 1-2 y. Mucosal lesions may be more persistent and recalcitrant to treatment.

1 Inflammatory Diseases of the Epidermis

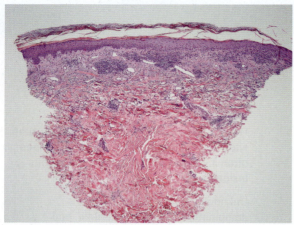

Figure 1.15.1 Lichenoid drug eruption. Hyperkeratosis and focal parakeratosis with a lichenoid dermal infiltrate extending deeper into the dermis around the superficial and mid-dermal vessels.

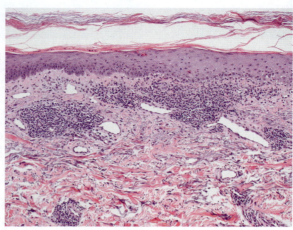

Figure 1.15.2 Lichenoid drug eruption. Focal parakeratosis and interface vacuolar change with necrotic keratinocytes in upper levels of the epidermis and along the basal zone.

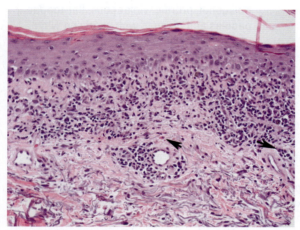

Figure 1.15.3 Lichenoid drug eruption. Lichenoid infiltrate of lymphocytes with occasional eosinophils and plasma cells (arrows).

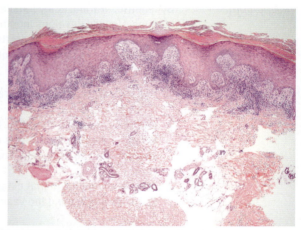

Figure 1.15.4 Lichen planus. Orthohyperkeratosis without parakeratosis. Epidermal hyperplasia with tapered rete ridges. A lichenoid infiltrate obscuring the dermal-epidermal interface without appreciable extension around deeper vascular plexus.

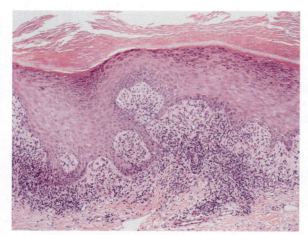

Figure 1.15.5 Lichen planus. Orthohyperkeratosis overlying epidermal hyperplasia with tapered ("sawtooth") rete ridges, glassy eosinophilic keratinocytes, and wedge-shaped hypergranulosis. A lichenoid infiltrate with interface vacuolation and necrotic keratinocytes along the basal zone.

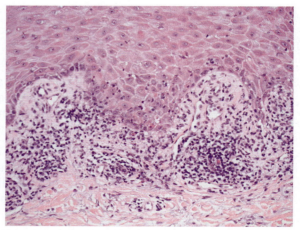

Figure 1.15.6 Lichen planus. A lichenoid infiltrate of lymphocytes and histiocytes associated with vacuolar change and necrotic keratinocytes ("Civatte bodies").

1.16 LICHEN PLANUS VS LICHEN SCLEROSUS

	Lichen Planus	**Lichen Sclerosus**
Age	Middle-aged adults.	Bimodal age distribution in prepubertal and postmenopausal women; middle-aged men.
Location	Flexor surfaces of extremities primarily, other sites less frequently. Oral and genital mucosa often involved, with or without cutaneous lesions.	Predilection for anogenital region including vulva, perineum, and perianal skin in women. In men, glans penis and foreskin are typically involved. Extragenital locations in less than 10% of cases with the most common locations of breasts, thighs, buttocks, back, neck, and chest.
Etiology	Unknown, theorized to be due to a combination of immune, genetic, and environmental factors.	Not entirely known. Autoimmune mechanisms, genetic factors, hormonal influence, trauma, and irritation, as well as localized infection have been proposed as components in the etiology.
Presentation	Polygonal, pruritic, violaceous, flat-topped papules and plaques with overlying white, lacy, reticular lines (Wickham striae).	Porcelain-white papules and plaques with follicular dells, hyperkeratosis, telangiectasia, and a cellophane paper appearance. Late-stage lesions are atrophic and may have erosions, purpura, and fissuring.
Histology	1. Compact orthohyperkeratosis *(Fig. 1.16.1)*. 2. Mild epidermal hyperplasia with tapered ("sawtooth") rete ridges and wedge-shaped hypergranulosis *(Figs. 1.16.1 and 1.16.2)*. 3. Lichenoid band of lymphocytes that obscures the dermal-epidermal junction *(Figs. 1.16.1 and 1.16.2)*. 4. Vacuolar change of the basal zone with necrotic/apoptotic keratinocytes ("Civatte", "cytoid", or "colloid" bodies) *(Figs. 1.16.2 and 1.16.3)*.	1. Compact hyperkeratosis *(Fig. 1.16.4)*. 2. Epidermal atrophy with occasional dell formation. 3. Interface vacuolar change with occasional necrotic basal keratinocytes *(Fig. 1.16.5)*. 4. Homogenization and sclerosis of superficial dermal collagen with telangiectasia *(Fig. 1.16.6)*. 5. Band of lymphomononuclear inflammation below the zone of sclerosis *(Figs. 1.16.4 and 1.16.6)*. May have eosinophils (associated with poor response to therapy).
Special studies	DIF reveals staining of colloid bodies with IgM, IgG, or IgA and a shaggy band with fibrinogen along the dermal-epidermal junction.	None.
Treatment	High-potency topical or intralesional corticosteroids are first-line therapy. Topical calcineurin inhibitors for mucosal disease. Systemic glucocorticoids, phototherapy, and oral retinoids for severe, widespread disease.	Ultrapotent or potent topical corticosteroids coupled with avoidance of irritants and treatment of any concomitant infection. Long-term surveillance.

(continued)

	Lichen Planus	**Lichen Sclerosus**
Prognosis	Resolution of lesions generally within 1-2 y. Mucosal lesions may be more persistent and recalcitrant to treatment.	Improvement in clinical signs with treatment but typically a chronic disease with only approximately 25% of patients showing complete resolution. Progression of disease with scarring and fusion particularly with delay in diagnosis or noncompliance in therapy. Increased risk for well-differentiated vulvar intraepithelial neoplasia (VIN) and squamous cell carcinoma.

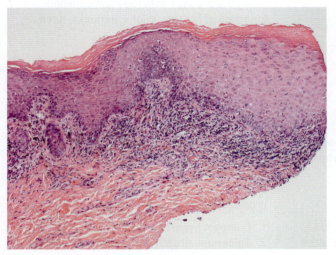

Figure 1.16.1 Lichen planus. Compact hyperkeratosis with epidermal hyperplasia and tapered rete ridges. Keratinocytes have glassy, eosinophilic cytoplasm with wedge-shaped hypergranulosis.

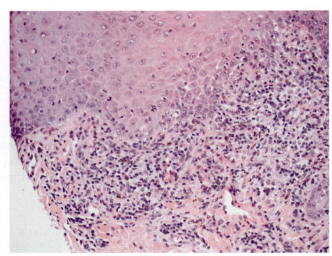

Figure 1.16.2 Lichen planus. Interface vacuolar change with degenerated/necrotic basal keratinocytes ("Civatte bodies"). Dermal melanophages representing pigment dropout due to interface destruction.

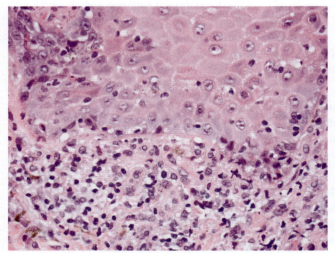

Figure 1.16.3 Lichen planus. A lichenoid lymphomononuclear infiltrate with tapered rete ridge. No appreciable sclerosis of the papillary dermis.

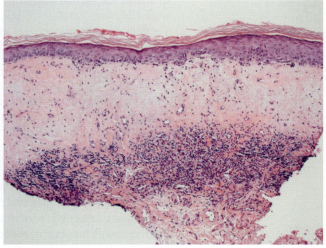

Figure 1.16.4 Lichen sclerosus. Epidermal thinning and effacement of the rete ridge architecture with overlying orthokeratosis. Edema and homogenization of the superficial dermis with underlying band of inflammation.

1.16 Lichen Planus vs Lichen Sclerosus

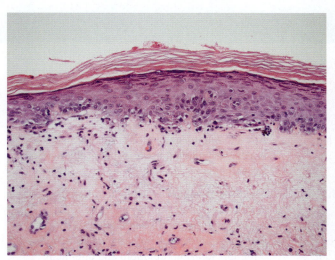

Figure 1.16.5 Lichen sclerosus. Interface vacuolation with exocytosis of lymphocytes and occasional necrotic basal keratinocytes.

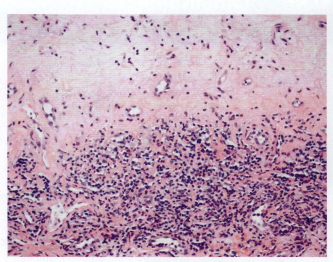

Figure 1.16.6 Lichen sclerosus. Homogenization and sclerosis of collagen in the superficial dermis associated with telangiectasia. A moderately dense band of lymphocytes beneath the sclerosis.

1.17 HYPERTROPHIC LICHEN PLANUS VS SQUAMOUS CELL CARCINOMA

	Hypertrophic Lichen Planus	**Squamous Cell Carcinoma**
Age	Adults.	Adults.
Location	Extremities, especially anterior lower legs and interphalangeal joints.	Any site but typically areas with chronic sun exposure including scalp, orbital region, nose, lip, and ear.
Etiology	T-cell–mediated immune disorder with inflammatory degradation of basal keratinocytes in skin and mucosa. Contributing factors include genetic predisposition, infection, and injury (Koebner phenomenon).	Multistep process involving mutations in multiple genes, notably p53, and exposure to risk factors including UVR, immunosuppression, human papillomavirus infection, ionizing radiation, and chemical carcinogens.
Presentation	Multiple, symmetric, intensely pruritic, hyperkeratotic, red-brown to violaceous plaques with follicular accentuation. Presentation as multiple lesions helpful in distinguishing from squamous cell carcinoma.	Solitary erythematous plaque or nodule with keratotic surface.
Histology	1. Marked compact hyperkeratosis; may have focal areas of parakeratosis, especially if traumatized *(Figs. 1.17.1* and *1.17.2)*. 2. Pseudoepitheliomatous epidermal hyperplasia with wedge-shaped hypergranulosis. Rete ridges are elongate and rounded *(Figs. 1.17.1* and *1.17.2)*. 3. A dense lichenoid infiltrate of lymphocytes and often numerous eosinophils *(Figs. 1.17.3* and *1.17.4)*. 4. Interface vacuolar change with individual and clustered necrotic keratinocytes along the basal zone and the dermal-epidermal junction (colloid bodies) *(Figs. 1.17.3* and *1.17.4)*. Interface changes accentuated at tips of rounded rete ridges. 5. Thickened collagen bundles may be present within papillae.	1. Hyperkeratosis and parakeratosis *(Fig. 1.17.5)*. 2. Irregular epidermal acanthosis with uniform or diminished granular layer *(Fig. 1.17.5)*. 3. Infiltrative islands of atypical squamous cells with enlarged, hyperchromatic nuclei and dyskeratosis *(Figs. 1.17.6* and *1.17.7)*. 4. Patchy inflammation that does not have predilection for tips of rete ridges and not associated with interface vacuolar change *(Figs. 1.17.5* and *1.17.7)*. Eosinophils are generally not prominent.
Special studies	DIF shows globular IgM deposition correlating with colloid bodies and shaggy fibrin deposition along the basement membrane zone.	None.

1.17 Hypertrophic Lichen Planus vs Squamous Cell Carcinoma

	Hypertrophic Lichen Planus	**Squamous Cell Carcinoma**
Treatment	High-potency topical corticosteroids and intralesional corticosteroids are first-line therapy. Second-line therapy includes systemic glucocorticoids, oral retinoids, topical or systemic immunomodulators, and phototherapy.	Excision.
Prognosis	More resistant to therapy than classic lichen planus, thereby requiring longer and more potent therapies. Reports of risk of development of squamous cell carcinoma.	Generally excellent with complete excision.

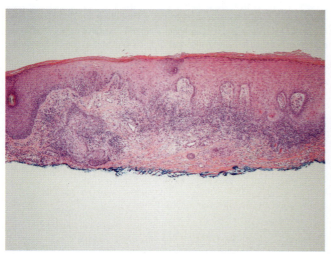

Figure 1.17.1 Hypertrophic lichen planus. Compact orthokeratosis with irregular epidermal hyperplasia and a lichenoid inflammatory infiltrate.

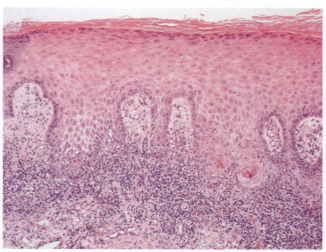

Figure 1.17.2 Hypertrophic lichen planus. Compact hyperkeratosis, wedge-shaped hypergranulosis, and a lichenoid inflammatory infiltrate concentrated at the tips of rete ridges.

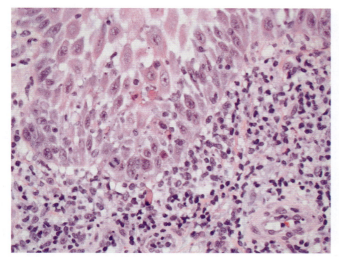

Figure 1.17.3 Hypertrophic lichen planus. Interface vacuolar change at tip of rete ridge with degenerated basal keratinocytes ("Civatte bodies") and lichenoid inflammation.

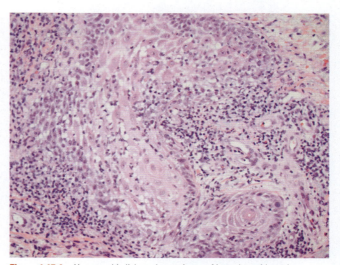

Figure 1.17.4 Hypertrophic lichen planus. Areas of irregular epidermal hyperplasia with mild reactive atypia of keratinocytes and associated lichenoid inflammation with vacuolar interface change.

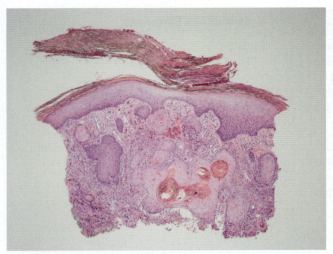

Figure 1.17.5 Squamous cell carcinoma. Confluent parakeratosis overlying irregular epidermal hyperplasia and infiltrative islands of atypical squamous epithelium.

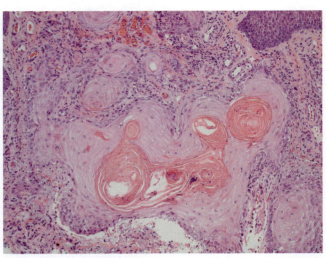

Figure 1.17.6 Squamous cell carcinoma. Infiltrative islands of atypical squamous epithelium with patchy inflammation that is not concentrated at tips of rete ridges.

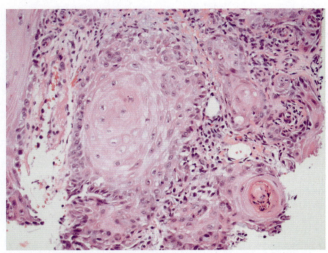

Figure 1.17.7 Squamous cell carcinoma. Infiltrative islands of squamous epithelium with enlarged, hyperchromatic nuclei and dyskeratosis ("squamous pearl").

1.18 LICHEN NITIDUS VS LICHEN STRIATUS

	Lichen Nitidus	**Lichen Striatus**
Age	Children and young adults.	Most commonly, children between ages of 1 and 15 y. Occasionally, adults between ages of 40 and 45 y.
Location	Neck, trunk, upper extremities, abdomen, and penile shaft. May be generalized.	Unilateral on extremities. Less commonly on head, neck, and trunk.
Etiology	Unknown. Immune reaction postulated.	Unknown. Thought to be a combination of genetic and environmental factors.
Presentation	Asymptomatic, monomorphous, 1-2 mm, flat-topped, tan-pink papules. Often shows Koebner phenomenon. Nail involvement in generalized form presents with longitudinal furrowing and ridging of nail plate.	Asymptomatic, 1-2 mm, pink or skin-colored, monomorphous papules coalescing into a linear plaque along Blaschko's lines.
Histology	1. Discrete collections of lymphocytes, histiocytes, Langerhans cells, and multinucleate giant cells within dermal papillae *(Figs. 1.18.1* and *1.18.2).* 2. The rete ridges surrounding the infiltrate are elongated creating a "ball-in-claw" configuration *(Figs. 1.18.1* and *1.18.2).* 3. The overlying epidermis is thinned and has basal vacuolar change with rare degenerated keratinocytes *(Fig. 1.18.3).*	1. A dense perivascular and lichenoid lymphohistiocytic infiltrate *(Figs. 1.18.4* and *1.18.5).* 2. The infiltrate involves eccrine sweat glands in the deep dermis *(Fig. 1.18.7).* 3. Vacuolar interface change with necrotic keratinocytes and overlying parakeratosis *(Fig. 1.18.6).*
Special studies	None.	None.
Treatment	Typically no treatment necessary. If symptomatic or cosmetically problematic, topical steroids or calcineurin inhibitors may be used.	Generally not required. Topical steroids may accelerate resolution.
Prognosis	Self-limiting and generally spontaneously resolves in months to a year.	Excellent. Resolves spontaneously with no long-term sequelae.

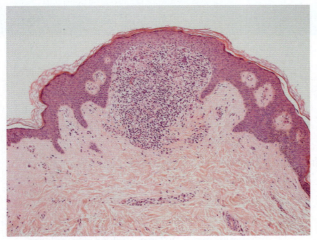

Figure 1.18.1 Lichen nitidus. A discrete lymphohistiocytic infiltrate that expands the dermal papilla ("ball and claw"). Epidermis overlying the infiltrate is thinned.

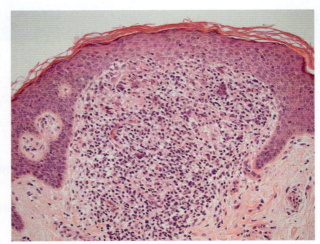

Figure 1.18.2 Lichen nitidus. Dermal papillae expanded by an infiltrate predominated by lymphocytes and histiocytes, but also including multinucleate giant cells.

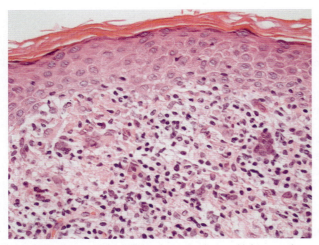

Figure 1.18.3 Lichen nitidus. Mild basal vacuolar change with few necrotic keratinocytes at dermal-epidermal interface.

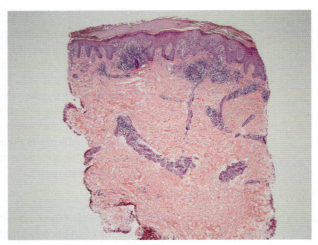

Figure 1.18.4 Lichen striatus. A superficial and deep perivascular infiltrate. The superficial lichenoid component shows contiguous involvement across multiple papillae.

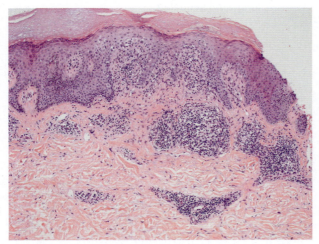

Figure 1.18.5 Lichen striatus. Slight parakeratosis and epidermal hyperplasia associated with a lichenoid lymphocytic infiltrate and interface vacuolar change.

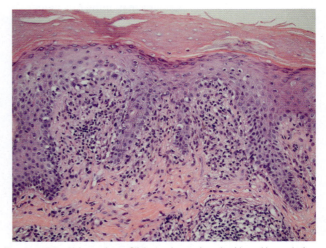

Figure 1.18.6 Lichen striatus. Slight parakeratosis and epidermal hyperplasia associated with a lichenoid lymphocytic infiltrate, interface vacuolar change, and slight spongiosis. Histiocytes and multinucleate giant cells not present.

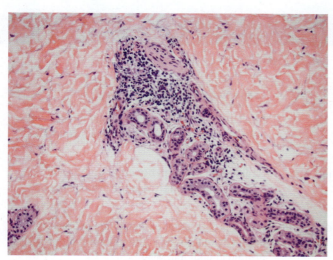

Figure 1.18.7 Lichen striatus. Perieccrine lymphocytic inflammation.

1.19 LICHEN NITIDUS VS LANGERHANS CELL HISTIOCYTOSIS

	Lichen Nitidus	**Langerhans Cell Histiocytosis**
Age	Children and young adults.	Most commonly in newborns and infants with peak incidence 1–3 y of age; less frequently in adults.
Location	Neck, trunk, upper extremities, abdomen, and penile shaft. May be generalized.	Scalp often involved but other cutaneous sites, including intertriginous areas, may be affected.
Etiology	Unknown. Immune reaction postulated.	Clonal proliferation of myeloid precursor cells driven by mutations in the mitogen-activated protein kinase pathway.
Presentation	Asymptomatic, monomorphous, 1-2 mm, flat-topped, tan-pink papules. Often shows Koebner phenomenon. Nail involvement in generalized form presents with longitudinal furrowing and ridging of nail plate.	Erythematous, brown-violaceous, scaly papules and plaques with areas of crust. Other organs may be involved, including bone and lungs.
Histology	1. Discrete collections of lymphocytes, histiocytes, Langerhans cells, and multinucleate giant cells within dermal papillae *(Figs. 1.19.1* and *1.19.2)*. 2. The rete ridges surrounding the infiltrate are elongated creating a "ball-in-claw" configuration *(Figs. 1.19.1* and *1.19.2)*. 3. The overlying epidermis in thinned and has basal vacuolar change with rare degenerated keratinocytes *(Fig. 1.19.3)*.	1. Stratum corneum thickened by parakeratosis and a serum crust *(Fig. 1.19.4)*. 2. A superficial dermal infiltrate of Langerhans cells, small lymphocytes, other types of histiocytes, and eosinophils *(Fig. 1.19.5)*. 3. Langerhans cells have a moderate amount of wispy light eosinophilic cytoplasm and nuclei that appear folded ("coffee bean" shape) *(Fig. 1.19.6)*. 4. Langerhans cells highlighted by CD1a *(Fig. 1.19.7)*, CD207 (langerin), and S100 protein.
Special studies	None.	Lesional cells show immunoreactivity for CD1a, CD207 (langerin), S100 protein.
Treatment	Typically no treatment necessary. If symptomatic or cosmetically problematic, topical steroids or calcineurin inhibitors may be used.	Treatment depends upon the extent of cutaneous and extracutaneous involvement. The single-system disease may be treated with systemic corticosteroids with or without chemotherapy. The multisystem disease is treated with induction chemotherapy followed by assessment of response and continuation of therapy based upon status.
Prognosis	Self-limiting and generally spontaneously resolves in months to a year.	Depends upon the extent of involvement of skin and other organ systems (particularly bone marrow, liver, spleen). The single-system disease has an excellent prognosis, while the multisystem disease has a potential risk of mortality. Initial response to therapy is prognostic.

1.19 Lichen Nitidus vs Langerhans Cell Histiocytosis

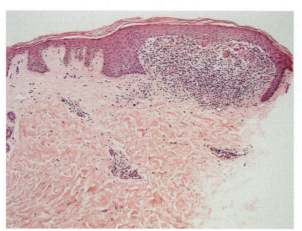

Figure 1.19.1 Lichen nitidus. A discrete infiltrate of lymphocytes and histiocytes expanding dermal papilla ("ball and claw").

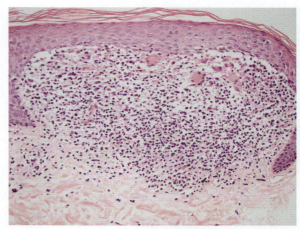

Figure 1.19.2 Lichen nitidus. An infiltrate composed of small lymphocytes, histiocytes with wispy cytoplasm, and multinucleate giant cells.

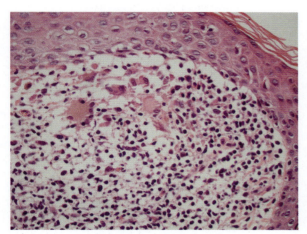

Figure 1.19.3 Lichen nitidus. Vacuolar change along the basal zone overlying the infiltrate. Histiocytes have a moderate amount of wispy, eosinophilic cytoplasm and round-oval nuclei.

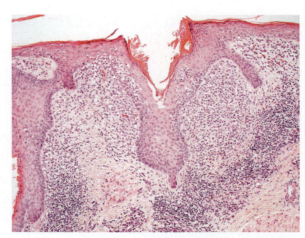

Figure 1.19.4 Langerhans cell histiocytosis. A moderately dense lichenoid infiltrate of lymphocytes, Langerhans cells, and eosinophils. Clusters of Langerhans cells within the epidermis associated with epidermal hyperplasia and hyperkeratosis.

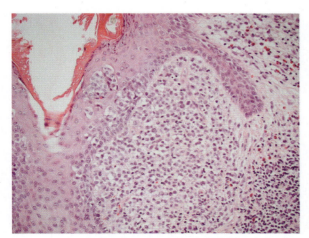

Figure 1.19.5 Langerhans cell histiocytosis. A superficial dermal infiltrate of Langerhans cells with extension into the epidermis. A background infiltrate of small lymphocytes and eosinophils (right).

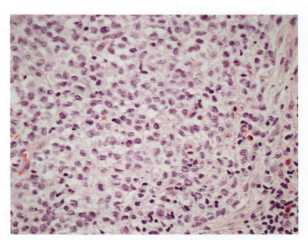

Figure 1.19.6 Langerhans cell histiocytosis. Langerhans cells with moderate amount of wispy light eosinophilic cytoplasm and nuclei that appear folded ("coffee bean" shape).

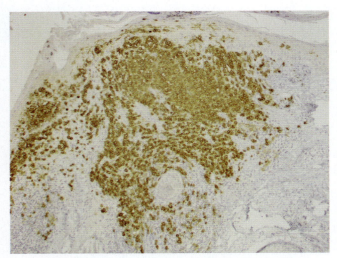

Figure 1.19.7 Langerhans cell histiocytosis. Immunohistochemical stain for CD1a highlighting Langerhans cells within the epidermis and the dermis.

1.20 PITYRIASIS LICHENOIDES ET VARIOLIFORMIS ACUTA VS PITYRIASIS LICHENOIDES CHRONICA

	Pityriasis Lichenoides et Varioliformis Acuta	Pityriasis Lichenoides Chronica
Age	Children and young adults, most commonly in the second or third decades of life.	Any age, primarily young adults and children.
Location	Trunk, proximal extremities, and flexural surfaces most commonly.	Trunk, proximal extremities, and buttocks primarily.
Etiology	Unknown. Theorized to be a T-cell dyscrasia or abnormal immune response to infections organisms.	Unknown. Theorized to be a T-cell dyscrasia or abnormal immune response to infections organisms.
Presentation	Abrupt onset of multiple erythematous macules that progress into papules or papulovesicles with overlying scale. The papule rapidly develops a hemorrhagic crust. Individual lesions resolve within weeks with scarring and dyspigmentation. New lesions often develop as others resolve resulting in lesions of different ages at any one time.	Indolent eruption of multiple asymptomatic red-brown papules with fine, mica-like scale. Lesions at various stages may be present at any given time. Lesions resolve with dyspigmentation but no scarring.
Histology	1. Confluent parakeratosis with entrapped serum and neutrophils *(Figs. 1.20.1-1.20.3)*. 2. Slight acanthosis with ballooning of keratinocytes and vacuolar interface alteration with necrotic keratinocytes in all levels of epidermis *(Fig. 1.20.3)*. 3. Exocytosis of small lymphocytes throughout epidermis *(Fig. 1.20.3)*. 4. A moderately dense, wedge-shaped lymphocytic infiltrate extending into the reticular dermis *(Fig. 1.20.1)*. 5. Erythrocyte extravasation within the epidermis and the superficial dermis *(Fig. 1.20.3)*.	1. Mounds of "wafer-like" parakeratosis without serum or neutrophils *(Figs. 1.20.4 and 1.20.5)*. 2. Interface vacuolar change with few necrotic keratinocytes and no ballooning *(Figs. 1.20.5 and 1.20.6)*. 3. Few lymphocytes within the epidermis *(Fig. 1.20.6)*. 4. A relatively sparse superficial perivascular infiltrate; no significant deep dermal involvement *(Fig. 1.20.4)*. 5. No extravasated erythrocytes. 6. Features overlap with those of pityriasis lichenoides et varioliformis acuta but are less pronounced.
Special studies	None.	None.
Treatment	Surveillance without treatment for many cases. If therapy is desired, systemic antibiotics (doxycycline, minocycline, erythromycin, azithromycin) and phototherapy are first-line treatments. Topical corticosteroids may be prescribed for symptomatic relief.	No therapy is necessary. If treatment is desired, first-line therapies include topical corticosteroids, oral antibiotics, and phototherapy.
Prognosis	Self-limited disease that waxes and wanes with a duration that is variable and lasting from several weeks to years. May progress to pityriasis lichenoides chronica. Rare reports of progression to cutaneous T-cell lymphoma.	A benign disease. Individual lesions resolve spontaneously over several weeks. Disease may persist for months to years, with remissions and exacerbations. Rare reports of progression to cutaneous T-cell lymphoma.

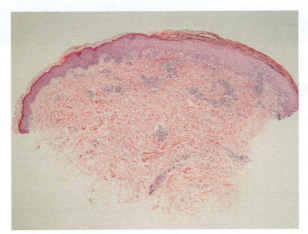

Figure 1.20.1 Pityriasis lichenoides et varioliformis acuta. A wedge-shaped superficial and deep lichenoid and perivascular infiltrate. Mild epidermal hyperplasia with blunted rete ridge pattern and overlying confluent parakeratosis.

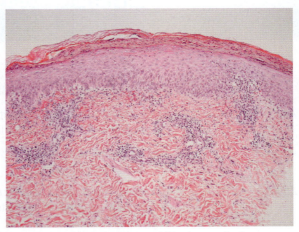

Figure 1.20.2 Pityriasis lichenoides et varioliformis acuta. Confluent parakeratosis with entrapped serum and neutrophils. Interface vacuolar change with lichenoid lymphocytic inflammation, exocytosis of lymphocytes, and erythrocyte extravasation.

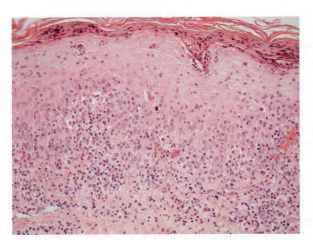

Figure 1.20.3 Pityriasis lichenoides et varioliformis acuta. Confluent parakeratosis with entrapped serum and neutrophils. Interface vacuolar change with necrotic keratinocytes and prominent lymphocytic exocytosis. Erythrocyte extravasation within dermal papillae.

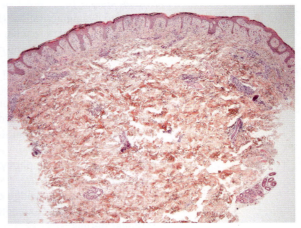

Figure 1.20.4 Pityriasis lichenoides chronica. Focal parakeratosis with slight epidermal hyperplasia and a patchy superficial to mid-perivascular and lichenoid inflammatory infiltrate.

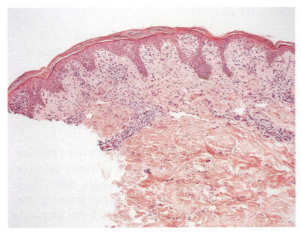

Figure 1.20.5 Pityriasis lichenoides chronica. Delicate "wafer-like" parakeratosis without serum or neutrophils. Vacuolar interface alteration with a superficial lichenoid lymphocytic infiltrate.

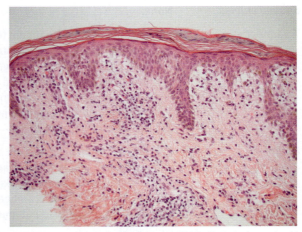

Figure 1.20.6 Pityriasis lichenoides chronica. "Wafer-like" parakeratosis with interface vacuolar change associated with rare degenerated keratinocytes and mild lymphocytic exocytosis.

1.21 PITYRIASIS LICHENOIDES ET VARIOLIFORMIS ACUTA VS LYMPHOMATOID PAPULOSIS

	Pityriasis Lichenoides et Varioliformis Acuta	**Lymphomatoid Papulosis**
Age	Children and young adults, most commonly in the second or third decades of life.	Any age, peak incidence in the fifth decade of life.
Location	Trunk, proximal extremities, and flexural surfaces most commonly.	Trunk and extremities. Mucosa spared.
Etiology	Unknown. Theorized to be a T-cell dyscrasia or abnormal immune response to infections organisms.	Unknown. Viral etiology postulated.
Presentation	Abrupt onset of multiple erythematous macules that progress into papules or papulovesicles with overlying scale. The papule rapidly develops a hemorrhagic crust. Individual lesions resolve within weeks with scarring and dyspigmentation. New lesions often develop as others resolve resulting in lesions of different ages at any one time.	Crops of multiple, asymptomatic, red to violaceous papulonodules that may become necrotic and hemorrhagic. Lesions spontaneously regress but recur. Resolve with dyspigmentation and scarring. Lesions at various stages may be present at any given time.
Histology	1. Confluent parakeratosis with a small amount of entrapped serum and neutrophils *(Figs. 1.21.1* and *1.21.2)*. 2. Slight acanthosis with vacuolar interface alteration and occasional necrotic keratinocytes *(Figs. 1.21.2* and *1.21.3)*. 3. Exocytosis of small lymphocytes throughout epidermis *(Fig. 1.21.3)*. 4. A moderately dense, wedge-shaped reactive lymphocytic infiltrate extending into the reticular dermis. No appreciable lymphocytic atypia *(Figs. 1.21.2* and *1.21.3)*. 5. Erythrocyte extravasation *(Fig. 1.21.3)*.	1. A wedge-shaped, moderate to dense infiltrate within the dermis *(Fig. 1.21.4)*. 2. The infiltrate is mixed composition with population of atypical lymphocytes with enlarged, irregular, and hyperchromatic nuclei *(Figs. 1.21.5* and *1.21.6)*. Mitoses may be present. 3. The infiltrate has admixed reactive inflammatory cells including neutrophils, eosinophils, and plasma cells *(Fig. 1.21.6)*. 4. Atypical lymphocytes show immunoreactivity for CD30 *(Fig. 1.21.7)*.
Special studies	Immunohistochemistry for lymphocyte markers show lymphocytes are primarily CD3- and CD8-positive T cells that are CD4- and CD30-negative.	The atypical lymphocytes are typically CD3, CD4, and CD30 positive and CD8 negative with immunohistochemical stains.
Treatment	Surveillance without treatment for many cases. If therapy is desired, systemic antibiotics (doxycycline, minocycline, erythromycin, azithromycin) and phototherapy are first-line treatments. Topical corticosteroids may be prescribed for symptomatic relief.	Watchful waiting given that most lesions show spontaneous resolution. If treatment desired, topical steroids, phototherapy, low-dose methotrexate, and bexarotene may be used.
Prognosis	Self-limited disease that waxes and wanes with a duration that is variable from several weeks to years. May progress to pityriasis lichenoides chronica. Rare reports of progression to cutaneous T-cell lymphoma.	Good. Most individuals have a chronic, indolent course. Up to 25% patients may have associated malignancy, primarily malignant lymphoma; therefore, long-term surveillance is recommended.

1 Inflammatory Diseases of the Epidermis

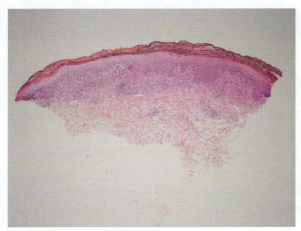

Figure 1.21.1 Pityriasis lichenoides et varioliformis acuta. Confluent parakeratosis, mild epidermal hyperplasia, and a wedge-shaped dermal infiltrate.

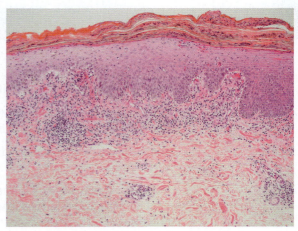

Figure 1.21.2 Pityriasis lichenoides et varioliformis acuta. Confluent parakeratosis with entrapped serum and neutrophils. Interface vacuolar change with prominent exocytosis of small lymphocytes without atypical forms.

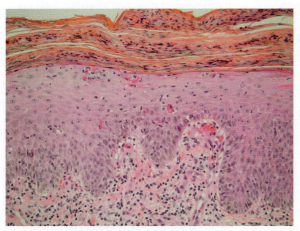

Figure 1.21.3 Pityriasis lichenoides et varioliformis acuta. Interface vacuolar change with occasional necrotic keratinocytes and prominent exocytosis of mature-appearing lymphocytes. A lichenoid infiltrate of small lymphocytes with erythrocyte extravasation.

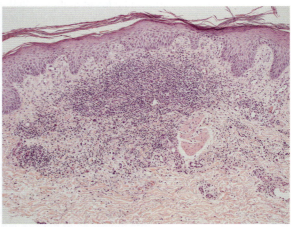

Figure 1.21.4 Lymphomatoid papulosis. A moderately dense, lichenoid dermal infiltrate with reactive epidermal changes and parakeratosis.

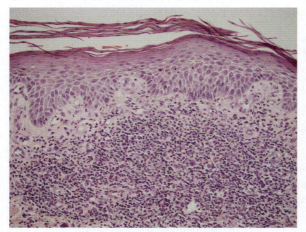

Figure 1.21.5 Lymphomatoid papulosis. Reactive epidermal changes with mild intercellular edema and exocytosis of rare inflammatory cells. No interface vacuolar change or necrotic keratinocytes.

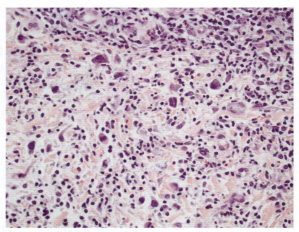

Figure 1.21.6 Lymphomatoid papulosis. A dermal infiltrate composed of large, atypical lymphocytes with irregular, hyperchromatic nuclei. Background of small lymphocytes with occasional eosinophils and plasma cells.

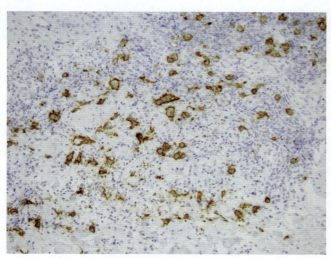

Figure 1.21.7 Lymphomatoid papulosis. Large, atypical lymphocytes show immunoreactivity for CD30.

1.22 ERYTHEMA MULTIFORME VS PITYRIASIS LICHENOIDES ET VARIOLIFORMIS ACUTA

	Erythema Multiforme	**Pityriasis Lichenoides et Varioliformis Acuta**
Age	Any age.	Children and young adults, most commonly in the second or third decades of life.
Location	Begins symmetrically on extensor surfaces of extremities and spreads centripetally to trunk. May involve mucosae.	Trunk, proximal extremities, and flexural surfaces most commonly.
Etiology	Cell-mediated immune response most often triggered by infection, especially herpes simplex virus and *Mycoplasma pneumoniae*, and medications.	Unknown. Theorized to be a T-cell dyscrasia or abnormal immune response to infections organisms.
Presentation	Pink-red papules that evolve into targetoid plaques with three concentric rings. May be accompanied by burning or pruritus.	Abrupt onset of multiple erythematous macules that progress into papules or papulovesicles with overlying scale. The papules rapidly develops a hemorrhagic crust. Individual lesions resolve within weeks with scarring and dyspigmentation. New lesions often develop as others resolve resulting in lesions of different ages at any one time.
Histology	1. A normal basket-weave stratum corneum (Figs. 1.22.1 and 1.22.2). 2. An epidermis of normal thickness and rete ridge architecture (Fig. 1.22.1). 3. Vacuolar interface alteration with numerous necrotic keratinocytes (Fig. 1.22.2). 4. A sparse, superficial perivascular lymphocytic infiltrate (Figs. 1.22.2 and 1.22.3).	1. Confluent parakeratosis with entrapped serum and neutrophils (Figs. 1.22.4 and 1.22.5). 2. Slight acanthosis with vacuolar interface alteration and occasional necrotic keratinocytes (Figs. 1.22.5 and 1.22.6). 3. Exocytosis of small lymphocytes throughout epidermis (Fig. 1.22.5). 4. A moderately dense, wedge-shaped lymphocytic infiltrate extending into the reticular dermis (Fig. 1.22.4). 5. Erythrocyte extravasation (Fig. 1.22.6).
Special studies	None.	None.
Treatment	Depends upon underlying etiology and severity. Treatment of triggering infection or removal of the offending drug. Topical corticosteroids and antihistamines for relief of symptoms. High-potency or systemic corticosteroids for mucosal involvement or severe cases.	Surveillance without treatment for many cases. If therapy is desired, systemic antibiotics (doxycycline, minocycline, erythromycin, azithromycin) and phototherapy are first-line treatments. Topical corticosteroids may be prescribed for symptomatic relief.
Prognosis	Generally resolves within 2 w, although may persist for several weeks.	Self-limited disease that waxes and wanes with a duration that is variable from several weeks to years. May progress to pityriasis lichenoides chronica. Rare reports of progression to cutaneous T-cell lymphoma.

1.22 Erythema Multiforme vs Pityriasis Lichenoides et Varioliformis Acuta

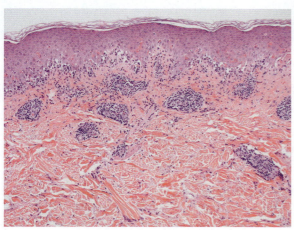

Figure 1.22.1 Erythema multiforme. A basket-weave orthokeratotic stratum corneum, interface vacuolar change, and a superficial perivascular lymphocytic infiltrate. Note that there is no parakeratosis.

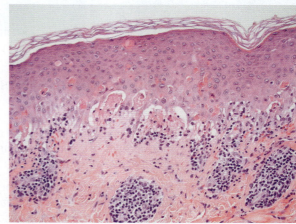

Figure 1.22.2 Erythema multiforme. A basket-weave orthokeratotic stratum corneum with numerous necrotic keratinocytes and exocytosis of lymphocytes along the basal zone.

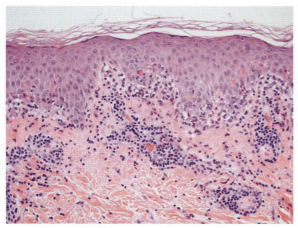

Figure 1.22.3 Erythema multiforme. Interface vacuolar change with necrotic keratinocytes and a relatively sparse superficial lymphocytic infiltrate.

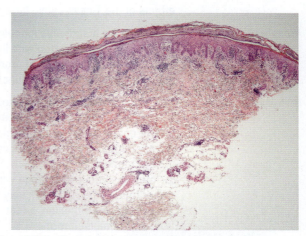

Figure 1.22.4 Pityriasis lichenoides et varioliformis acuta. Confluent parakeratosis with entrapped serum and neutrophils. A wedge-shaped superficial and deep dermal infiltrate.

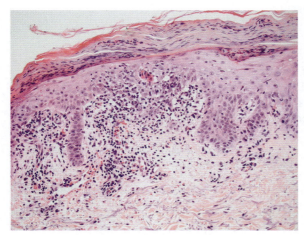

Figure 1.22.5 Pityriasis lichenoides et varioliformis acuta. Confluent parakeratosis with small collections of serum and neutrophils. Interface vacuolar change with clustered necrotic keratinocytes and prominent exocytosis of lymphocytes throughout the epidermis.

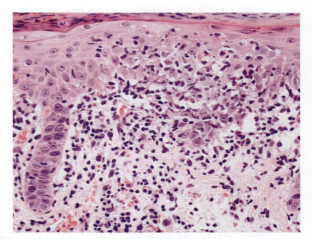

Figure 1.22.6 Pityriasis lichenoides et varioliformis acuta. Vacuolar interface change with prominent exocytosis of lymphocytes and extravasation of erythrocytes within the papillary dermis.

1.23 GRAFT-VERSUS-HOST DISEASE, ACUTE VS ERYTHEMA MULTIFORME

	Graft-Versus-Host Disease (GVHD), Acute	**Erythema Multiforme**
Age	Any age.	Any age.
Location	Begins on face, neck, ears, and acral skin, then spreads to trunk and extremities and may become generalized.	Begins symmetrically on extensor surfaces of extremities and spreads centripetally to trunk. May involve mucosae.
Etiology	Immune-mediated reaction after allogeneic hematopoietic stem cell transplantation. Related to HLA mismatch in which donor T-cell lymphocytes activate and proliferate. Tissue damage from chemotherapy/radiotherapy increases recognition of host's antigens by the donor T cells. The cytotoxic effects of the T cells cause host cell death.	Cell-mediated immune response most often triggered by infection, especially herpes simplex virus and *M. pneumoniae*, and medications.
Presentation	Erythematous blanchable macules and papules. Often associated with liver and gastrointestinal involvement producing diarrhea and abnormal liver function tests.	Pink-red papules that evolve into targetoid plaques with three concentric rings. May be accompanied by burning or pruritus.
Histology	1. A normal basket-weave orthokeratotic stratum corneum *(Figs. 1.23.1 and 1.23.2)*. 2. The epidermis is normal in thickness and rete ridge pattern. Keratinocytes have mild nuclear atypia *(Figs. 1.23.2 and 1.23.3)*. 3. Interface vacuolar change with necrotic keratinocytes *(Fig. 1.23.2)*; may also occur in follicular epithelium, a feature not seen in erythema multiforme. 4. Necrotic keratinocytes associated with two or more lymphocytes ("satellite cell necrosis") *(Figs. 1.23.2 and 1.23.3)*. 5. A superficial perivascular lymphocytic infiltrate; rare eosinophils may be present *(Fig. 1.23.1)*.	1. A stratum corneum composed of normal basket-weave orthokeratin *(Fig. 1.23.4)*. 2. Mild spongiosis with vesiculation and ballooning of keratinocytes *(Fig. 1.23.5)*. 3. Interface vacuolar change with numerous necrotic keratinocytes *(Figs. 1.23.5 and 1.23.6)*. 4. A sparse, superficial perivascular lymphocytic infiltrate with mild papillary dermal edema and erythrocyte extravasation *(Fig. 1.23.6)*.
Special studies	None.	None.
Treatment	Dependent upon the grade and extent of the disease. For grade I acute GVHD, topical corticosteroids and calcineurin inhibitors. Systemic immunosuppressive therapy for grades II-IV acute GVHD.	Depends upon underlying etiology and severity. Treatment of triggering infection or removal of the offending drug. Topical corticosteroids and antihistamines for relief of symptoms. High-potency or systemic corticosteroids for mucosal involvement or severe cases.
Prognosis	Variable.	Generally resolves within 2 w, although may persist for several weeks.

1.23 Graft-Versus-Host Disease, Acute vs Erythema Multiforme

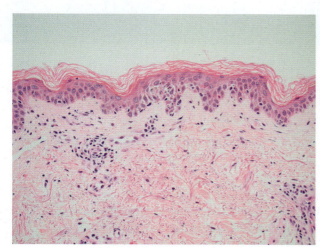

Figure 1.23.1 GVHD disease. Interface vacuolar change with occasional apoptotic, degenerated basal keratinocytes and a sparse superficial perivascular lymphocytic infiltrate.

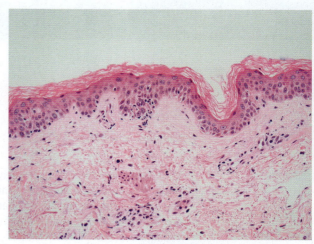

Figure 1.23.2 GVHD disease. Apoptotic, degenerated keratinocytes with closely associated lymphocytes ("satellite cell necrosis").

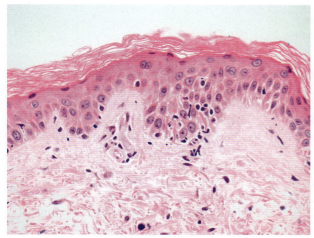

Figure 1.23.3 GVHD disease. Satellite cell necrosis with lymphocytes closely associated with apoptotic keratinocytes. Features may overlap with those of erythema multiforme and, therefore, clinical correlation is essential.

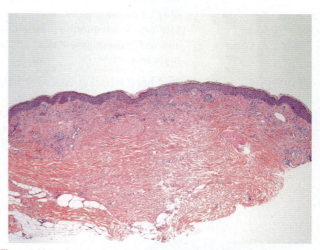

Figure 1.23.4 Erythema multiforme. Normal epidermal thickness with an overlying basket-weave stratum corneum and a sparse superficial perivascular and interstitial infiltrate.

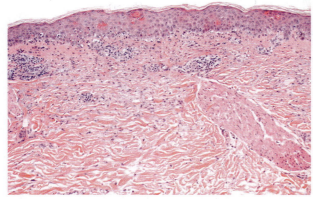

Figure 1.23.5 Erythema multiforme. Vacuolar interface change with numerous necrotic keratinocytes throughout the epidermis and a sparse superficial dermal infiltrate of lymphocytes.

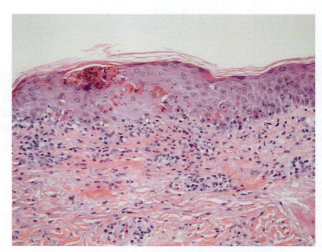

Figure 1.23.6 Erythema multiforme. Interface vacuolar change with numerous necrotic keratinocytes at all levels of the epidermis. Lymphocytic exocytosis along the zone. Although features may be indistinguishable from GVHD, no characteristic satellite cell necrosis is present.

1.24 FIXED DRUG ERUPTION VS ERYTHEMA MULTIFORME

	Fixed Drug Eruption	**Erythema Multiforme**
Age	Any age.	Any age.
Location	Genitals, lips, hands, and trunk.	Begins symmetrically on extensor surfaces of extremities and spreads centripetally to trunk.
Etiology	Localized cutaneous cellular delayed hypersensitivity reaction to a medication. Reaction is considered "fixed" because it recurs in same location if the drug is readministered.	Cell-mediated immune response most often triggered by infection, especially herpes simplex virus and *M. pneumoniae*, and medications.
Presentation	Well-circumscribed, round, dusky, red-brown macules and plaques that occur up to 2 w from the initial exposure to the drug. May be accompanied burning sensation or pruritus. Subsequent occurrences at same site with hyperpigmentation and surrounding erythema.	Pink-red papules that evolve into targetoid plaques with three concentric rings. May be accompanied by burning or pruritus.
Histology	1. A normal basket-weave orthokeratotic stratum corneum *(Fig. 1.24.1)*. 2. The epidermis is normal in thickness and rete ridge pattern *(Figs. 1.24.1 and 1.24.2)*. 3. Interface vacuolar change with necrotic keratinocytes *(Fig. 1.24.2)*. 4. A superficial and deep dermal infiltrate of eosinophils and neutrophils in addition to lymphocytes *(Figs. 1.24.2 and 1.24.3)*.	1. A normal basket-weave orthokeratotic stratum corneum *(Figs. 1.24.4 and 1.24.5)*. 2. The epidermis is normal in thickness and rete ridge pattern *(Figs. 1.24.4 and 1.24.5)*. 3. Interface vacuolar change with numerous necrotic keratinocytes *(Figs. 1.24.5 and 1.24.6)*. 4. A sparse superficial perivascular lymphocytic infiltrate *(Figs. 1.24.5 and 1.24.6)*. No appreciable eosinophils or neutrophils.
Special studies	None.	None.
Treatment	Avoidance of the offending medication; a short course of oral corticosteroids for severe cases; symptomatic treatment of pruritus with antihistamines.	Depends upon underlying etiology and severity. Treatment of triggering infection or removal of the offending drug. Topical corticosteroids and antihistamines for relief of symptoms. High-potency or systemic corticosteroids for mucosal involvement or severe cases.
Prognosis	Initial lesions persist from days to weeks and slowly resolve with hyperpigmentation. Each recurrence appears with more rapid onset and exhibits increased severity and longevity.	Generally resolves within 2 w, although may persist for several weeks.

1.24 Fixed Drug Eruption vs Erythema Multiforme

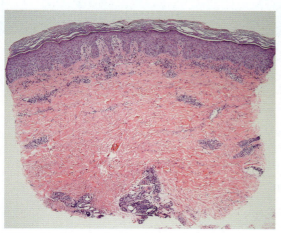

Figure 1.24.1 Fixed drug eruption. An epidermis of normal thickness and rete ridge architecture, with an overlying basket-weave orthokeratotic stratum corneum and a moderately dense superficial and deep perivascular dermal inflammatory infiltrate.

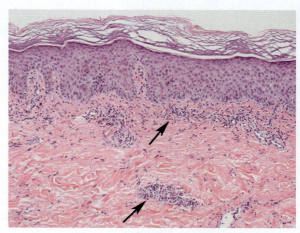

Figure 1.24.2 Fixed drug eruption. Vacuolar interface alteration with individual necrotic keratinocytes in lower portion of the epidermis. A dermal infiltrate includes eosinophils (arrows).

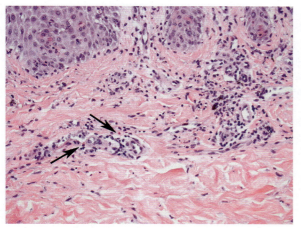

Figure 1.24.3 Fixed drug eruption. A dermal infiltrate containing eosinophils (arrows) and lymphocytes. Melanophages in the superficial dermis.

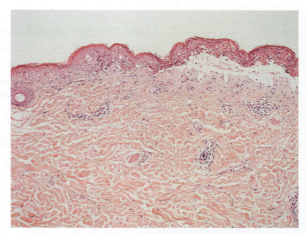

Figure 1.24.4 Erythema multiforme. An epidermis of normal thickness and rete ridge architecture, with an overlying basket-weave orthokeratotic stratum corneum. Interface alteration with focal separation of the epidermis from the dermis. A sparse superficial perivascular dermal inflammatory infiltrate.

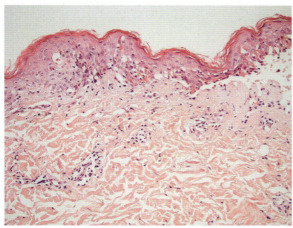

Figure 1.24.5 Erythema multiforme. Interface alteration with focal separation of the epidermis from the dermis. A sparse superficial perivascular dermal lymphocytic infiltrate. Note that there are no eosinophils or deep extension of the inflammation.

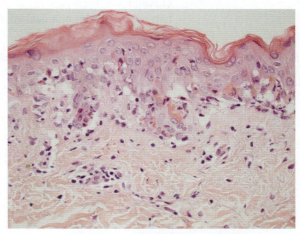

Figure 1.24.6 Erythema multiforme. Vacuolar interface alteration with numerous individual necrotic keratinocytes. A very sparse superficial lymphocytic dermal infiltrate.

1.25 ERYTHEMA MULTIFORME VS MORBILLIFORM DRUG ERUPTION

	Erythema Multiforme	**Morbilliform Drug Eruption**
Age	Any age.	Any age.
Location	Begins symmetrically on extensor surfaces of extremities and spreads centripetally to trunk. May involve mucosae.	Primarily develops on trunk and upper extremities and then spreads to lower extremities. Spares the face and mucosae.
Etiology	Cell-mediated immune response most often triggered by infection, especially herpes simplex virus and *M. pneumoniae*, and medications.	Delayed, T-cell–mediated reaction.
Presentation	Pink-red papules that evolve into targetoid plaques with three concentric rings. May be accompanied by burning or pruritus.	Erythematous macules, papules, and patches that coalesce. Occurs up to 2 w following first exposure to drug and 1-2 d after starting drug on subsequent episodes.
Histology	1. A normal basket-weave orthokeratotic stratum corneum *(Figs. 1.25.1 and 1.25.2)*. 2. The epidermis is normal in thickness and rete ridge pattern *(Figs. 1.25.1 and 1.25.2)*. 3. Interface vacuolar change with necrotic keratinocytes *(Figs. 1.25.2 and 1.25.3)*. 4. A sparse superficial perivascular lymphocytic infiltrate *(Figs. 1.25.1 and 1.25.1)*.	1. The stratum corneum usually consists of basket-weave orthokeratosis but may have subtle parakeratosis *(Fig. 1.25.4)*. 2. Subtle interface vacuolar change and mild spongiosis *(Figs. 1.25.4 and 1.25.5)*. Very rare degenerated keratinocytes along the basal zone *(Fig. 1.25.6)*. 3. A superficial perivascular and interstitial infiltrate of lymphocytes, eosinophils, and/or neutrophils *(Figs. 1.25.5 and 1.25.6)*. 4. Mild papillary dermal edema and erythrocyte extravasation *(Fig. 1.25.6)*.
Special studies	None.	None.
Treatment	Depends upon underlying etiology and severity. Treatment of triggering infection or removal of the offending drug. Topical corticosteroids and antihistamines for relief of symptoms. High-potency or systemic corticosteroids for mucosal involvement or severe cases.	Removal of the offending medication. Topical corticosteroids and antihistamine for symptomatic relief.
Prognosis	Generally resolves within 2 w, although may persist for several weeks.	Resolves 1-2 w after cessation of drug.

1.25 Erythema Multiforme vs Morbilliform Drug Eruption

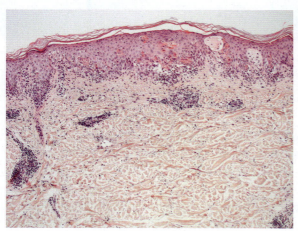

Figure 1.25.1 Erythema multiforme. A normal basket-weave orthokeratotic stratum corneum overlying the epidermis with interface vacuolar change and focal spongiosis. A sparse superficial perivascular lymphocytic infiltrate.

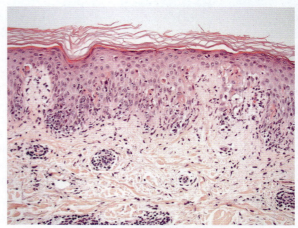

Figure 1.25.2 Erythema multiforme. Interface vacuolar alteration with numerous necrotic keratinocytes and mild lymphocytic exocytosis. A relatively sparse dermal infiltrate of lymphocytes; no eosinophils.

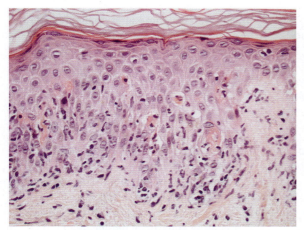

Figure 1.25.3 Erythema multiforme. Numerous necrotic keratinocytes in mid-epidermis associated with mild lymphocytic exocytosis.

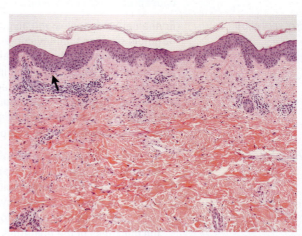

Figure 1.25.4 Morbilliform drug eruption. An epidermis of normal thickness with an overlying basket-weave stratum corneum and focal, subtle interface vacuolar change (arrow).

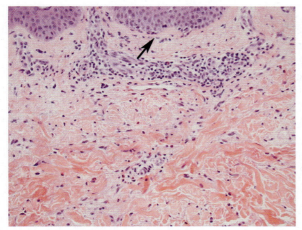

Figure 1.25.5 Morbilliform drug eruption. A superficial perivascular and interstitial infiltrate with slight interface vacuolar change (arrow) and exocytosis of rare lymphocytes along the basal zone. Eosinophils within a superficial dermal infiltrate.

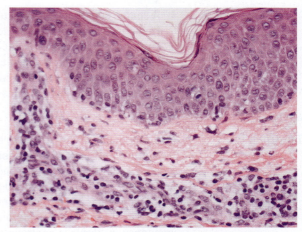

Figure 1.25.6 Morbilliform drug eruption. Slight epidermal spongiosis and interface inflammation. Reactive vascular changes with mild erythrocyte extravasation associated with a superficial dermal infiltrate.

1.26 TOXIC EPIDERMAL NECROLYSIS VS STAPHYLOCOCCAL SCALDED SKIN SYNDROME

	Toxic Epidermal Necrolysis	**Staphylococcal Scalded Skin Syndrome**
Age	Any age.	Children less than 6 y of age; rare in adults.
Location	Starts on face and chest before spreading to other sites in a symmetric fashion. Mucosal lesions are invariably present and may precede or follow the skin lesions.	Starts on face and intertriginous areas (neck, axillae, inguinal folds) and proceeds to trunk. Does not involve mucosa.
Etiology	Considered to be a type IV hypersensitivity reaction with an abnormal immune response resulting from HLA interactions with the offending drug and subsequent T-cell activation. This produces a cytotoxic response against keratinocytes that induces widespread keratinocyte necrosis.	Denudation of the skin by an epidermolytic exotoxin-producing strain of staphylococcus causing infection at a distant site, such as pharyngitis, otitis, and conjunctivitis. The exotoxin targets desmoglein 1 in the superficial epidermis causing acantholysis.
Presentation	Erythematous macules and atypical targetoid plaques that develop and spread rapidly. Vesicles and bullae develop with skin sloughing within a week of initial presentation. Eruption usually begins 1-2 w after administration of the causal drug. May have systemic symptoms including fever, sore throat, headache, and cytopenia.	Begins with widespread erythema followed by development of tender flaccid vesicles and bullae. These rupture and form erosions. Typically has a prodrome of irritability and fever.
Histology	1. A normal basket-weave orthokeratotic stratum corneum *(Figs. 1.26.1* and *1.26.2)*. 2. Vacuolar interface change with numerous necrotic keratinocytes *(Fig. 1.26.2)*. Necrosis progresses to involve full thickness of the epidermis with detachment of the epidermis from the dermis *(Fig. 1.26.3)*. 3. Interface changes may involve adnexal structures. 4. A sparse superficial perivascular lymphocytic infiltrate *(Figs. 1.26.2* and *1.26.3)*. 5. Distinction from staphylococcal scalded skin syndrome is often a clinical query. Histologically, the level of cleavage aids in distinguishing the two entities.	1. A normal basket-weave orthokeratotic stratum corneum *(Figs. 1.26.4* and *1.26.5)*. 2. Acantholysis of the superficial epidermis forming a subcorneal split *(Figs. 1.26.5* and *1.26.6)*. 3. A sparse superficial perivascular polymorphous infiltrate *(Figs. 1.26.4* and *1.26.6)*. 4. Bacteria are not present within the vesicle formed by acantholysis.
Special studies	None.	Culture of the suspected site of infection.
Treatment	Discontinuation of the offending drug. Supportive care, often in burn centers, with monitoring for fluid/electrolyte imbalance and sepsis. Intravenous immunoglobulin (IVIG) sometimes used for treatment but use of systemic corticosteroids and immunosuppressive is controversial.	Systemic antibiotics to treat staphylococcal infection. Emollients to prevent fluid loss and promote reepithelialization.

1.26 Toxic Epidermal Necrolysis vs Staphylococcal Scalded Skin Syndrome

	Toxic Epidermal Necrolysis	**Staphylococcal Scalded Skin Syndrome**
Prognosis	Can be life-threatening with high mortality rates if widespread and untreated.	Good prognosis in children if diagnosed early and treated appropriately. Eruption improves within a few days of treatment and shows complete resolution within 2 w. Worse prognosis in adults with a higher mortality rate due to sepsis.

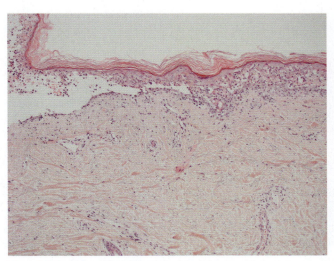

Figure 1.26.1 Toxic epidermal necrolysis. A basket-weave orthokeratotic stratum corneum and interface vacuolar change with numerous individual necrotic keratinocytes and an underlying sparse superficial perivascular lymphocytic infiltrate. Areas of full-thickness epidermal necrosis leading to detachment of the epidermis from the dermis (left).

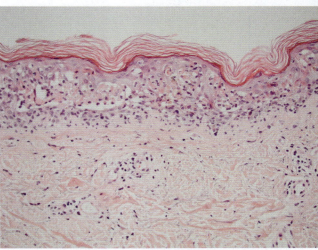

Figure 1.26.2 Toxic epidermal necrolysis. Interface vacuolar change with numerous necrotic keratinocytes at all levels of the epidermis. A sparse superficial dermal lymphocytic infiltrate.

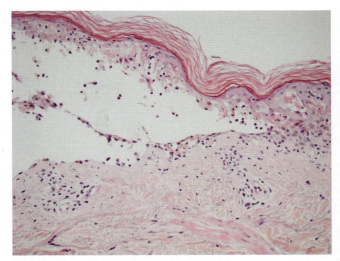

Figure 1.26.3 Toxic epidermal necrolysis. Areas of full-thickness epidermal necrosis with detachment of the epidermis from the dermis.

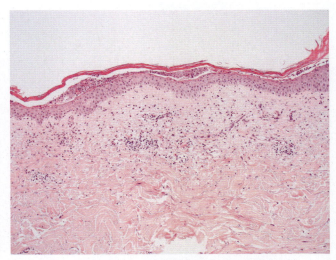

Figure 1.26.4 Staphylococcal scalded skin syndrome. Intraepidermal, subcorneal neutrophilic aggregates with a polymorphous dermal infiltrate.

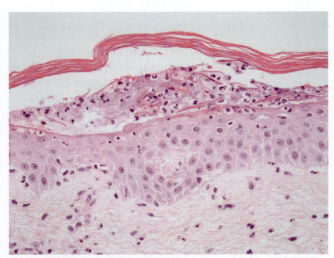

Figure 1.26.5 Staphylococcal scalded skin syndrome. Subcorneal split containing few neutrophils and degenerated acantholytic cells.

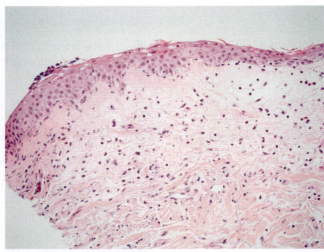

Figure 1.26.6 Staphylococcal scalded skin syndrome. Denuded stratum corneum with occasional acantholytic cells on surface of epidermis and exocytosis of rare neutrophils.

1.27 RADIATION DERMATITIS, CHRONIC VS LICHEN SCLEROSUS

	Radiation Dermatitis, Chronic	**Lichen Sclerosus**
Age	Any age but primarily adults undergoing treatment of cancer.	Bimodal age distribution in prepubertal and postmenopausal women; middle-aged men.
Location	Any location treated with radiation. Face, neck, upper back, and upper chest most susceptible to radiation dermatitis.	Predilection for anogenital region including vulva, perineum, and perianal skin in women. In men, glans penis and foreskin are typically involved. Extragenital locations in less than 10% of cases with the most common locations of breasts, thighs, buttocks, back, neck, and chest.
Etiology	Ionizing radiation generates free radicals and reactive oxygen intermediates that damage the dividing cells of the epidermal basal layer and the superficial dermis. This leads to alterations in proteins, lipids, and carbohydrates of the skin as well as DNA damage. Acute effects, arising within 90 d of the initiation of therapy, are a result of direct tissue injury and local inflammatory reactions. Chronic effects, typically present months to years after exposure, are due to changes in the vasculature and connective tissue of the dermis as a consequence of injury to endothelial cells and fibroblasts.	Not entirely known. Autoimmune mechanisms, genetic factors, hormonal influence, trauma, and irritation, as well as localized infection have been proposed as components in the etiology.
Presentation	Acute—erythema, dryness, alopecia, and desquamation. Chronic—epidermal thinning, dermal atrophy, telangiectasia, dyspigmentation, and induration.	Porcelain-white papules and plaques with follicular dells, hyperkeratosis, telangiectasia, and a cellophane paper appearance. Late-stage lesions are atrophic and may have erosions, purpura, and fissuring.
Histology	1. Epidermal atrophy with interface vacuolar change (Figs. 1.27.1 and 1.27.2). 2. Dermal edema with vascular ectasia and a sparse perivascular lymphocytic infiltrate (Fig. 1.27.2). Melanophages in the superficial dermis. 3. Light eosinophilic, homogenized, dermal sclerosis with atypical fibroblasts (Fig. 1.27.3). 4. Absence of adnexal structures (Fig. 1.27.1).	1. Compact hyperkeratosis (Fig. 1.27.4). 2. Epidermal thinning with effacement of rete ridges (Figs. 1.27.4 and 1.27.6). 3. Interface vacuolar change with occasional necrotic basal keratinocytes (Fig. 1.27.5). 4. Homogenization and sclerosis of superficial dermal collagen with telangiectasia (Fig. 1.27.6). No atypical fibroblasts. 5. Band of lymphomononuclear inflammation below the zone of sclerosis (Figs. 1.27.5 and 1.27.6).
Special studies	None.	None.
Treatment	Management depends upon the degree of skin damage. For dryness and pruritus, moisturizers and mid-potency corticosteroids may be used. Semitransparent films for dressing skin to promote healing and reepithelialization. Antimicrobials for any superinfection.	Ultrapotent or potent topical corticosteroids coupled with avoidance of irritants and treatment of any concomitant infection. Long-term surveillance.

(continued)

	Radiation Dermatitis, Chronic	Lichen Sclerosus
Prognosis	Dependent upon the degree of skin damage. Severe damage may be associated with wound formation and superinfection. Dystrophic calcification may occur in damaged skin and be associated with increased morbidity. There is an increased risk of nonmelanoma cutaneous malignancies.	Improvement in clinical signs with treatment but typically a chronic disease with only approximately 25% of patients showing complete resolution. Progression of disease with scarring and fusion particularly with delay in diagnosis or noncompliance in therapy. Increased risk for well-differentiated VIN and squamous cell carcinoma.

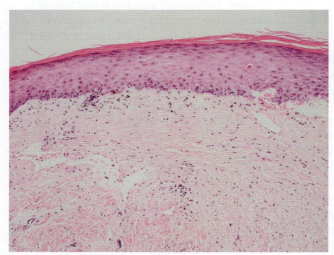

Figure 1.27.1 Radiation dermatitis. An epidermis of variable thickness with hyperkeratosis. Epidermal keratinocytes have reactive changes with hypergranulosis. The dermis is sclerotic with sparse inflammation and telangiectasia.

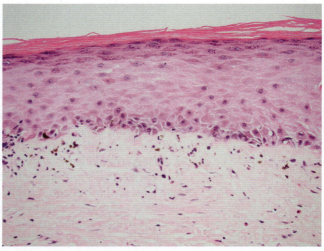

Figure 1.27.2 Radiation dermatitis. Interface vacuolar change with squamatization of the basal zone. Edema and homogenization of superficial dermal collagen with pigment incontinence.

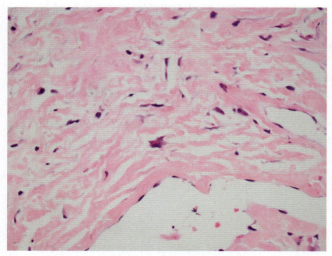

Figure 1.27.3 Radiation dermatitis. Light eosinophilic, edematous, and sclerotic collagen with atypical fibroblasts within the reticular dermis. Telangiectasia but no significant inflammation.

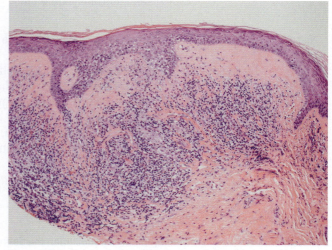

Figure 1.27.4 Lichen sclerosus. Mild compact orthohyperkeratosis with diminished rete ridge pattern. The dermis has superficial sclerosis with underlying dense band of inflammation.

1.27 Radiation Dermatitis, Chronic vs Lichen Sclerosus

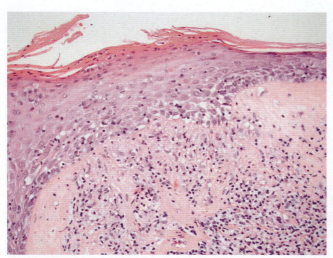

Figure 1.27.5 Lichen sclerosus. Focal parakeratosis with interface vacuolar change and occasional necrotic keratinocytes.

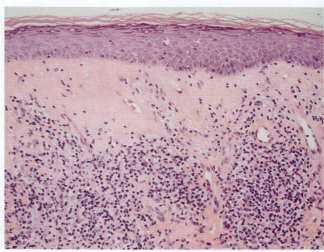

Figure 1.27.6 Lichen sclerosus. Expansion of the papillary dermis by sclerotic collagen with mild telangiectasia and underlying dense band of lymphocytes.

1.28 DERMATOMYOSITIS VS LUPUS ERYTHEMATOSUS (DISCOID)

	Dermatomyositis	**Lupus Erythematosus (Discoid)**
Age	Juvenile form onset between 4 and 14 y of age; adult form onset between 40 and 60 y of age.	Predominantly women in fourth and fifth decades of life.
Location	Heliotrope rash—periorbital; Gottron papules—overlying metacarpal phalangeal and intercarpal phalangeal joints; Gottron sign—extensor surfaces of fingers, elbows, knees, and ankles; shawl sign—upper back, posterior shoulders, and neck; V sign—anterior neck and upper chest; holster sign—hips and lateral thighs.	Face, scalp, ears, and neck commonly. Less frequently involving upper trunk. Localized form above the neck and disseminated form both above and below the neck. Involvement of hands and feet uncommon.
Etiology	Unknown but appears to be a combination of genetic, environmental, and immune mechanisms. There is an increased frequency in individuals with certain HLA alleles. Postulated environmental triggers include viral infections, medications, smoking, and UV radiation. The inflammatory changes in tissues of various organs, including skin, are thought to result from autoimmunity.	An autoimmune disease hypothesized to be caused by overstimulation of the immune system by repeated exposure to antigens and a loss of immune tolerance.
Presentation	Erythematous to violaceous macules, patches, or plaques with edema (especially periorbital skin) that are typically pruritic or burning. Sun-exposed areas demonstrate poikiloderma with mottled pigmentation, atrophy, and telangiectasia.	Discrete, erythematous, scaly plaques with follicular plugging. Older lesions have central scars with atrophy, telangiectasia, and hyper- or hypopigmentation.
Histology	1. Hyperkeratosis with epidermal atrophy *(Fig. 1.28.1)*. 2. Vacuolar interface alteration with occasional necrotic keratinocytes *(Figs. 1.28.2 and 1.28.3)*. 3. Dermal edema with a relatively sparse superficial perivascular lymphocytic infiltrate and telangiectasia *(Fig. 1.28.3)*. 4. Superficial dermal melanophages *(Fig. 1.28.3)*. 5. Dermal mucin deposition on colloidal iron stain *(Fig. 1.28.4)*.	1. Hyperkeratosis with follicular plugging *(Figs. 1.28.5 and 1.28.6)*. 2. Basal layer vacuolar alteration with occasional necrotic keratinocytes *(Figs. 1.28.6 and 1.28.7)*. 3. Basement membrane thickening *(Fig. 1.28.7)*. 4. A moderately dense perivascular and periadnexal mononuclear infiltrate *(Figs. 1.28.5 and 1.28.6)*. 5. Mucin deposition between collagen bundles in the reticular dermis with colloidal iron stain *(Fig. 1.28.8)*.
Special studies	Colloidal iron or Alcian Blue stain to detect dermal mucin. Muscle enzymes, serology for muscle-specific antibodies, and muscle biopsy to confirm diagnosis.	PAS stain to detect basement membrane thickening. Colloidal iron or Alcian Blue stain to demonstrate mucin deposition.

1.28 Dermatomyositis vs Lupus Erythematosus (Discoid)

	Dermatomyositis	**Lupus Erythematosus (Discoid)**
Treatment	Initial therapy begins with systemic corticosteroids with addition of azathioprine or methotrexate. Rituximab and IVIG for resistant disease.	Sun protection and topical corticosteroids are first-line therapeutic modalities. Other therapies include topical calcineurin inhibitors, intralesional corticosteroids, and antimalarials.
Prognosis	Highly variable. Spontaneous remission is seen in up to 20% of patients. Approximately 5% of individuals have a progressive course and mortality from disease. Those with less severe disease may have morbidity from muscle weakness and systemic involvement. There is an association with malignancy and approximately 25% of patients have or will develop an underlying malignancy.	A variable course with unpredictable prognosis. Usually a chronic course with remissions and exacerbations. Worse prognosis for cases with systemic involvement, particularly central nervous system and renal disease.

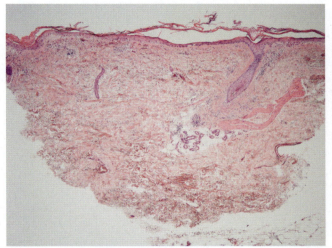

Figure 1.28.1 Dermatomyositis. Epidermal atrophy with hyperkeratosis and a sparse, patchy predominately superficial dermal infiltrate.

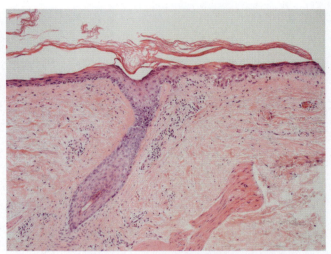

Figure 1.28.2 Dermatomyositis. Epidermal atrophy with interface vacuolar alteration and squamatization of the basal zone. A sparse superficial dermal infiltrate.

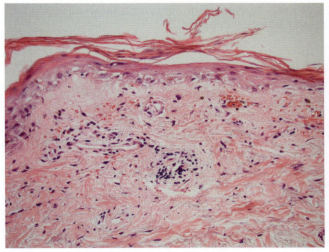

Figure 1.28.3 Dermatomyositis. Parakeratosis with epidermal atrophy and interface vacuolar change with few necrotic basal keratinocytes. The dermis has sparse lymphocytic inflammation, melanophages, and telangiectasia.

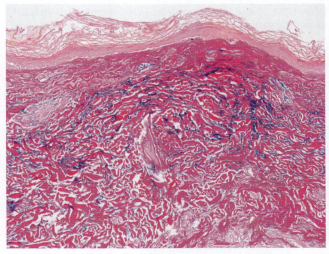

Figure 1.28.4 Dermatomyositis. Colloid iron stain showing abundant mucin deposition in the reticular dermis.

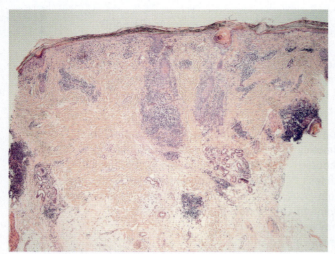

Figure 1.28.5 Discoid lupus erythematosus. Epidermal atrophy with hyperkeratosis and a moderately dense superficial and deep perivascular and periadnexal inflammatory infiltrate.

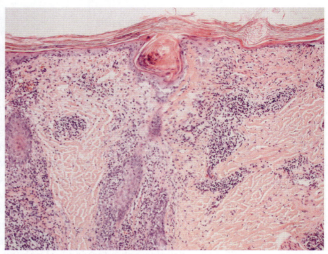

Figure 1.28.6 Discoid lupus erythematosus. Interface vacuolar change with atrophy, parakeratosis, and follicular plugging. A moderately dense perivascular and perifollicular lymphocytic infiltrate. Overlapping features with dermatomyositis but density and depth of inflammation, as well as follicular plugging, favor lupus erythematosus.

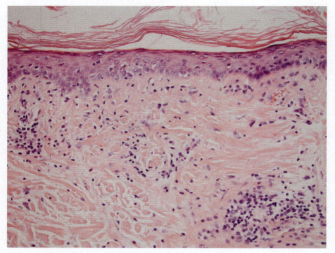

Figure 1.28.7 Discoid lupus erythematosus. Epidermal atrophy with interface vacuolar alteration and occasional necrotic keratinocytes.

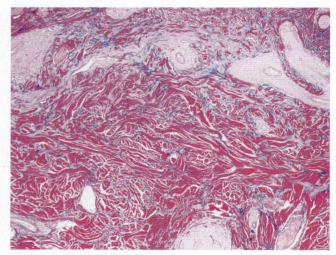

Figure 1.28.8 Discoid lupus erythematosus. Colloid iron showing mucin deposition within the reticular dermis.

1.29 LUPUS ERYTHEMATOSUS (SUBACUTE CUTANEOUS) VS POLYMORPHOUS LIGHT ERUPTION

	Lupus Erythematosus (Subacute Cutaneous)	**Polymorphous Light Eruption**
Age	Middle-aged adults; 4:1 women to men.	Onset typically in the second to third decade of life; women > men.
Location	Sun-exposed regions including upper back, shoulders, extensor surface of arms, neck, and upper chest. Face is generally spared.	Sun-exposed areas with preference for chest, extensor surface of arms, legs, upper back, and face.
Etiology	Autoimmune disease with contributions from genetic and environmental factors. Some cases may be drug-induced.	Resistance to UV radiation-induced immunosuppression and delayed hypersensitivity reaction to photoantigens.
Presentation	Erythematous macules that evolve into annular or psoriasiform plaques. Exacerbated by sun exposure.	Variable morphology including erythema, papules, papulovesicles, and plaques. Associated with pruritus and burning sensation. Occurs within hours or days of acute UV exposure, primarily in spring or early summer.
Histology	1. Compact orthohyperkeratosis and parakeratosis *(Figs. 1.29.1* and *1.29.2)*. 2. Vacuolar interface change with necrotic basal keratinocytes *(Figs. 1.29.2* and *1.29.3)*. Interface change may involve follicular units. 3. Smudging of basement membrane *(Fig. 1.29.3)*. 4. A superficial and deep perivascular and periadnexal lymphocytic infiltrate *(Fig. 1.29.1)*. 5. Mucin deposition within reticular dermis on colloidal iron stain *(Fig. 1.29.4)*.	1. A normal basket-weave orthokeratotic stratum corneum *(Figs. 1.29.5* and *1.29.6)*. 2. Variable epidermal spongiosis with vesicle formation *(Fig. 1.29.6)*. No interface vacuolar change or necrotic keratinocytes. 3. Marked papillary dermal edema *(Figs. 1.29.6* and *1.29.7)*. 4. A superficial and deep perivascular lymphocytic infiltrate *(Figs. 1.29.5-1.29.7)*.
Special studies	PAS and colloidal iron/Alcian Blue stains to demonstrate basement membrane thickening and mucin deposition, respectively. DIF shows granular deposits of immunoglobulins and complement at the dermal-epidermal junction. Serologies including ANA; anti-dsDNA, anti-Sm, and anti-rRNP; and anti-Ro, anti-La in systemic disease.	None.
Treatment	Sun avoidance. Topical corticosteroids and/or calcineurin inhibitors. Oral antimalarials are first-line for systemic therapy.	Prophylactic UVB therapy and sun protection. Symptomatic treatment with topical corticosteroids and antipruritics.
Prognosis	A chronic, relapsing course.	Transient eruption. Typically subsides within days if further UV exposure is avoided.

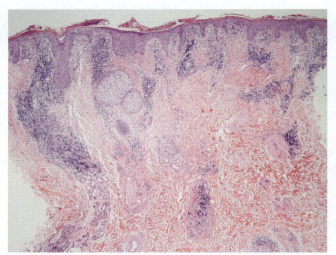

Figure 1.29.1 Lupus erythematosus. A superficial and deep perivascular and periadnexal lymphocytic infiltrate with mild epidermal hyperplasia and parakeratosis.

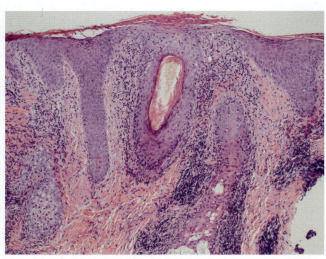

Figure 1.29.2 Lupus erythematosus. Follicular plugging with interface vacuolar change involving follicular epithelium and interfollicular epidermis.

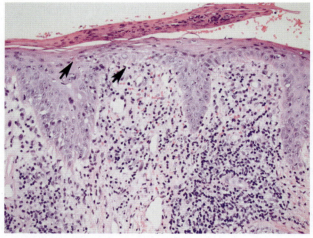

Figure 1.29.3 Lupus erythematosus. Interface vacuolar change with occasional necrotic keratinocytes (arrows).

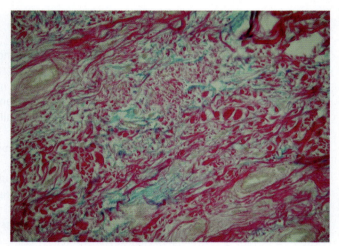

Figure 1.29.4 Lupus erythematosus. Colloidal iron stain demonstrating mucin deposition within the deep reticular dermis.

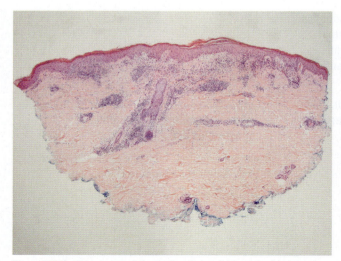

Figure 1.29.5 Polymorphous light eruption. A superficial and deep perivascular lymphocytic infiltrate with papillary dermal edema.

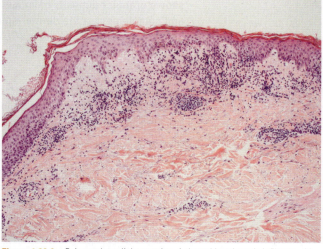

Figure 1.29.6 Polymorphous light eruption. A dermal lymphocytic infiltrate with mild spongiosis, lymphocytic exocytosis, and focally prominent papillary dermal edema.

1.29 Lupus Erythematosus (Subacute Cutaneous) vs Polymorphous Light Eruption

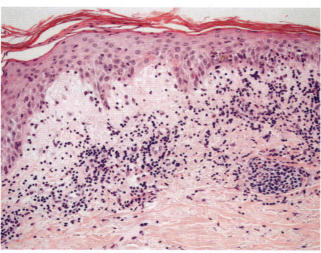

Figure 1.29.7 Polymorphous light eruption. A dermal lymphocytic infiltrate with mild spongiosis and prominent papillary dermal edema. Exocytosis of lymphocytes into the lower epidermis (early spongiosis) but no interface alteration or degenerated keratinocytes.

SUGGESTED READINGS

Chapter 1.1

Ale IS, Maibacht HA. Diagnostic approach in allergic and irritant contact dermatitis. *Expert Rev Clin Immunol.* 2010;6(2):291-310.

Nassau S, Fonacier L. Allergic contact dermatitis. *Med Clin North Am.* 2020;104(1):61-76.

Novak-Bilić G, Vučić M, Japundžić I, Meštrović-Štefekov J, Stanić-Duktaj S, Lugović-Mihić L. Irritant and allergic contact dermatitis–skin lesion characteristics. *Acta Clin Croat.* 2018;57(4):713-720.

Chapter 1.2

Bylaite M, Grigaitiene J, Lapinskaite GS. Photodermatoses: classification, evaluation and management. *Br J Dermatol.* 2009;161(suppl 3):61-68.

Glatz M, Hofbauer G F L. Phototoxic and photoallergic cutaneous drug reactions. *Chem Immunol Allergy.* 2012;97:167-179.

Monteiro AF, Rato M, Martins C. Drug-induced photosensitivity: photoallergic and phototoxic reactions. *Clin Dermatol.* 2016;34(5):571-581.

Montgomery S, Worswick S. Photosensitizing drug reactions. *Clin Dermatol.* 2022;40(1):57-63.

Yashar SS, Lim HW. Classification and evaluation of photodermatoses. *Dermatol Ther.* 2003;16:1-7.

Chapters 1.3–1.12

Al-Amiri A, Chatrath V, Bhawan J, Stefanato CM. The periodic acid-Schiff stain in diagnosing tinea: should it be used routinely in inflammatory skin diseases? *J Cutan Pathol.* 2003;30(10):611-615.

Alavi A, Skotnicki S, Sussman G, Sibbald RG. Diagnosis and treatment of hand dermatitis. *Adv Skin Wound Care.* 2012;25(8):371-380; quiz 381-382.

Balan R, Grigoraş A, Popovici D, Amălinei C. The histopathological landscape of the major psoriasiform dermatoses. *Arch Clin Cases.* 2019;6(3):59-68.

Bikowski JB. Hand eczema: diagnosis and management. *Cutis.* 2008;82(suppl 4):9-15.

Boehncke WH, Schön MP. Psoriasis. *Lancet.* 2015;386(9997):983-994.

Boehner A, Neuhauser R, Zink A, Ring J. Figurate erythemas – update and diagnostic approach. *J Dtsch Dermatol Ges.* 2021;19(7):963-972.

Bonamonte D, Foti C, Vestita M, Ranieri LD, Angelini G. Nummular eczema and contact allergy: a retrospective study. *Dermatitis.* 2012;23(4):153-157.

Cerroni L. Mycosis fungoides-clinical and histopathologic features, differential diagnosis, and treatment. *Semin Cutan Med Surg.* 2018;37(1):2-10.

Dessinioti C, Katsambas A. Seborrheic dermatitis: etiology, risk factors, and treatments—facts and controversies. *Clin Dermatol.* 2013;31(4):343-351.

Eastham AB. Pityriasis Rubra Pilaris. *JAMA Dermatol.* 2019;155(3):404.

Engin B, Aşkın Ö, Tüzün Y. Palmoplantar psoriasis. *Clin Dermatol.* 2017;35(1):19-27.

Galili E, Levy SR, Tzanani I, Segal O, Lyakhovitsky A, Barzilai A, Baum S. New-onset guttate psoriasis: a long-term follow-up study. *Dermatology.* 2022;239:1-7.

Gottlieb GJ, Ackerman AB. The "sandwich sign" of dermatophytosis. *Am J Dermatopathol.* 1986;8(4):347-350.

Griffiths CEM, Armstrong AW, Gudjonsson JE, Barker JNWN. Psoriasis. *Lancet.* 2021;397(10281):1301-1315.

Gru AA, Salavaggione AL. Common spongiotic dermatoses. *Semin Diagn Pathol.* 2017;34(3):226-236.

Halevy S, Kardaun SH, Davidovici B, Wechsler J, EuroSCAR and RegiSCAR study group. The spectrum of histopathological features in acute generalized exanthematous pustulosis: a study of 102 cases. *Br J Dermatol.* 2010;163(6):1245-1252.

Heath CR, Usatine RP. Seborrheic dermatitis. *Cutis.* 2021;108(5):297-298.

Hoegler KM, John AM, Handler MZ, Schwartz RA. Generalized pustular psoriasis: a review and update on treatment. *J Eur Acad Dermatol Venereol.* 2018;32(10):1645-1651.

Ju T, Vander Does A, Mohsin N, Yosipovitch G. Lichen simplex chronicus itch: an update. *Acta Derm Venereol.* 2022;102:adv00796.

Kardaun SH, Kuiper H, Fidler V, Jonkman MF. The histopathological spectrum of Acute Generalized Exanthematous Pustulosis (AGEP) and its differentiation from generalized pustular psoriasis. *J Cutan Pathol.* 2010;37(12):1220-1229.

Kim BY, Choi JW, Kim BR, Youn SW. Histopathological findings are associated with the clinical types of psoriasis but not with the corresponding lesional psoriasis severity index. *Ann Dermatol.* 2015;27(1):26-31.

Klein A, Landthaler M, Karrer S. Pityriasis rubra pilaris: a review of diagnosis and treatment. *Am J Clin Dermatol.* 2010;11(3):157-170.

Langan SM, Irvine AD, Weidinger S. Atopic dermatitis. *Lancet.* 2020;396(10247):345-360.

Leung AKC, Lam JM, Leong KF, Hon KL. Pityriasis rosea: an updated review. *Curr Pediatr Rev.* 2021;17(3):201-211.

Leung AKC, Lam JM, Leong KF, Leung AAM, Wong AHC, Hon KL. Nummular eczema: an updated review. *Recent Pat Inflamm Allergy Drug Discov.* 2020;14(2):146-155.

Litchman G, Nair PA, Le JK. *Pityriasis Rosea.* StatPearls Publishing; 2022.

Lotti T, Buggiani G, Prignano F. Prurigo nodularis and lichen simplex chronicus. *Dermatol Ther.* 2008;21(1):42-46.

Lyons JJ, Milner JD, Stone KD. Atopic dermatitis in children: clinical features, pathophysiology, and treatment. *Immunol Allergy Clin North Am.* 2015;35(1):161-183.

Masuda-Kuroki K, Murakami M, Kishibe M, Kobayashi S, Okubo Y, Yamamoto T, Terui T, Sayama K. Diagnostic histopathological features distinguishing palmoplantar pustulosis from pompholyx. *J Dermatol.* 2019;46(5):399-408.

Monteagudo B, Usero-Bárcena T, Vázquez-Bueno JÁ, Durana C. Annually recurring erythema annulare centrifugum: a case report and review of the literature. *Actas Dermosifiliogr.* 2022;113(8):835-837.

Muylaert BPB, Borges MT, Michalany AO, Scuotto CRC. Lichen simplex chronicus on the scalp: exuberant clinical, dermoscopic, and histopathological findings. *An Bras Dermatol.* 2018;93(1):108-110.

Park JH, Park YJ, Kim SK, Kwon JE, Kang HY, Lee ES, Choi JH, Kim YC. Histopathological differential diagnosis of psoriasis and Seborrheic dermatitis of the scalp. *Ann Dermatol.* 2016;28(4):427-432.

Ringin SA, Daniel BS. Treatment modalities for pityriasis rubra pilaris subtypes: a review. *J Dermatolog Treat.* 2022;33(1):587-588.

Roenneberg S, Biedermann T. Pityriasis rubra pilaris: algorithms for diagnosis and treatment. *J Eur Acad Dermatol Venereol.* 2018;32(6):889-898.

Ständer S. Atopic Dermatitis. *N Engl J Med.* 2021;384(12):1136-1143.

Szatkowski J, Schwartz RA. Acute Generalized Exanthematous Pustulosis (AGEP): a review and update. *J Am Acad Dermatol.* 2015;73(5):843-848.

Wang D, Chong V C L, Chong W S, Oon H H. A review on pityriasis rubra pilaris. *Am J Clin Dermatol.* 2018;19(3):377-390.

Wick MR. Psoriasiform dermatitides: a brief review. *Semin Diagn Pathol.* 2017;34(3):220-225.

Willemze R. Mycosis fungoides variants-clinicopathologic features, differential diagnosis, and treatment. *Semin Cutan Med Surg.* 2018;37(1):11-17.

Wollina U. Pompholyx: a review of clinical features, differential diagnosis, and management. *Am J Clin Dermatol.* 2010;11(5):305-314.

Chapters 1.13–1.17

Ameri AH, Foreman RK, Vedak P, Chen S, Miller DM, Demehri S. Hypertrophic lichen planus with histological features of squamous cell carcinoma associated with immune checkpoint blockade therapy. *Oncologist.* 2020;25(5):366-368.

Attili VR, Attili SK. Clinical and histopathological spectrum of genital lichen sclerosus in 133 cases: focus on the diagnosis of pre-sclerotic disease. *Indian J Dermatol Venereol Leprol.* 2022;88(6):774-780.

Cheraghlou S, Levy LL. Fixed drug eruptions, bullous drug eruptions, and lichenoid drug eruptions. *Clin Dermatol.* 2020;38(6):679-692.

Fistarol SK, Itin PH. Diagnosis and treatment of lichen sclerosus: an update. *Am J Clin Dermatol.* 2013;14(1):27-47.

Idriss MH, Barbosa N, Chang MB, Gibson L, Baum CL, Vidal NY. Concomitant hypertrophic lichen planus and squamous cell carcinoma: clinical features and treatment outcomes. *Int J Dermatol.* 2022;61(12):1527-1531.

Knackstedt TJ, Collins LK, Li Z, Yan S, Samie FH. Squamous cell carcinoma arising in hypertrophic lichen planus: a review and analysis of 38 cases. *Dermatol Surg.* 2015;41(12):1411-1418.

Lage D, Juliano PB, Metze K, de Souza EM, Cintra ML. Lichen planus and lichenoid drug-induced eruption: a histological and immunohistochemical study. *Int J Dermatol.* 2012;51(10):1199-1205.

Pogorzelska-Antkowiak A. Lichen planus-like keratosis: what do we know about it? *Clin Exp Dermatol.* 2022;47(11):1923-1927.

Puza C, Cardones AR. Concepts and controversies in the treatment of cutaneous lichen planus. *G Ital Dermatol Venereol.* 2017;152(6):607-614.

Sharma A, Białynicki-Birula R, Schwartz RA, Janniger CK. Lichen planus: an update and review. *Cutis.* 2012;90(1):17-23.

Totonchy MB, Leventhal JS, Ko CJ, Leffell DJ. Hypertrophic lichen planus and well-differentiated squamous cell carcinoma: a diagnostic conundrum. *Dermatol Surg.* 2018;44(11):1466-1470.

Tziotzios C, Lee JYW, Brier T, et al. Lichen planus and lichenoid dermatoses: clinical overview and molecular basis. *J Am Acad Dermatol.* 2018;79(5):789-804.

Van den Haute V, Antoine JL, Lachapelle JM. Histopathological discriminant criteria between lichenoid drug eruption and idiopathic lichen planus: retrospective study on selected samples. *Dermatologica.* 1989;179(1):10-13.

West AJ, Berger TG, LeBoit PE. A comparative histopathologic study of photodistributed and nonphotodistributed lichenoid drug eruptions. *J Am Acad Dermatol.* 1990;23(4 pt 1):689-693.

Chapters 1.18–1.19

Allen CE, Merad M, McClain KL. Langerhans-cell histiocytosis. *N Engl J Med.* 2018;379(9):856-868.

Arizaga AT, Gaughan MD, Bang RH. Generalized lichen nitidus. *Clin Exp Dermatol.* 2002;27(2):115-117.

Graham JN, Hossler EW. Lichen striatus. *Cutis.* 2016;97:86;120;122.

Johnson M, Walker D, Galloway W, Gardner JM, Shalin SC. Interface dermatitis along Blaschko's lines. *J Cutan Pathol.* 2014;41(12):950-954.

Krooks J, Minkov M, Weatherall AG. Langerhans cell histiocytosis in children: History, classification, pathobiology, clinical manifestations, and prognosis. *J Am Acad Dermatol.* 2018;78(6):1035-1044.

Lozano Masdemont B, Gómez-Recuero Muñoz L, Villanueva Álvarez-Santullano A, Parra Blanco V, Campos Domínguez M. Langerhans cell histiocytosis mimicking lichen nitidus with bone involvement. *Australas J Dermatol.* 2017;58(3):231-233.

Shockman S, Lountzis N. Lichen nitidus. *Cutis.* 2013;92(288):297-298.

Tilly JJ, Drolet BA, Esterly NB. Lichenoid eruptions in children. *J Am Acad Dermatol.* 2004;51(4):606-624.

Zhang Y, McNutt NS. Lichen striatus. Histological, immunohistochemical, and ultrastructural study of 37 cases. *J Cutan Pathol.* 2001;28(2):65-71.

Chapters 1.20–1.25

Fernandes NF, Rozdeba PJ, Schwartz RA, Kihiczak G, Lambert WC. Pityriasis lichenoides et varioliformis acuta: a disease spectrum. *Int J Dermatol.* 2010;49(3):257-261.

Fischer A, Jakubowski AA, Lacouture ME, et al. Histopathologic features of cutaneous acute graft-versus-host disease in t-cell-depleted peripheral blood stem cell transplant recipients. *Am J Dermatopathol.* 2015;37(7):523-529.

Flowers H, Brodell R, Brents M, Wyatt JP. Fixed drug eruptions: presentation, diagnosis, and management. *South Med J.* 2014;107(11):724-727.

Geller L, Antonov NK, Lauren CT, Morel KD, Garzon MC. Pityriasis lichenoides in childhood: review of clinical presentation and treatment options. *Pediatr Dermatol.* 2015;32(5):579-592.

Gerson D, Sriganeshan V, Alexis JB. Cutaneous drug eruptions: a 5-year experience. *J Am Acad Dermatol.* 2008;59(6):995-999.

Grünwald P, Mockenhaupt M, Panzer R, Emmert S. Erythema multiforme, Stevens-Johnson syndrome/toxic epidermal necrolysis – diagnosis and treatment. *J Dtsch Dermatol Ges.* 2020;18(6):547-553.

Guitart J, Querfeld C. Cutaneous CD30 lymphoproliferative disorders and similar conditions: a clinical and pathologic prospective on a complex issue. *Semin Diagn Pathol.* 2009;26(3):131-140.

Hogan DJ. Morbilliform drug eruptions. *J Am Acad Dermatol.* 2009;61(1):152.

Kavand S, Lehman JS, Hashmi S, Gibson LE, El-Azhary RA. Cutaneous manifestations of graft-versus-host disease: role of the dermatologist. *Int J Dermatol.* 2017;56(2):131-140.

Kempf W, Kazakov DV, Palmedo G, Fraitag S, Schaerer L, Kutzner H. Pityriasis lichenoides et varioliformis acuta with numerous CD30(+) cells: a variant mimicking lymphomatoid papulosis and other cutaneous lymphomas. A clinicopathologic, immunohistochemical, and molecular biological study of 13 cases. *Am J Surg Pathol.* 2012;36(7):1021-1029.

Khachemoune A, Blyumin ML. Pityriasis lichenoides: pathophysiology, classification, and treatment. *Am J Clin Dermatol.* 2007;8(1):29-36.

Kim GY, Schmelkin LA, Davis MD, El-Azhary RA, Wieland CN, Leise MD, Meves A, Lehman JS. Clinical and histopathologic manifestations of solid organ transplantation-associated graft-versus-host disease involving the skin: a single-center retrospective study. *J Cutan Pathol.* 2018;45(11):817-823.

McClatchy J, Yap T, Nirenberg A, Scardamaglia L. Fixed drug eruptions – the common and novel culprits since 2000. *J Dtsch Dermatol Ges.* 2022;20(10):1289-1302.

Naim M, Weyers W, Metze D. Histopathologic features of exanthematous drug eruptions of the macular and papular type. *Am J Dermatopathol.* 2011;33(7):695-704.

Patel S, John AM, Handler MZ, Schwartz RA. Fixed drug eruptions: an update, emphasizing the potentially lethal generalized bullous fixed drug eruption. *Am J Clin Dermatol.* 2020;21(3):393-399.

Sokumbi O, Wetter DA. Clinical features, diagnosis, and treatment of erythema multiforme: a review for the practicing dermatologist. *Int J Dermatol.* 2012;51(8):889-902.

Waldman L, Reddy SB, Kassim A, Dettloff J, Reddy VB. Neutrophilic fixed drug eruption. *Am J Dermatopathol.* 2015;37(7):574-6.

Wetter DA, Davis MDP. Recurrent erythema multiforme: clinical characteristics, etiologic associations, and treatment in a series of 48 patients at Mayo Clinic, 2000 to 2007. *J Am Acad Dermatol.* 2010;62(1):45-53.

Willemze R, Scheffer E. Clinical and histologic differentiation between lymphomatoid papulosis and pityriasis lichenoides. *J Am Acad Dermatol.* 1985;13(3):418-428.

Chapter 1.26

Dobson CM, King CM. Adult staphylococcal scalded skin syndrome: histological pitfalls and new diagnostic perspectives. *Br J Dermatol.* 2003;148(5):1068-1069.

Dodiuk-Gad RP, Chung WH, Valeyrie-Allanore L, Shear NH. Stevens-Johnson syndrome and toxic epidermal necrolysis: an update. *Am J Clin Dermatol.* 2015;16(6):475-493.

Handler MZ, Schwartz RA. Staphylococcal scalded skin syndrome: diagnosis and management in children and adults. *J Eur Acad Dermatol Venereol.* 2014;28(11):1418-1423.

Liy-Wong C, Pope E, Weinstein M, Lara-Corrales I. Staphylococcal scalded skin syndrome: an epidemiological and clinical review of 84 cases. *Pediatr Dermatol.* 2021;38(1):149-153.

Owen CE, Jones JM. Recognition and management of severe cutaneous adverse drug reactions (including drug reaction with eosinophilia and systemic symptoms, stevens-johnson syndrome, and toxic epidermal necrolysis). *Med Clin North Am.* 2021;105(4):577-597.

Chapter 1.27

Arif T, Fatima R, Sami M. Extragenital lichen sclerosus: A comprehensive review. *Australas J Dermatol.* 2022;63(4):452-462.

Baklouti M, Sellami K, Rekik M, Bahloul E, Hammami F, Slim C, Masmoudi A, Sellami T, Turki H. Extragenital lichen sclerosus: a retrospective study of 17 patients. *Indian J Dermatol.* 2022;67(2):146-149.

Hegedus F, Mathew LM, Schwartz RA. Radiation dermatitis: an overview. *Int J Dermatol.* 2017;56(9):909-914.

Hivnor CM, Seykora JT, Junkins-Hopkins J, et al. Subacute radiation dermatitis. *Am J Dermatopathol.* 2004;26(3):210-212.

Kirtschig G. Lichen sclerosus-presentation, diagnosis and management. *Dtsch Arztebl Int.* 2016;113(19):337-343.

Chapter 1.28–1.29

Boonstra HE, van Weelden H, Toonstra J, van Vloten WA. Polymorphous light eruption: a clinical, photobiologic, and follow-up study of 110 patients. *J Am Acad Dermatol.* 2000;42(2 pt 1):199-207.

Fairley JL, Oon S, Saracino AM, Nikpour M. Management of cutaneous manifestations of lupus erythematosus: a systematic review. *Semin Arthritis Rheum.* 2020;50(1):95-127.

Gruber-Wackernagel A, Byrne SN, Wolf P. Polymorphous light eruption: clinic aspects and pathogenesis. *Dermatol Clin.* 2014;32(3):315-34, viii.

Jorizzo JL. Dermatomyositis: practical aspects. *Arch Dermatol.* 2002;138(1):114-116.

Magro CM, Segal JP, Crowson AN, Chadwick P. The phenotypic profile of dermatomyositis and lupus erythematosus: a comparative analysis. *J Cutan Pathol.* 2010;37(6):659-671.

Oakley AM, Ramsey ML. *Polymorphic Light Eruption*. StatPearls Publishing; 2022.

Obermoser G, Sontheimer RD, Zelger B. Overview of common, rare and atypical manifestations of cutaneous lupus erythematosus and histopathological correlates. *Lupus*. 2010;19(9):1050-1070.

Pincus LB, LeBoit PE, Goddard DS, Cho RJ, McCalmont TH. Marked papillary dermal edema—an unreliable discriminator between polymorphous light eruption and lupus erythematosus or dermatomyositis. *J Cutan Pathol*. 2010;37(4):416-425.

Sena P, Gianatti A, Gambini D. Dermatomyositis: clinicopathological correlations. *G Ital Dermatol Venereol*. 2018;153(2):256-264.

Sepehr A, Wenson S, Tahan SR. Histopathologic manifestations of systemic diseases: the example of cutaneous lupus erythematosus. *J Cutan Pathol*. 2010;37:112-124.

Smith ES, Hallman JR, DeLuca AM, Goldenberg G, Jorizzo JL, Sangueza OP. Dermatomyositis: a clinicopathological study of 40 patients. *Am J Dermatopathol*. 2009;31(1):61-67.

Stratigos AJ, Antoniou C, Katsambas AD. Polymorphous light eruption. *J Eur Acad Dermatol Venereol*. 2002;16(3):193-206.

Vincent JG, Chan MP. Specificity of dermal mucin in the diagnosis of lupus erythematosus: comparison with other dermatitides and normal skin. *J Cutan Pathol*. 2015;42(10):722-729.

2 Inflammatory Diseases of the Dermis

- **2.1** Granuloma Annulare vs Necrobiosis Lipoidica
- **2.2** Sarcoidosis vs Granulomatous Rosacea
- **2.3** Foreign Body Granuloma vs Sarcoidosis
- **2.4** Necrobiosis Lipoidica vs Necrobiotic Xanthogranuloma
- **2.5** Granuloma Annulare vs Eruptive Xanthoma
- **2.6** Interstitial Granulomatous Drug Reaction vs Interstitial Granuloma Annulare
- **2.7** Palisaded Neutrophilic Granulomatous Dermatitis vs Interstitial Granuloma Annulare
- **2.8** Subcutaneous Granuloma Annulare vs Rheumatoid Nodule
- **2.9** Arthropod Assault Reaction vs Allergic Contact Dermatitis
- **2.10** Arthropod Assault Reaction vs Urticaria
- **2.11** Erythema Chronicum Migrans vs Urticaria
- **2.12** Urticaria vs Urticarial Vasculitis
- **2.13** Leukocytoclastic Vasculitis vs IgA Vasculitis
- **2.14** Leukocytoclastic Vasculitis vs Cryoglobulinemic Vasculitis
- **2.15** Granulomatosis With Polyangiitis vs Eosinophilic Granulomatosis With Polyangiitis
- **2.16** Pigmented Purpuric Dermatitis vs Leukocytoclastic Vasculitis
- **2.17** Pigmented Purpuric Dermatitis vs Stasis Dermatitis
- **2.18** Sweet Syndrome vs Pyoderma Gangrenosum
- **2.19** Granuloma Faciale vs Sweet Syndrome
- **2.20** Erythema Elevatum Diutinum vs Granuloma Faciale
- **2.21** Behcet Disease vs Sweet Syndrome
- **2.22** Pernio vs Tumid Lupus Erythematosus
- **2.23** Plasma Cell Mucositis vs Lichen Sclerosus
- **2.24** Morphea vs Lichen Sclerosus

2.1 GRANULOMA ANNULARE VS NECROBIOSIS LIPOIDICA

	Granuloma Annulare	**Necrobiosis Lipoidica**
Age	Any age, but typically under the age of 30 years. Women affected more than men.	Any age, with an average age of onset in the fourth decade. Women affected more than men.
Location	Localized form often on dorsal hands and feet. Generalized form presents on trunk and extremities. Subcutaneous form, seen in children, develops on distal extremities.	Anterior shins predominantly; usually bilateral. Rare occurrences on upper extremities and head and neck.
Etiology	Unknown. Delayed-type hypersensitivity reaction to an undetermined antigen is postulated.	Unknown. Immune complex deposition and/or microangiopathic changes causing collagen degeneration is postulated.
Presentation	Asymptomatic, shiny, erythematous papules and plaques in a ring-like or annular configuration with central clearing.	Yellow-brown atrophic plaques with telangiectasia. Frequently multiple, bilateral, and ulcerated. Increased prevalence in individuals with diabetes mellitus.
Histology	1. Normal epidermis *(Fig. 2.1.1)*. 2. Palisaded granulomas within reticular dermis composed of histiocytes and occasional multinucleate giant cells *(Figs. 2.1.1-2.1.3)*. Upper part of dermis usually involved more than lower. 3. Granulomas surround areas of degenerated collagen *(Figs. 2.1.2 and 2.1.3)* with mucin accumulation as demonstrated on colloidal iron stain *(Fig. 2.1.4)*. 4. May have sparse perivascular lymphocytic infiltrate but no or very few plasma cells.	1. Palisaded and interstitial granulomas, formed by histiocytes and multinucleate giant cells, arranged in layers parallel to skin surface *(Figs. 2.1.5 and 2.1.6)*. 2. Granulomas involve entire dermis and extend into subcutis along septae *(Figs. 2.1.5 and 2.1.6)*. 3. Layers of necrobiotic and sclerotic collagen between granulomas *(Figs. 2.1.6 and 2.1.7)*. No mucin deposition. 4. Perivascular lymphoplasmacytic infiltrate with vasculopathy *(Fig. 2.1.8)*.
Special studies	Colloidal iron stain confirms presence of mucin.	None.
Treatment	Intralesional steroids for localized disease. Antimalarial drugs or phototherapy for widespread or generalized disease.	Topical corticosteroids, under occlusion, or intralesional corticosteroids for early lesions. Avoidance of trauma to prevent ulceration. Wound care for ulcerated lesions.
Prognosis	Benign condition that is self-limited. Lesions tend to resolve spontaneously but often recur.	Chronic, slowly progressive course with eventual stabilization. Complications of ulceration and, rarely, squamous cell carcinoma.

2 Inflammatory Diseases of the Dermis

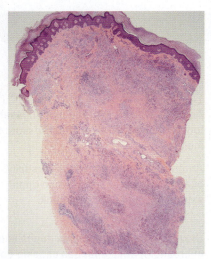

Figure 2.1.1 Granuloma annulare. Skin of distal extremity with serpiginous granulomas involving the reticular dermis.

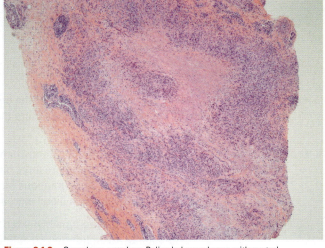

Figure 2.1.2 Granuloma annulare. Palisaded granulomas with central necrobiosis.

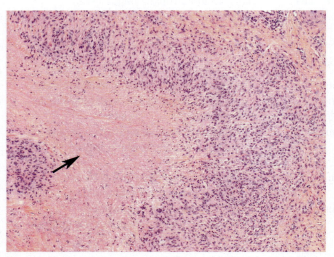

Figure 2.1.3 Granuloma annulare. Palisaded granuloma composed of histiocytes arranged loosely and in a perpendicular fashion to central necrobiotic collagen with mucin accumulation (arrow).

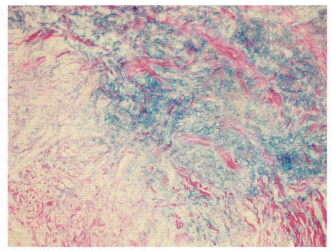

Figure 2.1.4 Granuloma annulare. Colloidal iron demonstrating mucin (blue stringy material) deposition in area of necrobiosis.

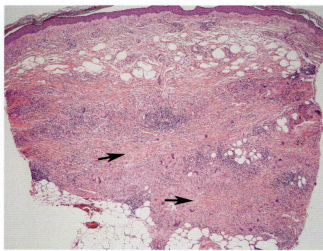

Figure 2.1.5 Necrobiosis lipoidica. Thinned epidermis with palisaded granulomas involving deep reticular dermis and superficial subcutis. Granulomas have a "layered cake" appearance with layers of histiocytes and multinucleate giant cells alternating with degenerated collagen (necrobiosis) (arrows).

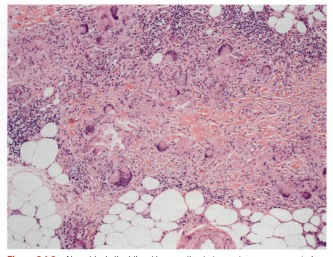

Figure 2.1.6 Necrobiosis lipoidica. Linear palisaded granulomas composed of epithelioid histiocytes and numerous multinucleate giant cells. Central zone of fragmented and degenerated collagen (necrobiosis).

2.1 Granuloma Annulare vs Necrobiosis Lipoidica

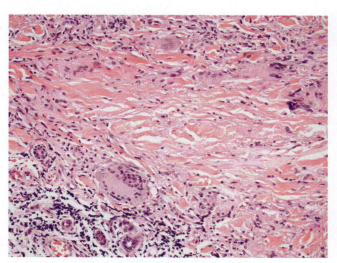

Figure 2.1.7 Necrobiosis lipoidica. Palisaded granuloma surrounding area of degenerated collagen (necrobiosis) without mucin accumulation.

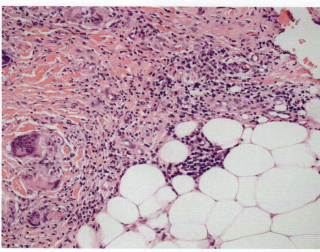

Figure 2.1.8 Necrobiosis lipoidica. Extension of granulomatous inflammation into superficial subcutis with accompanying plasma cells.

2.2 SARCOIDOSIS VS GRANULOMATOUS ROSACEA

	Sarcoidosis	**Granulomatous Rosacea**
Age	Any age. Typically presents in third to fourth decade.	Young adults between ages of 30 and 50 years; women more commonly affected than men.
Location	Central face, extremities, and areas of trauma.	Nose, cheeks, chin, forehead, lateral face, and neck below the mandible.
Etiology	Unknown. Pathogenesis postulated to involve dysregulation of the Th1 immune response to extrinsic antigens.	Unknown. Multifactorial etiology postulated with involvement of genetic factors, immune system dysregulation, vascular dysfunction, and *Demodex folliculorum* organisms. Triggers include stress, heat, alcohol, hot beverages, and spicy foods.
Presentation	Smooth macules or papules that may be violaceous, hyperpigmented, hypopigmented, or skin-colored.	Monomorphic, firm, red-brown papules and nodules. May or may not have concomitant flushing, erythema, and telangiectasia.
Histology	1. Normal epidermis *(Fig. 2.2.1)*. 2. Noncaseating granulomas composed of epithelioid histiocytes and multinucleate giant cells *(Figs. 2.2.1 and 2.2.2)*. May coalesce within the interstitium but are not perifollicular. 3. Granulomas are surrounded by a minimal to mild lymphocytic infiltrate ("naked granulomas") *(Figs. 2.2.1 and 2.2.2)*. 4. Asteroid bodies, Schaumann bodies (laminated calcific inclusions), and crystalline inclusions may be present *(Fig. 2.2.3)*.	1. Follicular dilatation with *Demodex* organisms *(Figs. 2.2.4 and 2.2.5)*. 2. Perifollicular noncaseating epithelioid granulomas *(Figs. 2.2.6 and 2.2.7)*. 3. Vascular ectasia with perivascular lymphoplasmacytic infiltrate *(Fig. 2.2.5)*.
Special studies	Polarization to detect foreign material. Histochemical stains to exclude microorganisms (PAS or GMS stain for fungus and AFB stain for mycobacteria).	None.
Treatment	Based upon extent and severity of disease. Topical and intralesional corticosteroids for limited disease. Systemic therapy for extensive disease or localized disease not responsive to therapy. Systemic therapies include antimalarial drugs, methotrexate, and tetracyclines.	Often requires combination of topical (ivermectin cream, pimecrolimus cream, or metronidazole gel) and oral tetracycline antibiotics (doxycycline or minocycline).
Prognosis	Chronic disorder; prognosis depends upon extent of cutaneous disease and involvement of other organ systems. Systemic involvement seen in approximately two-thirds of cases of cutaneous sarcoidosis. Involvement of the central face by erythematous plaques (lupus pernio variant) is associated with high risk of concomitant pulmonary disease.	Benign disease with chronic course. May have adverse effect on quality of life due to cosmetic issues. Granulomatous rosacea responds slower to therapy than other forms of rosacea and is more likely to be recalcitrant to standard treatments.

2.2 Sarcoidosis vs Granulomatous Rosacea

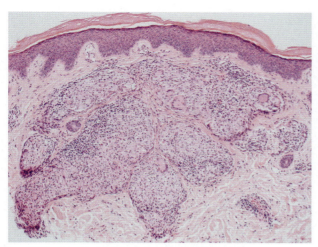

Figure 2.2.1 Sarcoidosis. Tight, discrete noncaseating granulomas without appreciable surrounding lymphocytic infiltrate ("naked"). Granulomas are not folliculocentric.

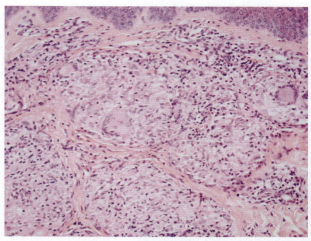

Figure 2.2.2 Sarcoidosis. Tight, discrete granulomas composed of epithelioid histiocytes and multinucleate giant cells. Minimal surrounding lymphocytic infiltrate and no central necrosis or suppuration.

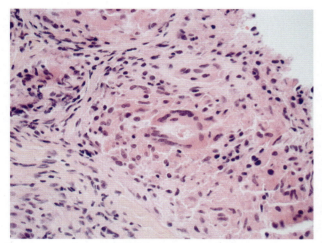

Figure 2.2.3 Sarcoidosis. Epithelioid histiocytes forming granuloma. Multinucleate cell with star-shaped eosinophilic inclusion ("asteroid body"), a finding that is not specific for sarcoidosis.

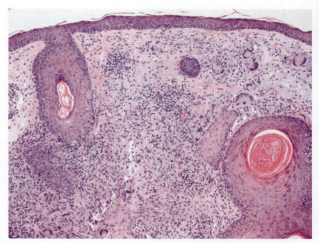

Figure 2.2.4 Granulomatous rosacea. Facial skin with mild follicular dilatation. Perivascular and perifollicular infiltrate of lymphocytes, plasma cells, histiocytes, and multinucleate giant cells. Background of solar damage with elastosis.

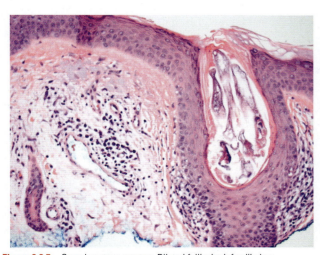

Figure 2.2.5 Granulomatous rosacea. Dilated follicular infundibulum with numerous *Demodex* mites. Telangiectatic vessel with perivascular and perifollicular lymphoplasmacytic infiltrate.

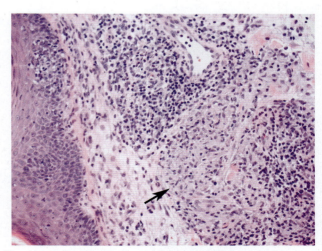

Figure 2.2.6 Granulomatous rosacea. Loose perifollicular noncaseating granuloma (arrow) with associated telangiectasia and lymphoplasmacytic infiltrate.

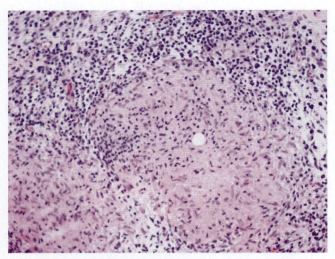

Figure 2.2.7 Granulomatous rosacea. Epithelioid noncaseating granuloma with central space (lipid from disrupted sebaceous gland) and surrounding lymphoplasmacytic infiltrate.

2.3 FOREIGN BODY GRANULOMA VS SARCOIDOSIS

	Foreign Body Granuloma	**Sarcoidosis**
Age	Any age.	Any age. Typically presents in third to fourth decade.
Location	Any location.	Central face, extremities, and areas of trauma.
Etiology	Histiocytic reaction to the introduction of a substance into the skin, either exogenous material or endogenous material that is altered in a fashion in which it is recognized as foreign. May be intentional, as in tattoos and cosmetic fillers, or unintentional.	Unknown. Pathogenesis postulated to involve dysregulation of the Th1 immune response to extrinsic antigens.
Presentation	Erythematous papules and nodules.	Smooth macules or papules that may be violaceous, hyperpigmented, hypopigmented, or skin-colored.
Histology	1. Nodular dermal infiltrate consisting of loose aggregates of histiocytes, multinucleate giant cells, lymphocytes, and neutrophils *(Figs. 2.3.1-2.3.3)*. 2. Foreign body–type giant cells have nuclei scattered irregularly throughout the cytoplasm *(Fig. 2.3.2)*. 3. Polarizable or nonpolarizable material present within giant cells and extracellularly *(Fig. 2.3.3)*.	1. Normal epidermis *(Fig. 2.3.4)*. 2. Discrete noncaseating granulomas composed of epithelioid histiocytes and multinucleate giant cells that coalesce within the interstitium *(Figs. 2.3.4 and 2.3.5)*. 3. Granulomas are surrounded by a minimal to mild lymphocytic infiltrate ("naked granulomas") *(Figs. 2.3.5 and 2.3.6)*. No neutrophils. 4. Asteroid bodies, Schaumann bodies (laminated calcific inclusions), and crystalline inclusions may be present. Important not to misdiagnose these bodies and inclusions as foreign material.
Special studies	Polarization of tissue sections aids in determining composition of foreign material. Histochemical stains to detect microorganisms may be indicated to exclude secondary infection.	Polarization to detect foreign material. Histochemical stains to exclude microorganisms (PAS or GMS stain for fungus and AFB stain for mycobacteria).
Treatment	Most removed by simple excision. Other therapies include topical corticosteroids, intralesional corticosteroid injections, and topical imiquimod. Laser therapy for foreign body granulomas due to tattoo ink.	Based upon extent and severity of disease. Topical and intralesional corticosteroids for limited disease. Systemic therapy for extensive disease or localized disease not responsive to therapy. Systemic therapies include antimalarial drugs, methotrexate, and tetracyclines.
Prognosis	Depends upon type of foreign material. Some regress spontaneously while others may persist indefinitely. Complications include abscess formation, secondary infection, and scarring.	Chronic disorder; prognosis depends upon extent of cutaneous disease and involvement of other organ systems. Systemic involvement seen in approximately two-thirds of cases of cutaneous sarcoidosis. Involvement of the central face by erythematous plaques (lupus pernio variant) is associated with high risk of concomitant pulmonary disease.

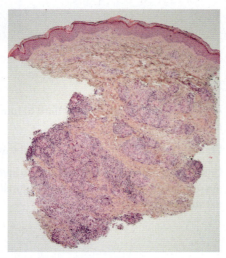

Figure 2.3.1 Foreign body granuloma. Dermal granulomas with variable lymphocytic infiltrate.

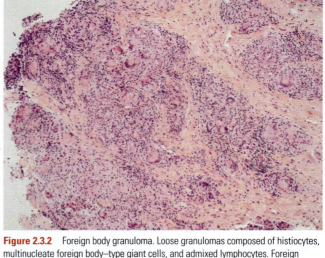

Figure 2.3.2 Foreign body granuloma. Loose granulomas composed of histiocytes, multinucleate foreign body–type giant cells, and admixed lymphocytes. Foreign body–type giant cells have irregular distribution of nuclei within cytoplasm.

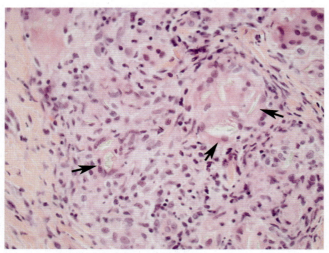

Figure 2.3.3 Foreign body granuloma. Multinucleate histiocytes with cytoplasmic refractile foreign material (arrows).

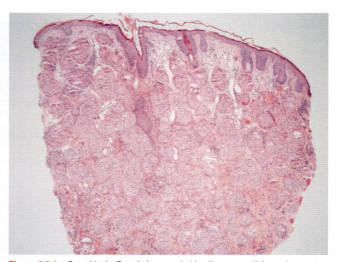

Figure 2.3.4 Sarcoidosis. Dermis is expanded by discrete, well-formed, noncaseating granulomas without appreciable lymphocytic inflammation.

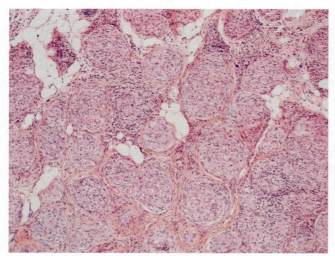

Figure 2.3.5 Sarcoidosis. Tight collections of epithelioid histiocytes and multinucleate cells with no significant lymphocytic infiltrate ("naked granulomas"). No polarizable or nonpolarizable material within histiocytes.

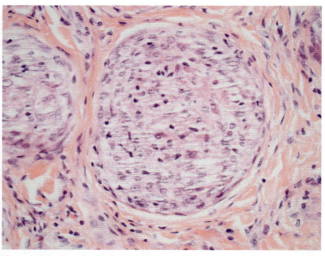

Figure 2.3.6 Sarcoidosis. Discrete, noncaseating granuloma without surrounding inflammation or foreign material.

2.4 NECROBIOSIS LIPOIDICA VS NECROBIOTIC XANTHOGRANULOMA

	Necrobiosis Lipoidica	**Necrobiotic Xanthogranuloma**
Age	Any age, with an average age of onset in the fourth decade. Women affected more than men.	Adults, 20-85 years of age.
Location	Anterior shins predominantly; usually bilateral. Rare occurrences on upper extremities and head and neck.	Periorbital region is the most common site, with other parts of the face, trunk, and extremities involved less frequently.
Etiology	Unknown. Immune complex deposition and/or microangiopathic changes causing collagen degeneration is postulated.	Precise etiology is unknown.
Presentation	Yellow-brown atrophic plaques with telangiectasia. Frequently multiple, bilateral, and ulcerated. Increased prevalence in individuals with diabetes mellitus.	Indurated, red-yellow-orange papules, nodules, or plaques that can be associated with atrophy, ulceration, and scarring.
Histology	1. Palisaded and interstitial granulomas, formed by histiocytes and multinucleate giant cells, arranged in layers parallel to skin surface *(Figs. 2.4.1, 2.4.3, 2.4.4)*. No significant population of foamy macrophages. 2. Granulomas involve entire dermis and extend into subcutis along septae *(Fig. 2.4.1)*. 3. Layers of necrobiotic and sclerotic collagen between granulomas *(Figs. 2.4.2 and 2.4.3)*. No mucin deposition or cholesterol cleft formation. 4. Perivascular lymphoplasmacytic infiltrate with vasculopathy *(Fig. 2.4.4)*.	1. Epidermis is normal or ulcerated *(Fig. 2.4.5)*. 2. Stellate palisaded granulomas with extensive necrobiotic collagen, often with cholesterol clefts *(Figs. 2.4.6 and 2.4.8)*. 3. Granulomas are composed of epithelioid histiocytes, foamy histiocytes, foreign body and Touton giant cells *(Figs. 2.4.7 and 2.4.9)*. 4. Surrounding lymphoplasmacytic infiltrate *(Fig. 2.4.6)*.
Special studies	None.	None.
Treatment	Topical corticosteroids, under occlusion, or intralesional corticosteroids for early lesions. Avoidance of trauma to prevent ulceration. Wound care for ulcerated lesions.	Combination of corticosteroids and immunosuppressive agents.
Prognosis	Chronic, slowly progressive course with eventual stabilization. Complications of ulceration and, rarely, squamous cell carcinoma.	Poor. Considered to be a paraneoplastic process associated with paraproteinemia, myeloma, lymphoma, and other lymphoproliferative disorders.

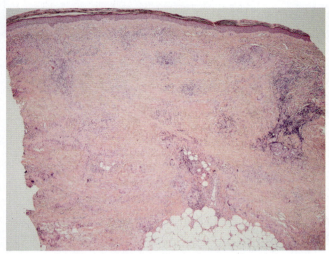

Figure 2.4.1 Necrobiosis lipoidica. Palisaded granulomatous inflammation arranged in incomplete horizontal layers with intervening zones of degenerated collagen (necrobiosis). Inflammation fills dermis and extends into the superficial subcutis.

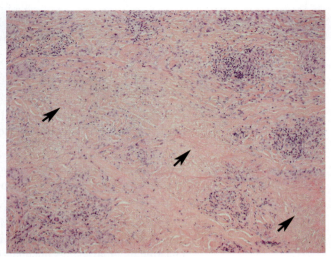

Figure 2.4.2 Necrobiosis lipoidica. Ill-defined interstitial infiltrate of histiocytes and lymphocytes surrounding areas of necrobiotic collagen (arrows).

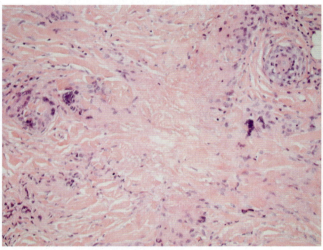

Figure 2.4.3 Necrobiosis lipoidica. Palisaded granulomas composed of histiocytes and multinucleate giant cells surrounding areas of degenerated, acellular collagen (necrobiosis).

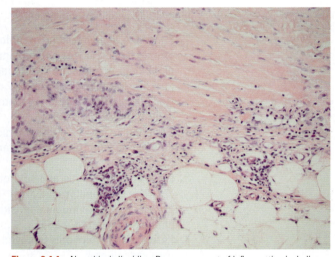

Figure 2.4.4 Necrobiosis lipoidica. Deep component of inflammation including histiocytes, multinucleate giant cells, and plasma cells. Inflammation extending into subcutis and associated with reactive vessels.

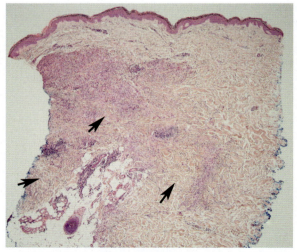

Figure 2.4.5 Necrobiotic xanthogranuloma. Perivascular and interstitial inflammatory infiltrate involving mid and deep dermis. Focal areas of necrobiosis (arrows).

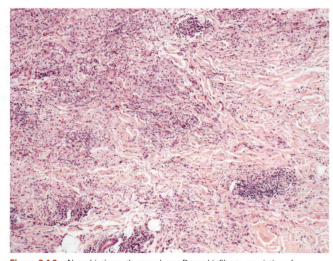

Figure 2.4.6 Necrobiotic xanthogranuloma. Dermal infiltrate consisting of histiocytes forming ill-defined granulomas accompanied by clusters of plasma cells.

2.4 Necrobiosis Lipoidica vs Necrobiotic Xanthogranuloma

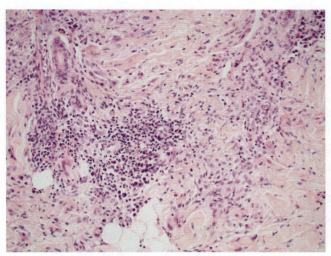

Figure 2.4.7 Necrobiotic xanthogranuloma. Loose aggregates of histiocytes, some foamy, accompanied by collections of plasma cells and occasional neutrophils.

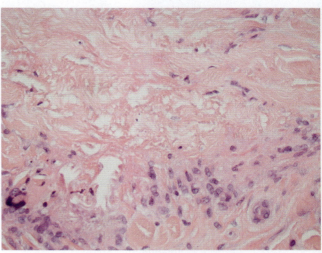

Figure 2.4.8 Necrobiotic xanthogranuloma. High-magnification image of necrobiosis surrounded by palisaded granulomatous inflammation.

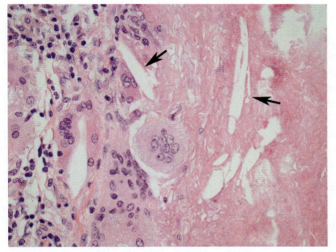

Figure 2.4.9 Necrobiotic xanthogranuloma. Cholesterol clefts (arrows) may be seen within areas of necrobiosis and granulomatous inflammation with foamy histiocytes and Touton giant cells.

2.5 GRANULOMA ANNULARE VS ERUPTIVE XANTHOMA

	Granuloma Annulare	**Eruptive Xanthoma**
Age	Any age, but typically under the age of 30 years. Women affected more than men.	Adults.
Location	Localized form often on dorsal hands and feet. Generalized form presents on trunk and extremities. Subcutaneous form, seen in children, develops on distal extremities.	Extensor surfaces of extremities and buttocks.
Etiology	Unknown. Delayed-type hypersensitivity reaction to an undetermined antigen is postulated.	Increased local extravasation of lipids from vasculature into interstitium of dermis. Phagocytosis of the excess lipid by histiocytes that accumulate in the dermis.
Presentation	Asymptomatic, erythematous, smooth papules and plaques in a ring-like or annular configuration with central clearing.	Crops of 1-4 mm white-yellow papules that arise abruptly.
Histology	1. Normal epidermis *(Fig. 2.5.1)*. 2. Palisaded granulomas within reticular dermis composed of histiocytes and occasional multinucleate giant cells *(Figs. 2.5.2 and 2.5.3)*. Note that histiocytes have eosinophilic, rather than foamy, cytoplasm. 3. Granulomas surround areas of altered collagen with mucin accumulation *(Figs. 2.5.2-2.5.4)*. No extracellular lipid material.	1. Loose aggregates of foamy histiocytes within the dermis *(Figs. 2.5.5-2.5.7)*. 2. Extracellular lipid accumulation *(Figs. 2.5.6 and 2.5.8)*. 3. No necrobiosis or mucin deposition.
Special studies	Colloidal iron stain confirms presence of mucin.	None.
Treatment	Intralesional steroids for localized disease. Antimalarial drugs or phototherapy for widespread or generalized disease.	May spontaneously resolve within a few weeks. If persistent, treatment of underlying lipid disorder with statins, fibrates, or niacin is indicated.
Prognosis	Benign condition that is self-limited. Lesions tend to resolve spontaneously but often recur.	Highly associated with hypertriglyceridemia and may signal chylomicronemia syndrome with risk of acute pancreatitis.

2.5 Granuloma Annulare vs Eruptive Xanthoma

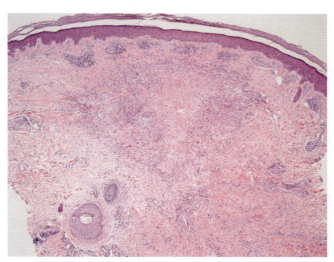

Figure 2.5.1 Granuloma annulare. Well-formed, palisaded granulomas surrounding areas of degenerated collagen in reticular dermis.

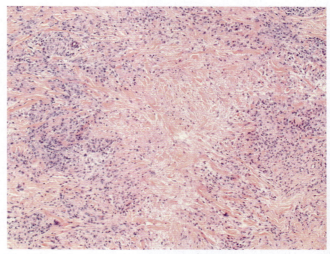

Figure 2.5.2 Granuloma annulare. Palisaded granuloma with histiocytes surrounding area of degenerated collagen. Histiocytes have eosinophilic, not foamy, cytoplasm.

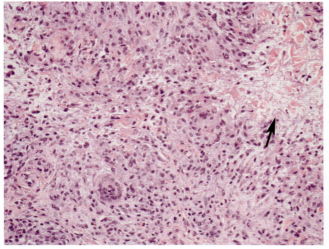

Figure 2.5.3 Granuloma annulare. Palisaded granuloma composed of histiocytes and occasional multinucleate giant cells with central area of necrobiosis (arrow). Stringy basophilic material resembling mucin associated with necrobiosis.

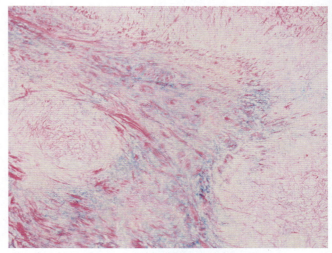

Figure 2.5.4 Granuloma annulare. Colloidal iron stain demonstrating extracellular mucin in central area of necrobiotic palisaded granuloma.

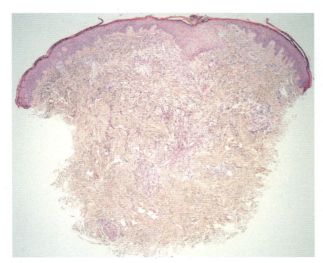

Figure 2.5.5 Eruptive xanthoma. Interstitial infiltrate of histiocytes within reticular dermis.

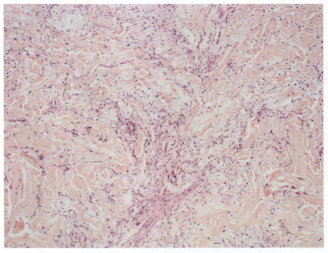

Figure 2.5.6 Eruptive xanthoma. Interstitial infiltrate of foamy histiocytes with pools of extracellular lipid.

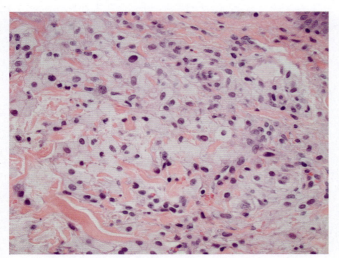

Figure 2.5.7 Eruptive xanthoma. Loose collections of foamy histiocytes with finely vacuolated cytoplasm.

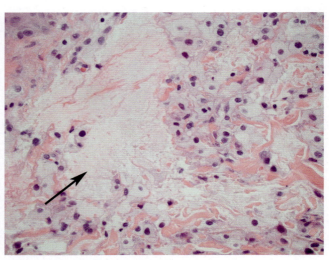

Figure 2.5.8 Eruptive xanthoma. Foamy histiocytes associated with pools of extracellular lipid (arrow).

2.6 INTERSTITIAL GRANULOMATOUS DRUG REACTION VS INTERSTITIAL GRANULOMA ANNULARE

	Interstitial Granulomatous Drug Reaction	**Interstitial Granuloma Annulare**
Age	Any age, but more common in adults.	Any age, but typically under the age of 30 years. Women affected more than men.
Location	Inner upper arms, medial upper thighs, trunk, buttocks, and intertriginous sites.	Localized form often on wrists, dorsal hands, and feet. Generalized form presents on trunk and extremities.
Etiology	Unknown but may involve type IVa delayed-type hypersensitivity reaction. Reported classes of drugs include calcium channel blockers, angiotensin-converting enzyme inhibitors, antihistamines, anticonvulsants, and antidepressants.	Unknown. Delayed-type hypersensitivity reaction to an undetermined antigen is postulated.
Presentation	Indurated, erythematous to violaceous plaques. Other morphologies include annular plaques, small skin-colored papules, ropelike cords, and subcutaneous nodules.	Localized form presents as asymptomatic, erythematous papules and plaques in a ring-like or annular configuration. Generalized form has widespread erythematous papules that may be annular.
Histology	1. Vacuolar interface change with occasional necrotic keratinocytes *(Fig. 2.6.2)*. 2. Interstitial infiltrate of histiocytes within superficial and deep reticular dermis *(Fig. 2.6.1)*. Infiltrate also includes lymphocytes, some atypical, and eosinophils *(Figs. 2.6.3 and 2.6.4)*. 3. Histiocytes surround foci of altered collagen *(Fig. 2.6.3)*. 4. Clusters of histiocytes form small granulomas surrounding degenerated collagen ("floating sign") *(Fig. 2.6.4)*. 5. No or minimal mucin deposition on colloidal iron stain. No vasculitis.	1. Normal epidermis *(Fig. 2.6.5)*. 2. Interstitial infiltrate composed of histiocytes and occasional multinucleate giant cells within superficial reticular dermis *(Figs. 2.6.6 and 2.6.7)*. 3. Histiocytes are embedded in mucin between altered and partially degenerated collagen bundles *(Figs. 2.6.6 and 2.6.7)*. 4. Mucin between collagen bundles in area of histiocytic infiltrate *(Fig. 2.6.8)* on colloidal iron stain.
Special studies	None.	Colloidal iron stain confirms presence of mucin.
Treatment	Removal of offending drug. Topical or intralesional corticosteroids, dapsone, and hydroxychloroquine are also used for management.	Intralesional steroids for localized disease. Antimalarial drugs or phototherapy for widespread or generalized disease.
Prognosis	Good prognosis but may take weeks to months to resolve following cessation of the culprit medication.	Benign condition that is self-limited. Lesions tend to resolve spontaneously but often recur. No definitive association with systemic diseases, malignancy, or medications.

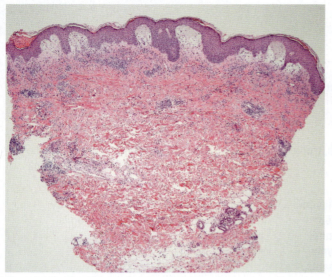

Figure 2.6.1 Interstitial granulomatous drug reaction. Perivascular and interstitial dermal inflammatory infiltrate with papillary dermal edema and focal scale crust.

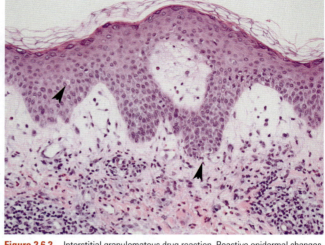

Figure 2.6.2 Interstitial granulomatous drug reaction. Reactive epidermal changes with focal interface vacuolar change and occasional necrotic keratinocytes (arrows).

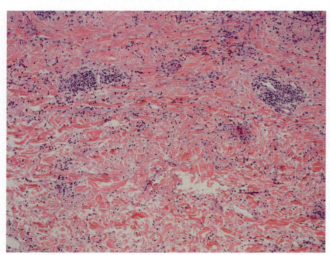

Figure 2.6.3 Interstitial granulomatous drug reaction. Histiocytes forming ill-defined interstitial granulomas with areas of degenerated collagen. Infiltrate includes lymphocytes and eosinophils.

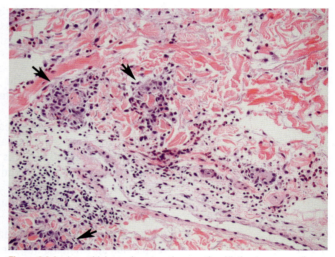

Figure 2.6.4 Interstitial granulomatous drug reaction. Histiocytes surrounding balls of degenerated collagen (arrows) with associated lymphocytes and eosinophils.

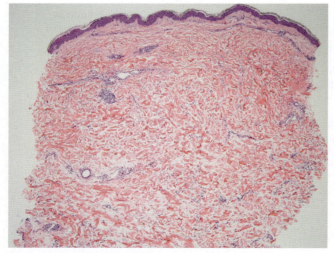

Figure 2.6.5 Interstitial granuloma annulare. Vague interstitial and perivascular dermal inflammatory infiltrate with normal overlying epidermis.

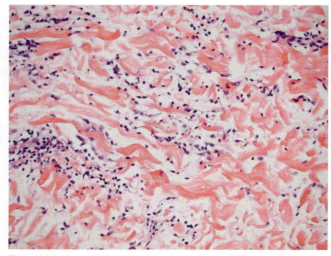

Figure 2.6.6 Interstitial granuloma annulare. Interstitial infiltrate of histiocytes and small lymphocytes associated with fragmented and mildly degenerated collagen bundles.

2.6 Interstitial Granulomatous Drug Reaction vs Interstitial Granuloma Annulare

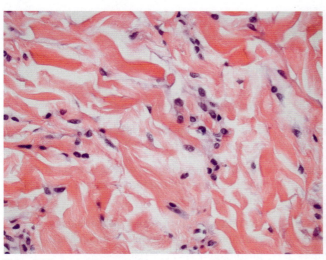

Figure 2.6.7 Interstitial granuloma annulare. Interstitial infiltrate of small histiocytes.

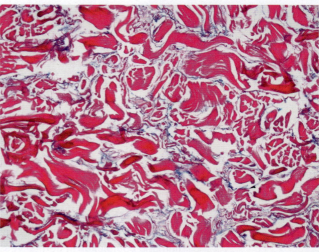

Figure 2.6.8 Interstitial granuloma annulare. Colloidal iron stain demonstrating extracellular mucin between fragmented collagen bundles in reticular dermis.

2.7 PALISADED NEUTROPHILIC GRANULOMATOUS DERMATITIS VS INTERSTITIAL GRANULOMA ANNULARE

	Palisaded Neutrophilic Granulomatous Dermatitis	**Interstitial Granuloma Annulare**
Age	Generally affects adults; rare in children. Women more frequently affected than men.	Any age, but typically under the age of 30 years. Women affected more than men.
Location	Trunk and extensor surfaces of extremities.	Localized form often on wrists, dorsal hands, and feet. Generalized form presents on trunk and extremities.
Etiology	Unknown. Theorized to involve an immune complex-mediated process. Deposition of immune complexes in dermal vessels leads to activation of complement and neutrophils. Degranulation of neutrophils causes damage to dermal collagen initiating a granulomatous response.	Unknown. Delayed-type hypersensitivity reaction to an undetermined antigen is postulated.
Presentation	Symmetric erythematous to violaceous papules and plaques. May present as linear cords on lateral trunk.	Localized form presents as asymptomatic, erythematous papules and plaques in a ring-like or annular configuration. Generalized form has widespread erythematous papules that may be annular.
Histology	1. Normal epidermis and stratum corneum *(Fig. 2.7.1)*. 2. Moderately dense perivascular and interstitial infiltrate of neutrophils and histiocytes with neutrophilic nuclear debris *(Figs. 2.7.1-2.7.3)*. 3. Degenerated collagen bundles surrounded by histiocytes *(Fig. 2.7.3)*. 4. Mild vasculitic changes may be present *(Fig. 2.7.4)*.	1. Normal epidermis *(Fig. 2.7.5)*. 2. Interstitial infiltrate composed of histiocytes and occasional multinucleate giant cells within superficial reticular dermis *(Figs. 2.7.6 and 2.7.7)*. No neutrophilic component. 3. Histiocytes are embedded in mucin between altered and partially degenerated collagen bundles *(Figs. 2.7.7 and 2.7.8)*.
Special studies	None.	Colloidal iron stain confirms presence of mucin.
Treatment	Most lesions resolve spontaneously or with treatment of associated immune-mediated disease and do not necessarily require therapy. Treatment modalities include topical corticosteroids, low-dose prednisone, and dapsone.	Intralesional steroids for localized disease. Antimalarial drugs or phototherapy for widespread or generalized disease.
Prognosis	Usually self-limited. Associated with a variety of systemic conditions including rheumatoid arthritis, lupus erythematosus, systemic vasculitis, and lymphoproliferative disorders.	Benign condition that is self-limited. Lesions tend to resolve spontaneously but often recur. No definitive association with systemic diseases, malignancy, or medications.

2.7 Palisaded Neutrophilic Granulomatous Dermatitis vs Interstitial Granuloma Annulare

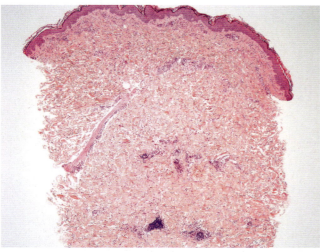

Figure 2.7.1 Palisaded neutrophilic granulomatous dermatitis. Patchy, moderately dense perivascular and interstitial dermal infiltrate involving majority of dermis.

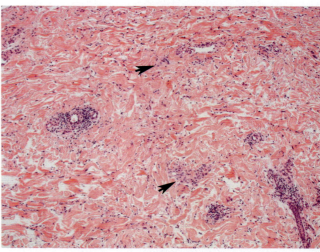

Figure 2.7.2 Palisaded neutrophilic granulomatous dermatitis. Perivascular and interstitial infiltrate with loose aggregates of histiocytes forming vague granulomas (arrow).

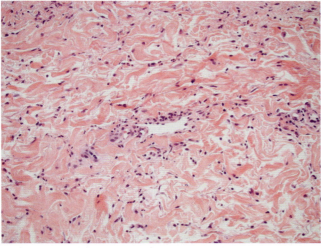

Figure 2.7.3 Palisaded neutrophilic granulomatous dermatitis. Interstitial neutrophils, with small amount of karyorrhectic nuclear debris, accompanied by small lymphocytes and histiocytes.

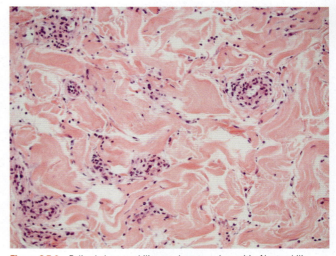

Figure 2.7.4 Palisaded neutrophilic granulomatous dermatitis. Neutrophilic infiltrate associated with mild vasculitic change consisting of intramural neutrophils and mild erythrocyte extravasation.

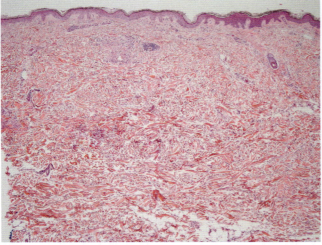

Figure 2.7.5 Interstitial granuloma annulare. Unremarkable epidermis with underlying perivascular and interstitial inflammatory infiltrate.

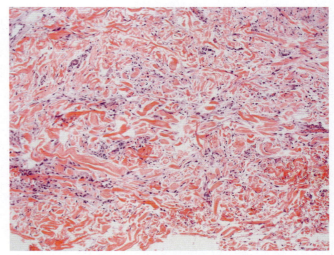

Figure 2.7.6 Interstitial granuloma annulare. Interstitial infiltrate of histiocytes surrounding swollen and fragmented collagen bundles. No neutrophils.

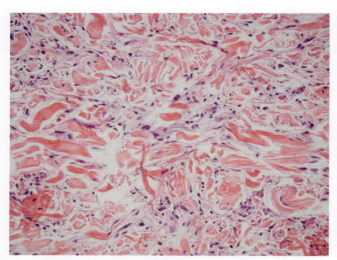

Figure 2.7.7 Interstitial granuloma annulare. Interstitial infiltrate of histiocytes associated with fragmented collagen bundles and stringy basophilic material.

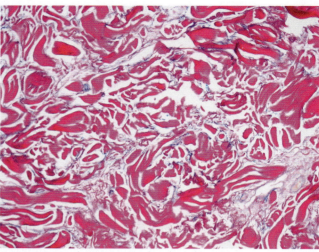

Figure 2.7.8 Interstitial granuloma annulare. Colloidal iron stain demonstrating mucin in area of interstitial granulomatous inflammation and degenerated collagen.

2.8 SUBCUTANEOUS GRANULOMA ANNULARE VS RHEUMATOID NODULE

	Subcutaneous Granuloma Annulare	Rheumatoid Nodule
Age	Children or young adults, typically before 20 years of age. Uncommon in older adults.	Adults.
Location	Lower extremities and scalp are sites of predilection. Upper extremities and trunk less frequently.	Most commonly on extensors surfaces, pressure points, and areas that are prone to trauma (such as olecranon process).
Etiology	Unknown. Delayed-type hypersensitivity reaction to an undetermined antigen is postulated.	Uncertain. Postulated to be caused by accumulation of immune complexes (rheumatoid factor) in areas of trauma leading to macrophage activation and IL-1 release. The inflammatory reaction triggers fibrin deposition and degradation of collagen with ultimate containment by histiocytes forming palisaded granulomas.
Presentation	Asymptomatic, slowly enlarging, firm subcutaneous nodule(s) measuring from 0.5-4 cm in greatest dimension. May be single or multiple.	Firm, nontender, skin-colored nodules that measure from few millimeters to several centimeters.
Histology	1. Epidermis and superficial dermis are unremarkable. 2. Palisaded granulomas within the deep reticular dermis and subcutaneous tissue *(Figs. 2.8.1-2.8.3)*. 3. Granulomas formed by histiocytes surrounding areas of basophilic degeneration of collagen (necrobiosis) with mucin accumulation *(Fig. 2.8.4)*.	1. Circumscribed palisaded granulomas within the reticular dermis and subcutis *(Fig. 2.8.5)*. 2. Granulomas are composed of epithelioid histiocytes and occasional multinucleate giant cells *(Fig. 2.8.7)*. 3. Central degenerated collagen with fibrin deposition *(Figs. 2.8.5 and 2.8.6)*.
Special studies	Colloidal iron or alcian blue stain to detect mucin deposition.	None.
Treatment	Treatment is generally not necessary as lesions usually resolve without therapy. Topical or intralesional corticosteroids may be used if treatment is desired.	No therapy is needed for asymptomatic nodules that do not interfere with function. If treatment is desired, intralesional corticosteroid injection is the first line of therapy. Surgical excision is indicated for nodules causing nerve compression, severe pain, or ulceration. Methotrexate and other systemic therapies are not proven due to paradoxical acceleration of nodule formation.
Prognosis	Excellent. Spontaneous resolution occurs in up to 50% of patients within 24 months.	Complications of nodules are generally effectively reduced by treatment methods. However, rheumatoid nodules are typically associated with a worse prognosis for rheumatoid arthritis manifestations. May also have visceral involvement involving pulmonary, cardiac, and central nervous systems.

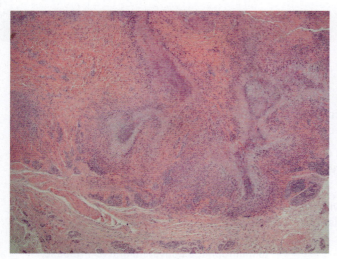

Figure 2.8.1 Subcutaneous granuloma annulare. Large, serpiginous palisaded granulomas surrounding degenerated collagen in the deep dermis and superficial subcutis.

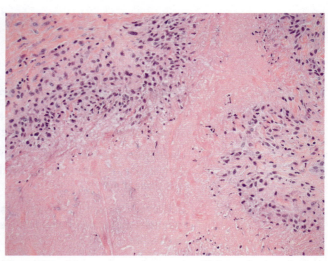

Figure 2.8.2 Subcutaneous granuloma annulare. Histiocytes forming palisaded granuloma surrounding area of necrobiotic collagen.

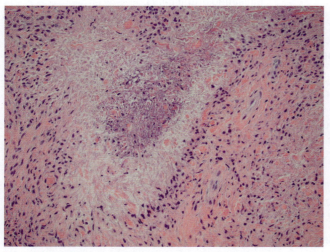

Figure 2.8.3 Subcutaneous granuloma annulare. Well-formed palisaded granuloma with central area of degenerated collagen and mucin accumulation.

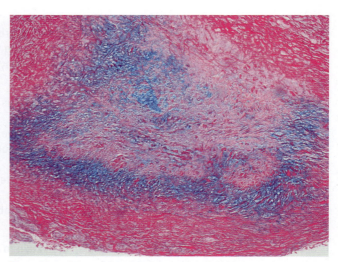

Figure 2.8.4 Subcutaneous granuloma annulare. Colloidal iron stain highlighting mucin in central necrobiotic area of palisaded granuloma.

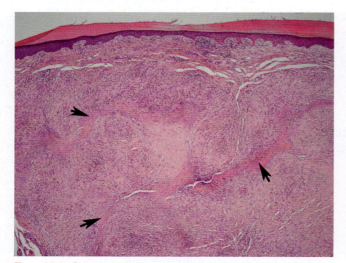

Figure 2.8.5 Rheumatoid nodule. Large, irregular palisaded granulomas within deep dermis and extending into subcutis. Granulomas surround areas of fibrinoid degeneration (arrows).

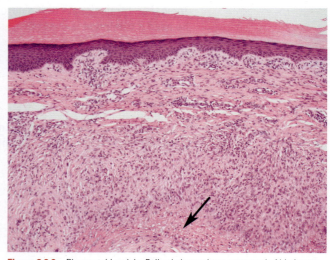

Figure 2.8.6 Rheumatoid nodule. Palisaded granuloma composed of histiocytes with central area of fibrinoid change (arrow).

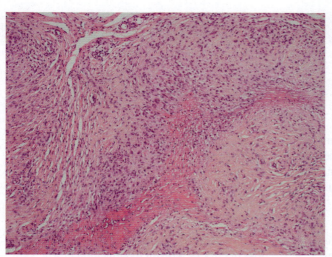

Figure 2.8.7 Rheumatoid nodule. Palisaded granuloma surrounding area of degenerated collagen and fibrin. Note that there is no mucin accumulation.

2.9 ARTHROPOD ASSAULT REACTION VS ALLERGIC CONTACT DERMATITIS

	Arthropod Assault Reaction	**Allergic Contact Dermatitis**
Age	Any age.	Any age.
Location	Any area of skin with some predilection depending upon type of arthropod. Flea bites usually on lower legs around ankles, chigger bites along sock and belt lines, mosquito bites on any area of exposed skin.	Hands and face, especially eyelids, most common sites of involvement, although any area of body may be affected. Distribution aids in diagnosis and identification of allergen. May also present in a generalized fashion.
Etiology	Local cutaneous reaction from the bite of arachnids and insects of the phylum Arthropoda. Bite wound is produced by mouth parts of insect.	Type IV delayed hypersensitivity reaction that occurs as a result of activation of a specific population of T cells by an allergen. Sensitization is the first phase when the individual is exposed to the allergen causing an immune response. This is followed by the elicitation phase during which re-exposure to the allergen causes a release of cytokines and inflammation that mediate the cutaneous symptoms.
Presentation	Pruritic, pink-red papules with central punctum; may have associated purpura. Sometimes present in groups ("breakfast, lunch, and dinner").	Pruritic scaly, erythematous papules and vesicles. Chronic lesions have lichenification and fissuring.
Histology	1. Epidermis has mild intercellular edema but no diffuse spongiosis *(Figs. 2.9.1 and 2.9.2)*. 2. Moderately dense superficial and deep inflammatory infiltrate in the dermis *(Figs. 2.9.1-2.9.3)*. Infiltrate has wedge shape with interstitial pattern superficially and perivascular pattern within the deep dermis. 3. Infiltrate composed of numerous eosinophils in addition to lymphocytes *(Fig. 2.9.3)*. 4. Subepidermal edema and mild extravasation of erythrocytes *(Fig. 2.9.2)*.	1. Parakeratosis and serum crust *(Fig. 2.9.4)*. 2. Epidermal hyperplasia with spongiosis and microvesicle formation in multiple foci *(Figs. 2.9.4 and 2.9.5)*. 3. Lymphocytic and eosinophilic exocytosis with aggregates of Langerhans cells *(Fig. 2.9.6)*. 4. Superficial perivascular infiltrate of lymphocytes and eosinophils *(Figs. 2.9.4 and 2.9.7)*. No extensive deep inflammation.
Special studies	None.	Patch testing to clinically identify allergen.
Treatment	Bite prevention by avoiding high-risk sites, protective clothing, and applying insect repellents. Symptomatic treatment of bites with topical corticosteroids and antihistamines for pruritus. Short course of systemic steroids for severe reactions.	Avoidance of offending allergen. Topical steroids are first-line treatment, and topical calcineurin inhibitors are second line. Antihistamines for itch and emollients to decrease dryness.
Prognosis	Excellent for most common types of insects.	Good prognosis if individual is able to avoid allergen.

2.9 Arthropod Assault Reaction vs Allergic Contact Dermatitis

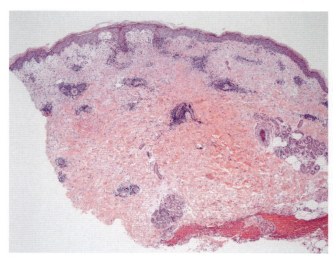

Figure 2.9.1 Arthropod assault reaction. Epidermis of normal thickness and rete architecture with overlying basket-weave orthokeratotic stratum corneum (acute process). Wedge-shaped superficial and deep, perivascular and interstitial inflammatory infiltrate with papillary dermal edema.

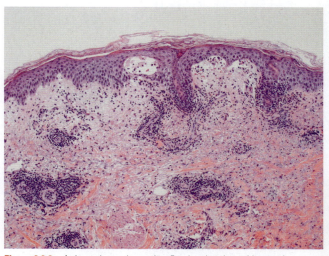

Figure 2.9.2 Arthropod assault reaction. Focal, rather than widespread, spongiosis with few degenerated keratinocytes correlating with site of arthropod mouth insertion into skin. Perivascular and interstitial infiltrate that includes eosinophils.

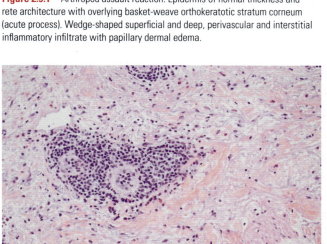

Figure 2.9.3 Arthropod assault reaction. Perivascular and interstitial infiltrate including numerous eosinophils in addition to lymphocytes.

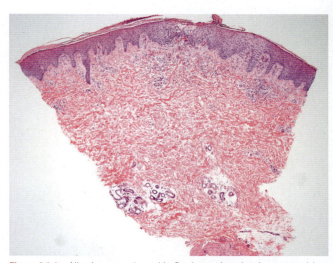

Figure 2.9.4 Allergic contact dermatitis. Parakeratosis and scale crust overlying hyperplastic epidermis with diffuse spongiosis (subacute process). Superficial dermal inflammatory infiltrate limited to the superficial plexus.

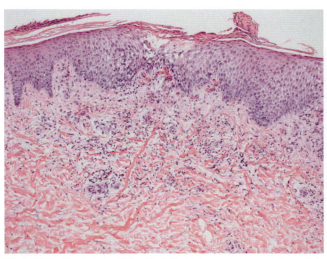

Figure 2.9.5 Allergic contact dermatitis. Epidermis has varying degrees of spongiosis with focal microvesicle formation and overlying parakeratosis and serum crust.

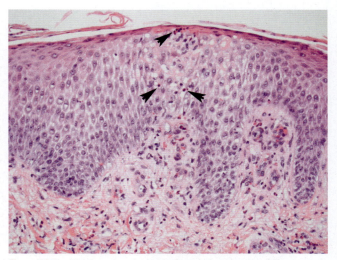

Figure 2.9.6 Allergic contact dermatitis. Spongiosis with eosinophilic exocytosis (arrows). Langerhans cells also present in area of spongiosis.

2 INFLAMMATORY DISEASES OF THE DERMIS

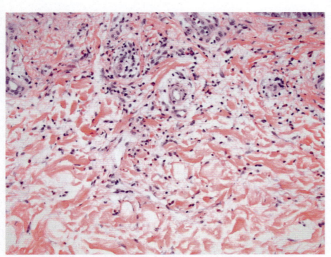

Figure 2.9.7 Allergic contact dermatitis. Superficial dermal infiltrate of small lymphocytes and eosinophils. No appreciable deep component.

2.10 ARTHROPOD ASSAULT REACTION VS URTICARIA

	Arthropod Assault Reaction	**Urticaria**
Age	Any age.	Any age.
Location	Any area of skin with some predilection depending upon type of arthropod. Flea bites usually on lower legs around ankles, chigger bites along sock and belt lines, mosquito bites on any area of exposed skin.	Any location.
Etiology	Local cutaneous reaction from the bite of arachnids and insects of the phylum Arthropoda. Bite wound is produced by mouth parts of insect.	Various triggers (including food, infection, medications as well as many others) cause release of histamine and other mediators from mast cells and basophils. Most commonly the reactions are mediated by IgE.
Presentation	Pruritic, pink-red papules with central punctum; may have associated purpura. Sometimes present in groups ("breakfast, lunch, and dinner").	Rapid onset of intensely pruritic erythematous and edematous plaques (wheals). Lesions may be annular or serpiginous and range from several millimeters to several centimeters. Individual lesions typically resolve within 24 hours without treatment but new lesions may occur. Individual lesions resolve without residua.
Histology	1. Epidermis may have mild diffuse intercellular edema *(Fig. 2.10.1)*. 2. Moderately dense superficial and deep inflammatory infiltrate in the dermis *(Figs. 2.10.1 and 2.10.2)*. Infiltrate has wedge shape with interstitial pattern superficially and perivascular pattern within the deep dermis. 3. Infiltrate composed of eosinophils in addition to lymphocytes *(Figs. 2.10.3 and 2.10.4)*. No appreciable neutrophilic component. 4. Subepidermal edema and mild extravasation of erythrocytes *(Fig. 2.10.2)*.	1. Skin may look normal at low magnification *(Fig. 2.10.5)*. 2. Normal epidermis and stratum corneum *(Fig. 2.10.6)*. 3. Sparse interstitial infiltrate including neutrophils and eosinophils *(Fig. 2.10.7)*. Basophilic degeneration of collagen due to neutrophil degranulation *(Fig. 2.10.8)*. 4. Mild diffuse dermal edema *(Fig. 2.10.6)*.
Special studies	None.	None.
Treatment	Bite prevention by avoiding high-risk sites, protective clothing, and applying insect repellents. Symptomatic treatment of bites with topical corticosteroids and antihistamines for pruritus. Short course of systemic steroids for severe reactions.	H1 antihistamines are first line of therapy. Short course of systemic corticosteroids for persistent symptoms or if associated with angioedema.
Prognosis	Excellent for most common types of insects.	Most cases are self-limited and resolve spontaneously.

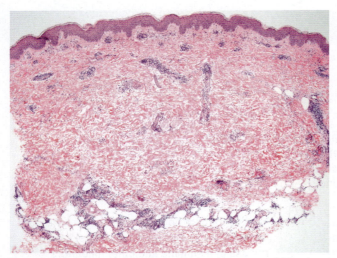

Figure 2.10.1 Arthropod assault reaction. Moderately dense superficial and deep, perivascular and interstitial inflammatory infiltrate.

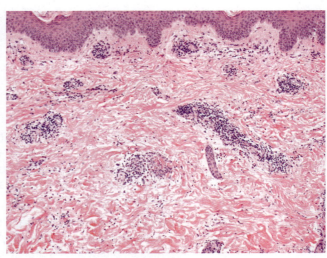

Figure 2.10.2 Arthropod assault reaction. Moderately dense infiltrate consisting of perivascular lymphocytes accompanied by perivascular and interstitial eosinophils.

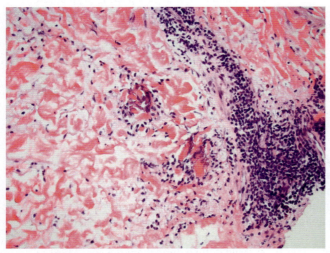

Figure 2.10.3 Arthropod assault reaction. Eosinophilic degranulation causing collagen degeneration and formation of "flame figures." Seen in a variety of eosinophil-rich inflammatory processes and not specific for arthropod assault reaction.

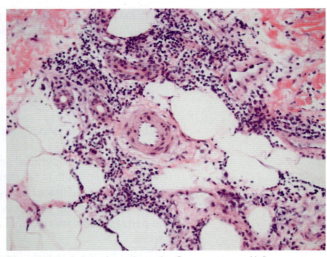

Figure 2.10.4 Arthropod assault reaction. Deep component of inflammatory infiltrate with eosinophils and lymphocytes in the vicinity of eccrine unit and medium-sized dermal vessel.

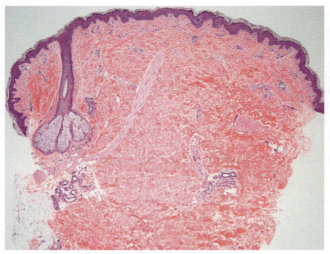

Figure 2.10.5 Urticaria. Normal epidermis and stratum corneum with very sparse perivascular and interstitial dermal inflammatory infiltrate.

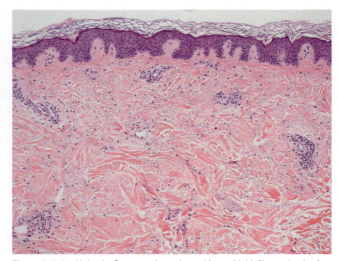

Figure 2.10.6 Urticaria. Sparse perivascular and interstitial infiltrate that is of mixed composition including eosinophils and neutrophils.

2.10 Arthropod Assault Reaction vs Urticaria

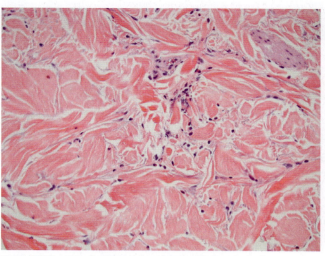

Figure 2.10.7 Urticaria. Neutrophils and eosinophils in area of collagen degeneration secondary to degranulation of neutrophils.

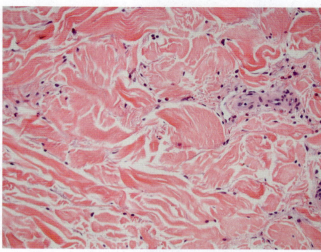

Figure 2.10.8 Urticaria. Dermal edema associated with sparse interstitial infiltrate of eosinophils and neutrophils.

2.11 ERYTHEMA CHRONICUM MIGRANS VS URTICARIA

	Erythema Chronicum Migrans	**Urticaria**
Age	Any age.	Any age.
Location	Any site but typically extremities and trunk.	Any location.
Etiology	Tick-borne disease caused by spirochete *Borrelia burgdorferi*. The spirochete is transmitted through the bite of a tick belonging to the genus *Ixodes*. The spirochete is transmitted from the infected tick when attachment to the skin lasts for 36-48 hours.	Various triggers (including food, infection, medications as well as many others) cause release of histamine and other mediators from mast cells and basophils. Most commonly the reactions are mediated by IgE.
Presentation	Erythematous, bluish-red macule or patch that expands over days to weeks after the tick bite. Characteristic lesion has bright red outer border with central clearing ("bull's-eye"). However, a large proportion of lesions do not have the typical concentric ring appearance. Multiple lesions are seen in a minority of cases. May be associated with low-grade fever, chills, fatigue, and joint pain.	Rapid onset of intensely pruritic erythematous and edematous plaques (wheals). Lesions may be annular or serpiginous and range from several millimeters to several centimeters. Individual lesions typically resolve within 24 hours without treatment, but new lesions may occur. Individual lesions resolve without residua.
Histology	1. Normal epidermis and stratum corneum *(Fig. 2.11.1)*. 2. Superficial and deep perivascular and interstitial dermal infiltrate *(Fig. 2.11.2)*. 3. Infiltrate is of mixed composition with central eosinophils and peripheral plasma cells *(Figs. 2.11.2* and *2.11.3)*. 4. Unconventional features may be seen including interface vacuolar change, spongiosis, and absence of plasma cells.	1. Skin may look normal at low magnification *(Fig. 2.11.4)*. 2. Normal epidermis and stratum corneum *(Fig. 2.11.5)*. 3. Sparse interstitial infiltrate including neutrophils and eosinophils *(Fig. 2.11.6)*. Notably, no plasma cells in infiltrate. 4. Mild diffuse dermal edema *(Fig. 2.11.6)*.
Special studies	Given that the histologic features are nonspecific, confirmation of the diagnosis by ancillary studies such as serology, polymerase chain reaction, or culture is essential.	None.
Treatment	Antibiotics including doxycycline, amoxicillin, and cefuroxime.	H1 antihistamines are first line of therapy. Short course of systemic corticosteroids for persistent symptoms or if associated with angioedema.
Prognosis	Good prognosis with early and appropriate antibiotic treatment. Untreated cases may be associated with long-term chronic affects.	Most cases are self-limited and resolve spontaneously.

2.11 Erythema Chronicum Migrans vs Urticaria

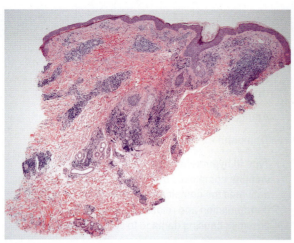

Figure 2.11.1 Erythema chronicum migrans. Moderately dense superficial and deep dermal infiltrate with relatively normal overlying epidermis.

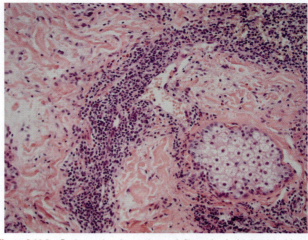

Figure 2.11.2 Erythema chronicum migrans. Infiltrate is of mixed composition including small lymphocytes, eosinophils, and plasma cells.

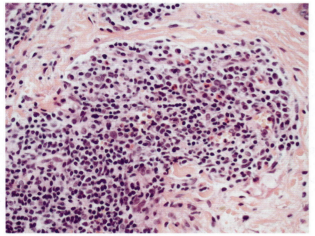

Figure 2.11.3 Erythema chronicum migrans. Mixed inflammatory infiltrate. Note plasma cells accompanying lymphocytes and eosinophils.

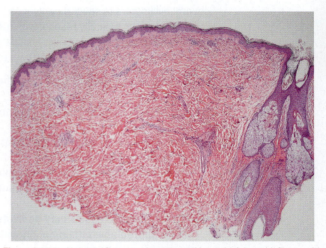

Figure 2.11.4 Urticaria. Sparse perivascular and interstitial dermal infiltrate with overlying normal epidermis.

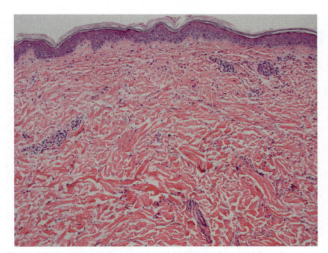

Figure 2.11.5 Urticaria. Sparse interstitial infiltrate of neutrophils and eosinophils with mild edema.

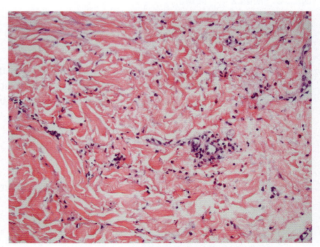

Figure 2.11.6 Urticaria. Sparse interstitial infiltrate of neutrophils and eosinophils. May have overlapping features with erythema chronicum migrans, but note absence of plasma cells.

2.12 URTICARIA VS URTICARIAL VASCULITIS

	Urticaria	**Urticarial Vasculitis**
Age	Any age.	Adults.
Location	Any location.	Trunk and extremities primarily.
Etiology	Various triggers (including food, infection, medications as well as many others) cause release of histamine and other mediators from mast cells and basophils. Most commonly the reactions are mediated by IgE.	Type III hypersensitivity reaction resulting in immune complexes that deposit in vessel walls. This activates the complement pathway causing mast cell degranulation and release of neutrophil proteolytic enzymes causing damage to vessels and edema.
Presentation	Rapid onset of intensely pruritic erythematous and edematous plaques (wheals). Lesions may be annular or serpiginous and range from several millimeters to several centimeters. Individual lesions typically resolve within 24 hours without treatment, but new lesions may occur. Individual lesions resolve without residua.	Rapid onset of painful and burning red-purple and edematous plaques (wheals). Lesions have associated purpura. Individual lesions often last greater than 24 hours and may resolve with purpura or hyperpigmentation.
Histology	1. Skin may look normal at low magnification *(Fig. 2.12.1)*. 2. Normal epidermis and stratum corneum *(Fig. 2.12.2)*. 3. Sparse interstitial infiltrate including neutrophils and eosinophils *(Fig. 2.12.3)*. No appreciable leukocytoclasis. Basophilic degeneration of collagen due to neutrophil degranulation. 4. Dermal edema. Vessels may be dilated but no appreciable inflammation within the vessel walls and minimal erythrocyte extravasation *(Fig. 2.12.4)*.	1. Skin may look normal at low magnification *(Fig. 2.12.5)*. 2. Normal epidermis and stratum corneum *(Fig. 2.12.6)*. 3. Sparse interstitial infiltrate including neutrophils and eosinophils *(Fig. 2.12.6)*. Leukocytoclasis and erythrocyte extravasation in vicinity of vessels *(Fig. 2.12.7)*. 4. Small vessels show vascular damage with endothelial hypertrophy, infiltration by neutrophils, and ragged walls *(Fig. 2.12.8)*.
Special studies	None.	Direct immunofluorescence shows granular deposits of immunoglobulin and/or complement and/or fibrinogen in vessel walls and at dermoepidermal junction.
Treatment	H1 antihistamines are first line of therapy. Short course of systemic corticosteroids for persistent symptoms or if associated with angioedema.	Antihistamines are usually ineffective but can be used for pruritus. Nonsteroidal anti-inflammatory drugs usually used for mild disease. Systemic corticosteroids with or without dapsone or antimalarial drugs for moderate disease. Other systemic anti-inflammatory agents for refractory or severe disease.
Prognosis	Most cases are self-limited and resolve spontaneously.	Unpredictable course. In individuals with normal complement levels, the disease lasts a few years and has no sequelae. Hypocomplementemia is associated with severe disease and increased likelihood of extracutaneous manifestations (musculoskeletal, pulmonary, renal, and gastrointestinal).

2.12 Urticaria vs Urticarial Vasculitis

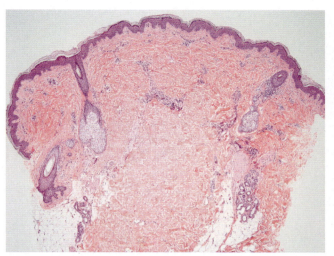

Figure 2.12.1 Urticaria. Very sparse perivascular and interstitial dermal infiltrate with normal epidermis.

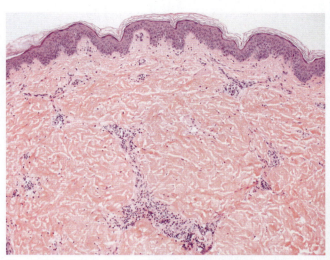

Figure 2.12.2 Urticaria. Sparse perivascular and interstitial mixed infiltrate including eosinophils and neutrophils with mild edema.

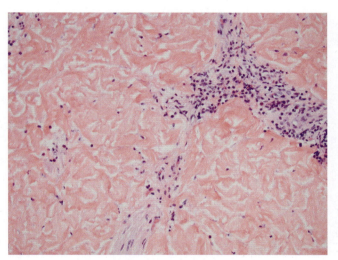

Figure 2.12.3 Urticaria. Sparse perivascular and interstitial mixed infiltrate including eosinophils and neutrophils.

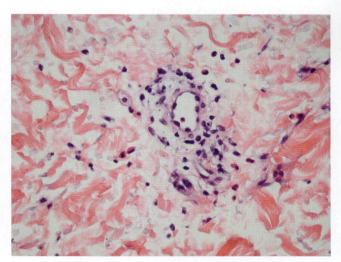

Figure 2.12.4 Urticaria. Eosinophils and neutrophils in the vicinity of an unremarkable dermal vessel.

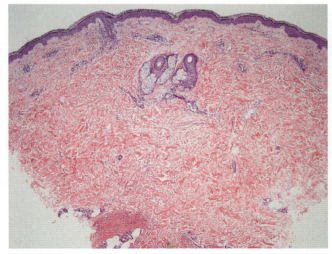

Figure 2.12.5 Urticarial vasculitis. Perivascular and interstitial infiltrate with vascular ectasia and mild edema (less than urticaria).

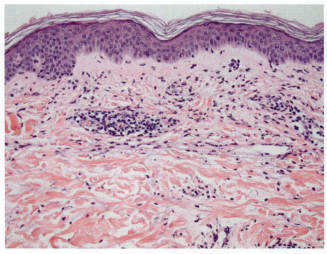

Figure 2.12.6 Urticarial vasculitis. Normal epidermis overlying dermal infiltrate of small lymphocytes, neutrophils, and occasional eosinophils.

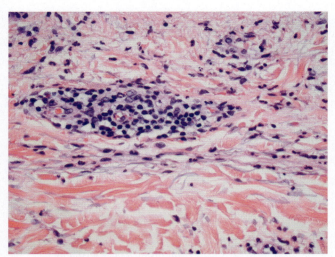

Figure 2.12.7 Urticarial vasculitis. Lymphocytes and neutrophils encroaching upon vessel with erythrocyte extravasation.

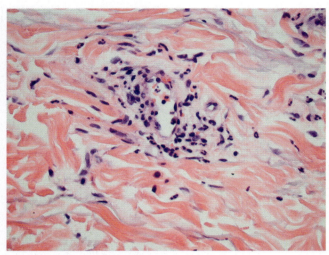

Figure 2.12.8 Urticarial vasculitis. Neutrophils within vessel wall associated with mild erythrocyte extravasation and leukocytoclasis.

2.13 LEUKOCYTOCLASTIC VASCULITIS VS IgA VASCULITIS

	Leukocytoclastic Vasculitis	**IgA Vasculitis**
Age	All ages but typically in adults.	Most common form of vasculitis in children (peak between 2-8 years). May occur in adults but less frequently than in children.
Location	Bilateral lower extremities and buttocks predominantly. Other regions may be involved but less frequently.	Generally lower extremities and buttocks.
Etiology	Many cases are idiopathic but may be associated with autoimmune disease, infection, malignancy, and medications. Caused by deposition of immune complexes in walls of small vessels leading to activation of complement, chemotaxis of neutrophils, and destruction of vessel walls.	IgA1-dominant immune complex deposition within vessels walls. Genetics, disrupted mucosal immunity, and environmental factors play a role in the pathogenesis. Infections, including viral upper respiratory and streptococcal pharyngitis, may be triggers.
Presentation	Erythematous nonblanching macules and palpable purpura. Lesions may be annular, papulonodular, vesiculobullous, or ulcerated. May be associated with pruritus, fever, malaise, myalgia, and arthralgia.	Palpable purpura (without thrombocytopenia or coagulopathy) often associated with postprandial diffuse abdominal pain and arthralgia. Purpura typically symmetrically distributed. Kidney involvement may present with hematuria with or without proteinuria.
Histology	1. Normal epidermis and stratum corneum *(Figs. 2.13.1* and *2.13.2)*. 2. Neutrophil-rich perivascular and interstitial infiltrate within dermis with leukocytoclasis *(Figs. 2.13.2* and *2.13.3)*. 3. Erythrocyte and fibrin extravasation *(Figs. 2.13.2* and *2.13.3)* 4. Fibrinoid necrosis of walls of small vessels *(Figs. 2.13.2* and *2.13.4)*. Thrombus formation in robust cases.	1. Indistinguishable from other forms of leukocytoclastic vasculitis by light microscopy *(Fig. 2.13.5)*. 2. Perivascular and interstitial dermal infiltrate of mature neutrophils with neutrophilic nuclear debris (leukocytoclasis) *(Fig. 2.13.6)*. 3. Small dermal vessels infiltrated by neutrophils and showing fibrinoid mural necrosis *(Fig. 2.13.7)*. 4. Erythrocyte and fibrin extravasation *(Fig. 2.13.6)*.
Special studies	Direct immunofluorescence may show deposition of fibrinogen, C3, and immunoglobulins (IgM, IgG) within vessels. No specific IgA deposition.	Direct immunofluorescence demonstrates granular IgA deposition in the walls of small vessels *(Fig. 2.13.8)*. Not specific finding for IgA vasculitis but supportive in the correct clinical context.
Treatment	Idiopathic cases may be treated with supportive therapies including leg elevation, rest, and compression stockings with the addition of nonsteroidal anti-inflammatory agents and antihistamines for pain and pruritus, respectively. Chronic or recurrent disease may be treated with systemic corticosteroids, colchicine, or dapsone.	Generally supportive care with hydration and symptomatic pain relief. Extracutaneous disease may require additional therapy depending upon signs and symptoms (such as gastrointestinal bleeding, peritonitis, hypertension).
Prognosis	Most idiopathic cases show spontaneous resolution within a month. A minority of patients will have persistent or recurrent disease, especially when associated with chronic conditions.	Disease is generally self-limited, but relapse is common. Morbidity and mortality generally associated with gastrointestinal and renal involvement. Advanced age impacts the severity of disease with increased risk of severe purpura and glomerulonephritis, while younger patients tend to have associated joint and gastrointestinal involvement.

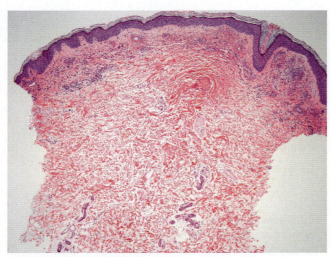

Figure 2.13.1 Leukocytoclastic vasculitis. Superficial perivascular and interstitial inflammatory infiltrate with erythrocyte extravasation.

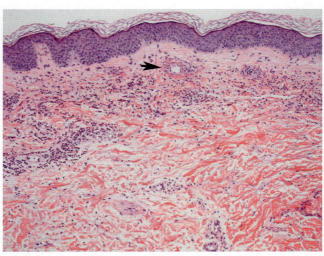

Figure 2.13.2 Leukocytoclastic vasculitis. Infiltrate composed primarily of mature neutrophils with leukocytoclasis (neutrophilic nuclear debris). Fibrinoid mural necrosis involving small vessel of superficial plexus (arrow).

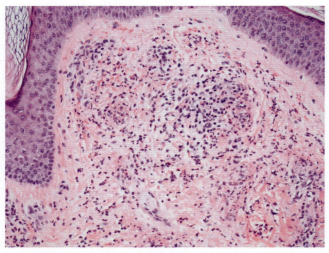

Figure 2.13.3 Leukocytoclastic vasculitis. Neutrophilic infiltrate with leukocytoclastic debris and extravasation of erythrocytes and fibrin.

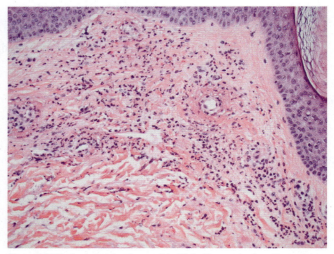

Figure 2.13.4 Leukocytoclastic vasculitis. Fibrinoid necrosis of small vessels with extravasation of red blood cells and leukocytoclasis.

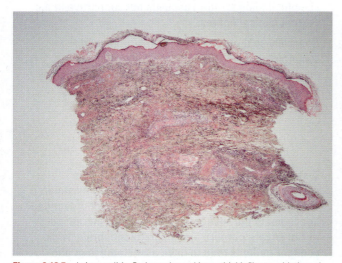

Figure 2.13.5 IgA vasculitis. Perivascular and interstitial infiltrate with dermal edema and extensive erythrocyte extravasation.

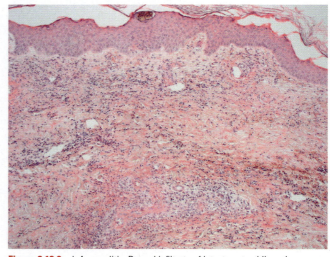

Figure 2.13.6 IgA vasculitis. Dermal infiltrate of intact neutrophils and neutrophilic nuclear debris (leukocytoclasis) with fibrinoid mural necrosis of vessels and prominent erythrocyte extravasation.

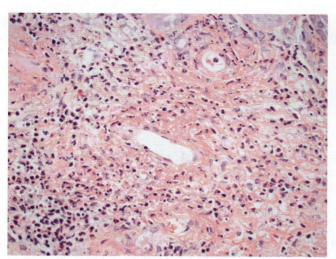

Figure 2.13.7 IgA vasculitis. Fibrinoid mural necrosis involving small vessels in deep dermis.

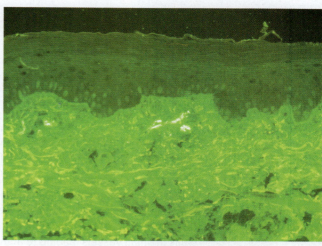

Figure 2.13.8 IgA vasculitis. Direct immunofluorescence demonstrating granular deposition of IgA in the walls of small vessels within the superficial dermis.

2.14 LEUKOCYTOCLASTIC VASCULITIS VS CRYOGLOBULINEMIC VASCULITIS

	Leukocytoclastic Vasculitis	**Cryoglobulinemic Vasculitis**
Age	All ages but typically in adults.	Onset typically in fourth to fifth decades; female:male 2-3:1.
Location	Bilateral lower extremities and buttocks. Other regions may be involved but less frequently.	Lower extremities, initially, but may extend to the lower trunk.
Etiology	Many cases are idiopathic but may be associated with autoimmune disease, infection, malignancy, and medications. Caused by deposition of immune complexes in walls of small vessels leading to activation of complement, chemotaxis of neutrophils, and destruction of vessel walls.	Abnormal immunoglobulins that precipitate in vessels at low temperatures and dissolve when the temperature is increased. There are three subtypes: type I characterized by a single monoclonal immunoglobulin (typically IgM); type II caused by polyclonal immunoglobulins that form immune complexes with one or more monoclonal immunoglobulins; type III involving only polyclonal immunoglobulins that form immune complexes. Complexes cause occlusion of the capillary lumen at lower temperatures. There is associated small vessel vasculitis in types II and III.
Presentation	Erythematous nonblanching macules and palpable purpura. Lesions may be annular, papulonodular, vesiculobullous, or ulcerated. May be associated with pruritus, fever, malaise, myalgia, and arthralgia.	Intermittent purpura with livedo reticularis, Raynaud phenomenon, cold-induced acrocyanosis, and distal extremity necrosis in type I. Presents in setting of myeloma, monoclonal gammopathy of unknown significance, leukemia, and lymphoma. Palpable purpura in types II and III. Presents in association with connective tissue disease and infection, most commonly hepatitis C.
Histology	1. Normal epidermis and stratum corneum *(Fig. 2.14.1)*. 2. Neutrophil-rich perivascular and interstitial infiltrate within dermis with leukocytoclasis *(Figs. 2.14.2 and 2.14.3)*. 3. Erythrocyte and fibrin extravasation *(Figs. 2.14.2 and 2.14.3)*. 4. Fibrinoid necrosis of walls of small vessels *(Figs. 2.14.1 and 2.14.2)*. Rare fibrin thrombus formation.	1. Normal epidermis *(Fig. 2.14.4)*. 2. Neutrophilic inflammation with neutrophilic nuclear debris (leukocytoclasis) (types II and III) *(Figs. 2.14.4 and 2.14.5)*. 3. Distention of vascular lumina by amorphous, eosinophilic globules (types I, II, II) *(Fig. 2.14.6)*. 4. Erythrocyte extravasation and hemosiderin deposition *(Fig. 2.14.4)*.
Special studies	Direct immunofluorescence may show deposition of fibrinogen, C3, and immunoglobulins (IgM, IgG) within vessels.	PAS stain positive in intravascular deposits and aids in distinguishing from fibrin *(Fig. 2.14.7)*. Direct immunofluorescence shows immunoglobulin deposition in vessels with a single type (usually IgM) in type I and multiple types (IgG and IgM most commonly) in types II and III. Testing of blood for cryoglobulins confirms the diagnosis.

(continued)

	Leukocytoclastic Vasculitis	**Cryoglobulinemic Vasculitis**
Treatment	Idiopathic cases may be treated with supportive therapies including leg elevation, rest, and compression stockings with the addition of nonsteroidal anti-inflammatory agents and antihistamines for pain and pruritus, respectively. Chronic or recurrent disease may be treated with systemic corticosteroids, colchicine, or dapsone.	Treatment depends upon underlying disease, severity, and extent of organ involvement. Treatment of underlying hematologic malignancy, connective tissue disease, or infection is first aim of therapy. Immunosuppression with rituximab or cyclophosphamide in combination with corticosteroids for cutaneous and systemic disease.
Prognosis	Most idiopathic cases show spontaneous resolution within a month. A minority of patients will have chronic or recurrent disease.	Variable and depends on associated disease and extent of involvement of extracutaneous organ systems. Hematologic malignancy associated with type I is associated with poor prognosis. Gastrointestinal, pulmonary, and renal involvement associated with poor prognosis.

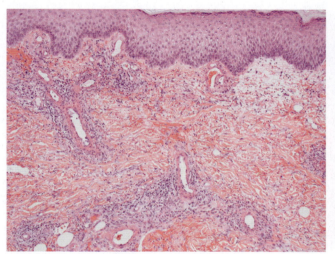

Figure 2.14.1 Leukocytoclastic vasculitis. Dermal neutrophilic infiltrate with erythrocyte extravasation and edema. Multiple small vessels showing prominent fibrinoid mural necrosis.

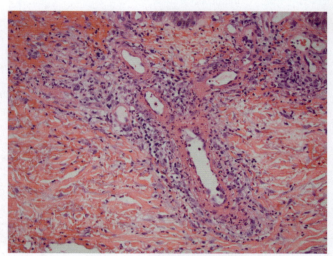

Figure 2.14.2 Leukocytoclastic vasculitis. Fibrinoid mural necrosis of small vessels associated with neutrophilic infiltrate, leukocytoclasis, and red blood cell extravasation.

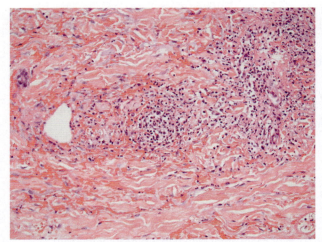

Figure 2.14.3 Leukocytoclastic vasculitis. Destruction of vessels by neutrophils resulting in erythrocyte and fibrin extravasation.

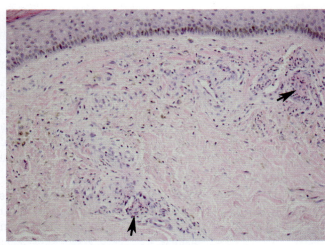

Figure 2.14.4 Cryoglobulinemic vasculitis. Sparse superficial neutrophilic infiltrate with focal fibrinoid mural necrosis of vessels (arrows), mild erythrocyte extravasation, and hemosiderin deposition.

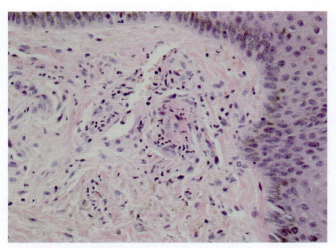

Figure 2.14.5 Cryoglobulinemic vasculitis. Sparse superficial neutrophilic infiltrate with focal fibrinoid mural necrosis of vessel, mild erythrocyte extravasation, and hemosiderin deposition.

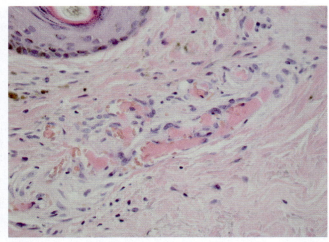

Figure 2.14.6 Cryoglobulinemic vasculitis. Eosinophilic hyaline thrombi with mild erythrocyte extravasation and hemosiderin deposition.

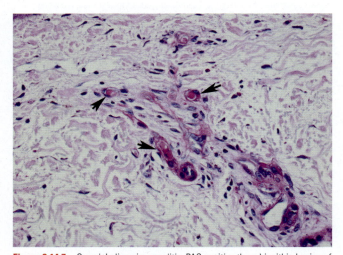

Figure 2.14.7 Cryoglobulinemic vasculitis. PAS-positive thrombi within lumina of small vessels (arrows).

2.15 GRANULOMATOSIS WITH POLYANGIITIS VS EOSINOPHILIC GRANULOMATOSIS WITH POLYANGIITIS

	Granulomatosis With Polyangiitis	Eosinophilic Granulomatosis With Polyangiitis
Age	Middle age, between 40 and 60 years of age.	Middle age, between 45 and 60 years of age.
Location	Lower extremities.	Extremities, including extensor surfaces of arms, hands, and lower legs. Scalp may also be involved.
Etiology	Systemic vasculitis that is associated with antineutrophil cytoplasmic autoantibodies (ANCAs) and affects small to medium-sized vessels.	Systemic vasculitis that is associated with ANCAs and affects small to medium-sized vessels.
Presentation	Palpable purpura, subcutaneous nodules, and papulonecrotic papules that ulcerate. Systemic involvement affecting lungs, kidneys, and eyes characterized by necrotizing granulomatous inflammation of respiratory tract, glomerulonephritis, and peripheral neuropathy.	Palpable purpura, urticarial plaques, hemorrhagic bullae, livedo, and subcutaneous nodules. Other manifestations include asthma, peripheral eosinophilia, mono- or polyneuropathy, paranasal sinus abnormalities, and pulmonary infiltrates. Minimal renal involvement.
Histology	1. Neutrophilic inflammation with leukocytoclasis *(Figs. 2.15.1* and *2.15.2)*. Eosinophilic infiltrate not present. 2. Fibrinoid necrosis of vessels, both small and medium sized, with erythrocyte extravasation *(Figs. 2.15.2* and *2.15.3)*. 3. Interstitial necrotizing granulomatous inflammation present in some cases and characterized by scattered multinucleate giant cells *(Fig. 2.15.4)*.	1. Neutrophilic infiltrate with leukocytoclasis and fibrinoid necrosis of small vessel walls *(Figs. 2.15.5* and *2.15.6)*. Eosinophils typically prominent. 2. Medium-sized vessels demonstrate inflammatory cell infiltrates into the media or adventitia *(Figs. 2.15.7* and *2.15.8)*. 3. Extravascular necrotizing granulomas characterized by degenerated collagen surrounded by palisading histiocytes ("red granulomas") *(Fig. 2.15.9)*.
Special studies	Serologic tests for ANCA with diffuse cytoplasmic staining (c-ANCA) in most cases.	Serologic test for ANCA, directed against myeloperoxidase (p-ANCA) is positive in most cases. Eosinophilia on complete blood count.
Treatment	Immunosuppressives including systemic corticosteroids, rituximab, or cyclophosphamide.	First-line therapy is systemic glucocorticoids. Additional immunosuppressive agents, such as cyclophosphamide, azathioprine, or methotrexate, may be added in severe or recalcitrant disease.
Prognosis	High rate of mortality if untreated. Substantial morbidity due to involvement of multiple organ systems.	Generally good prognosis with use of systemic glucocorticoids. Factors associated with poor prognosis include cardiac disease, gastrointestinal involvement, and advanced age.

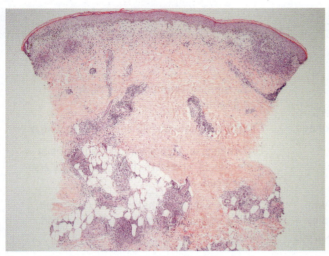

Figure 2.15.1 Granulomatosis with polyangiitis. Moderately dense perivascular infiltrate involving vessels in reticular dermis and subcutaneous tissue.

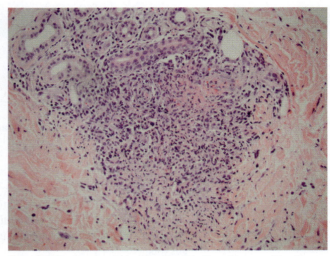

Figure 2.15.2 Granulomatosis with polyangiitis. Necrotizing vasculitis with fibrinoid necrosis and neutrophilic infiltrate with leukocytoclasis.

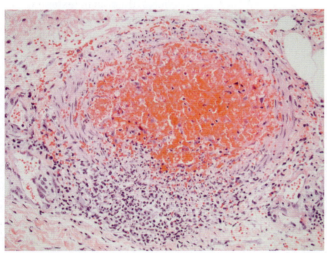

Figure 2.15.3 Granulomatosis with polyangiitis. Invasion of medium-sized vessel wall by neutrophils with partial destruction of wall and erythrocyte extravasation.

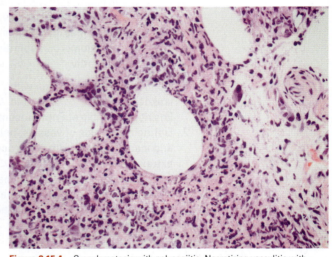

Figure 2.15.4 Granulomatosis with polyangiitis. Necrotizing vasculitis with histiocytes and scattered multinucleate giant cells associated with neutrophilic inflammation and karyorrhectic debris.

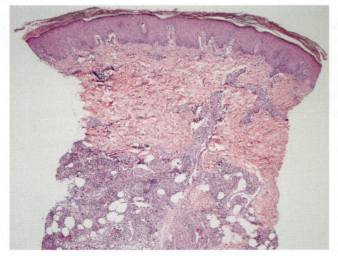

Figure 2.15.5 Eosinophilic granulomatosis with polyangiitis. Dense perivascular infiltrate involving vessels throughout the dermis but particularly in deep dermis and superficial subcutis.

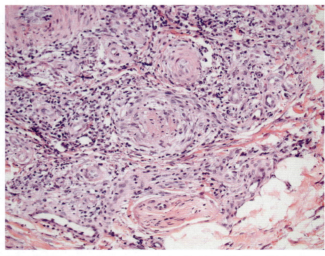

Figure 2.15.6 Eosinophilic granulomatosis with polyangiitis. Vasculitis involving small and medium-sized vessels with fibrinoid mural necrosis and a mixed dermal infiltrate of lymphocytes, neutrophils, and eosinophils.

2.15 Granulomatosis With Polyangiitis vs Eosinophilic Granulomatosis With Polyangiitis

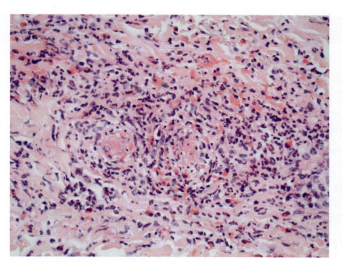

Figure 2.15.7 Eosinophilic granulomatosis with polyangiitis. Necrotizing vasculitis with eosinophil-rich infiltrate and erythrocyte extravasation.

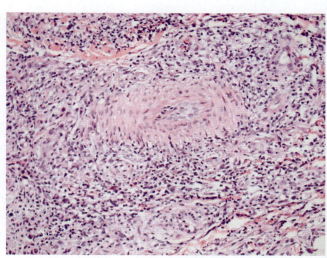

Figure 2.15.8 Eosinophilic granulomatosis with polyangiitis. Inflamed larger arteriole of deep dermis with associated eosinophil-rich inflammatory infiltrate.

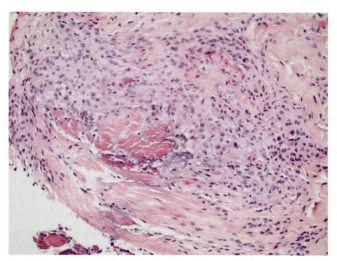

Figure 2.15.9 Eosinophilic granulomatosis with polyangiitis. Extravascular necrotizing granuloma characterized by collagen degeneration surrounded by palisading histiocytes ("red granuloma").

2.16 PIGMENTED PURPURIC DERMATITIS VS LEUKOCYTOCLASTIC VASCULITIS

	Pigmented Purpuric Dermatitis	**Leukocytoclastic Vasculitis**
Age	Any age, but mainly seen in middle-aged adults. Lichen aureus subtype seen in younger individuals.	All ages but typically in adults.
Location	Primarily involves the lower legs but may be seen on trunk and arms.	Bilateral lower extremities and buttocks.
Etiology	Unknown. Potential cofactors include venous hypertension, exercise, infection, gravitational dependency, systemic disease, and medications.	Many cases are idiopathic but may be associated with autoimmune disease, infection, malignancy, and medications. Caused by deposition of immune complexes in walls of small vessels leading to activation of complement, chemotaxis of neutrophils and destruction of vessel walls.
Presentation	Several clinical subtypes that are all characterized by symmetric petechiae and purpura. Schamberg disease presents with pinpoint red puncta resembling cayenne pepper. Lichenoid form of Gougerot and Blum consists of red-brown papules and plaques. Eczematoid form of Doucas and Kapetanakis has scaly purpuric macules and patches. Purpura annularis telangiectodes of Majocchi is characterized by annular purpuric patches with telangiectasia. Lichen aureus consists of golden-brown macules, papule, or plaques. The lesions are generally asymptomatic but may have associated pruritus.	Erythematous nonblanching macules and palpable purpura. Lesions may be annular, papulonodular, vesiculobullous, and ulcerated. May be associated with pruritus, fever, malaise, myalgia, and arthralgia.
Histology	1. Normal epidermis and stratum corneum *(Fig. 2.16.1)*. 2. Superficial interstitial infiltrate of small lymphocytes and occasional histiocytes *(Figs. 2.16.1 and 2.16.2)*. 3. Erythrocyte extravasation with variable hemosiderin deposition *(Figs. 2.16.3 and 2.16.4)*. 4. Vessels show mild endothelial cell swelling and ectasia but no fibrinoid necrosis or thrombus formation *(Fig. 2.16.3)*.	1. Normal epidermis and stratum corneum *(Fig. 2.16.5)*. 2. Neutrophil-rich perivascular and interstitial infiltrate within dermis with leukocytoclasis *(Figs. 2.16.6 and 2.16.7)*. 3. Erythrocyte and fibrin extravasation *(Figs. 2.16.6 and 2.16.7)*. 4. Fibrinoid necrosis of walls of small vessels *(Fig. 2.16.7)*.
Special studies	Iron stain may be used to demonstrate hemosiderin deposition.	Direct immunofluorescence may show deposition of fibrinogen, C3, and immunoglobulins (IgM, IgG) within vessels.
Treatment	No treatment necessary in most cases. Reducing exacerbating factors and topical steroids are first-line therapies for those desiring treatment.	Idiopathic cases may be treated with supportive therapies including leg elevation, rest, and compression stockings with the addition of nonsteroidal anti-inflammatory agents and antihistamines for pain and pruritus, respectively. Chronic or recurrent disease may be treated with systemic corticosteroids, colchicine, or dapsone.
Prognosis	Chronic, benign disease. Unpredictable course with exacerbation and remission, persistence, and spontaneous resolution reported. Rare occurrences of progression to mycosis fungoides.	Most idiopathic cases show spontaneous resolution within a month. A minority of patients will have chronic or recurrent disease.

2.16 Pigmented Purpuric Dermatitis vs Leukocytoclastic Vasculitis

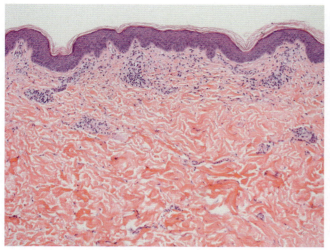

Figure 2.16.1 Pigmented purpuric dermatitis. Superficial interstitial lymphocytic infiltrate with overlying unremarkable epidermis and stratum corneum.

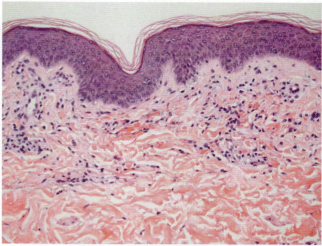

Figure 2.16.2 Pigmented purpuric dermatitis. Erythrocyte extravasation with infiltrate of small, mature lymphocytes.

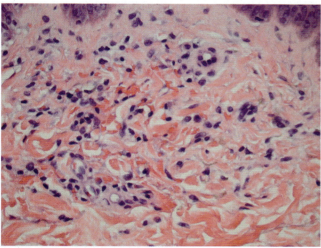

Figure 2.16.3 Pigmented purpuric dermatitis. Lymphocytic infiltrate and erythrocyte extravasation within papillary dermis. Note that the vessels are intact and not inflamed.

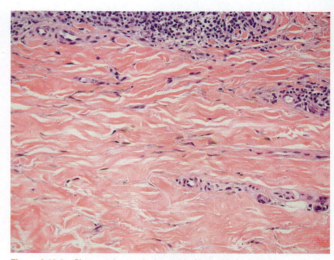

Figure 2.16.4 Pigmented purpuric dermatitis. Hemosiderin deposition correlating with red-brown clinical appearance of older lesions.

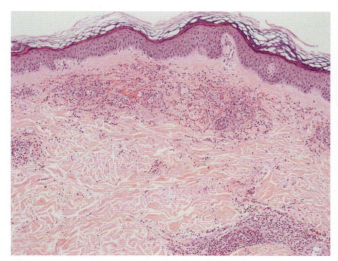

Figure 2.16.5 Leukocytoclastic vasculitis. Perivascular and interstitial infiltrate predominated by neutrophils with areas of erythrocyte extravasation.

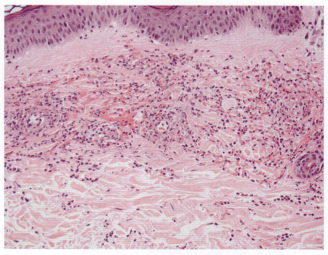

Figure 2.16.6 Leukocytoclastic vasculitis. Neutrophils and leukocytoclasis (neutrophilic nuclear debris) with fibrinoid mural necrosis of small vessels and erythrocyte extravasation.

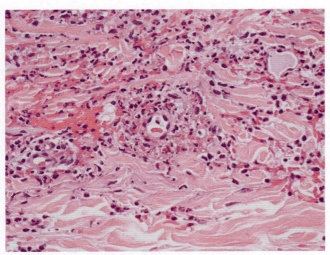

Figure 2.16.7 Leukocytoclastic vasculitis. Destruction of small vessel by neutrophils with extravasation of fibrin and red blood cells.

2.17 PIGMENTED PURPURIC DERMATITIS VS STASIS DERMATITIS

	Pigmented Purpuric Dermatitis	Stasis Dermatitis
Age	Any age, but mainly seen in middle-aged adults. Lichen aureus subtype seen in younger individuals.	Adults, principally over 65 years of age.
Location	Primarily involves the lower legs but may be seen on trunk and arms.	Lower extremities primarily. Upper extremities in setting of arteriovenous fistulas or malformations.
Etiology	Unknown. Potential cofactors include venous hypertension, exercise, infection, gravitational dependency, systemic disease, and medications.	Chronic venous stasis due to venous hypertension. Venous hypertension results from incompetent valves, venous outflow obstruction, or failure of venous pump.
Presentation	Several clinical subtypes that are all characterized by symmetric petechiae and purpura. Schamberg disease presents with pinpoint red puncta resembling cayenne pepper. Lichenoid form of Gougerot and Blum consists of red-brown papules and plaques. Eczematoid form of Doucas and Kapetanakis has scaly purpuric macules and patches. Purpura annularis telangiectodes of Majocchi is characterized by annular purpuric patches with telangiectasia. Lichen aureus consists of golden-brown macules, papule, or plaques. The lesions are generally asymptomatic but may have associated pruritus.	Erythematous, scaly plaques in setting of edema and varicosities. Late-stage lesions may have induration and mottled hyperpigmentation.
Histology	1. Normal epidermis and stratum corneum *(Fig. 2.17.1)*. 2. Superficial interstitial infiltrate of small lymphocytes and occasional histiocytes *(Figs. 2.17.2 and 2.17.3)*. 3. Erythrocyte extravasation with variable hemosiderin deposition *(Figs. 2.17.3 and 2.17.4)*. 4. Vessels show mild endothelial cell swelling but no wall thickening, fibrinoid necrosis, or thrombus formation *(Figs. 2.17.3 and 2.17.4)*. Vessels are not increased in number.	1. Epidermal acanthosis with hyperkeratosis and parakeratosis *(Fig. 2.17.5)*. 2. Epidermal spongiosis with lymphocytic exocytosis *(Figs. 2.17.5 and 2.17.6)*. 3. Proliferation of small-caliber blood vessels in superficial dermis *(Fig. 2.17.6)*. Vessels are grouped and have thick walls *(Fig. 2.17.7)*. 4. Erythrocyte extravasation and hemosiderin deposition *(Fig. 2.17.8)*.
Special studies	Iron stain may be used to demonstrate hemosiderin deposition.	None.
Treatment	No treatment necessary in most cases. Reducing exacerbating factors and topical steroids are first-line therapies for those desiring treatment.	Treatment of underlying venous hypertension and stasis is first step in therapy. This includes elevation of extremity and compression therapy. Skin care includes gentle cleansing, emollients, and topical corticosteroids. Treatment of any superinfection with antibiotics.
Prognosis	Chronic, benign disease. Unpredictable course with exacerbation and remission, persistence, and spontaneous resolution reported. Rare occurrences of progression to mycosis fungoides.	Mild forms respond to therapy to treat venous hypertension. Disease may become chronic and progress to lipodermatosclerosis. Risk factors for progression include older age, sedentary lifestyle, female sex, and obesity.

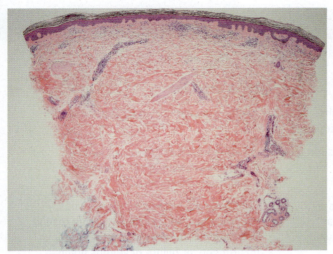

Figure 2.17.1 Pigmented purpuric dermatitis. Perivascular and interstitial infiltrate involving superficial and mid dermis.

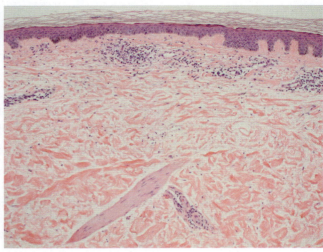

Figure 2.17.2 Pigmented purpuric dermatitis. Interstitial infiltrate of lymphocytes with normal distribution of small vessels showing mild reactive changes.

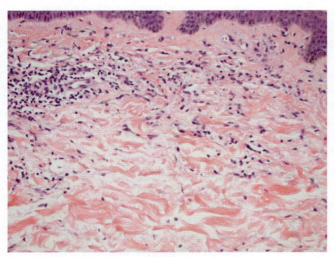

Figure 2.17.3 Pigmented purpuric dermatitis. Lymphocytic infiltrate with erythrocyte extravasation. Note that vessels are of normal number, distribution, and caliber.

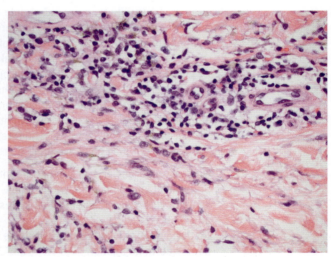

Figure 2.17.4 Pigmented purpuric dermatitis. Normal vessels associated with lymphocytic infiltrate, erythrocyte extravasation, and hemosiderin-laden macrophages.

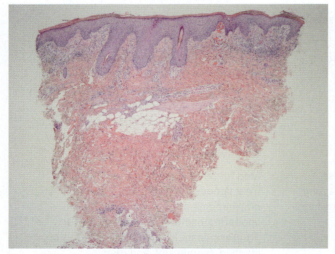

Figure 2.17.5 Stasis dermatitis. Mild epidermal hyperplasia with parakeratosis and a superficial interstitial infiltrate.

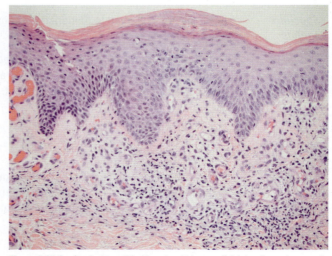

Figure 2.17.6 Stasis dermatitis. Vessels within superficial dermis are increased in number, grouped, and have thick walls with plump endothelial cells. Superficial lymphocytic infiltrate with mild spongiosis and parakeratosis.

2.17 Pigmented Purpuric Dermatitis vs Stasis Dermatitis

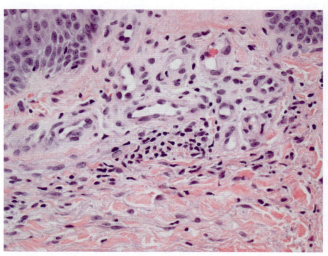

Figure 2.17.7 Stasis dermatitis. Grouped thick-walled vessels with endothelial cell hypertrophy.

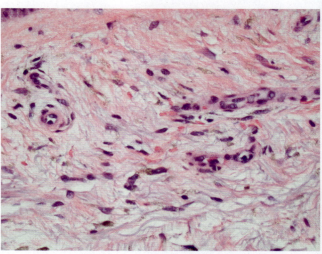

Figure 2.17.8 Stasis dermatitis. Vascular changes associated with extravasation of red blood cells and siderophages.

2.18 SWEET SYNDROME VS PYODERMA GANGRENOSUM

	Sweet Syndrome	**Pyoderma Gangrenosum**
Age	Any age, but typically between 30 and 60 years. Female predilection.	Any age, but predominately adults.
Location	Most commonly on upper extremities and also head and neck region, trunk, and lower extremities. Rarely oral or genital mucosal lesions.	Any location, but most commonly trunk and lower extremity.
Etiology	Most cases are idiopathic but may be associated with malignancy (most commonly myeloproliferative diseases), autoimmune disease, infection, and medications.	Associated with systemic inflammatory diseases, most commonly rheumatoid arthritis and inflammatory bowel disease. Etiology not fully known but postulated to involve systemic inflammation, neutrophil dysfunction, pathergy, and genetic factors.
Presentation	Acute onset of multiple tender erythematous plaques or nodules that may be pustular or bullous. Fever generally accompanies lesions and may have other constitutional symptoms.	Four morphologic subtypes: ulcerative, bullous, pustular, vegetative. Pustular subtype mimics Sweet syndrome and begins as painful, 2- to 5-mm erythematous, folliculocentric pustules. Associated fever and arthralgia in some cases. May progress to more common ulcerative form with rapid breakdown and rolled borders. Lesions demonstrate pathergy.
Histology	1. Reactive epidermal changes with tapered rete ridges and marked subepidermal edema *(Figs. 2.18.1* and *2.18.2)*. 2. Dense, diffuse superficial dermal infiltrate predominated by neutrophils *(Figs. 2.18.2* and *2.18.3)*. Not folliculocentric. 3. Leukocytoclasis but no fibrinoid necrosis of vessels walls *(Fig. 2.18.4)*.	1. Reactive epidermal changes with variable hyperplasia that may be pseudoepitheliomatous and undermine the adjacent epidermis *(Figs. 2.18.5* and *2.18.6)*. 2. Folliculocentric dense neutrophilic infiltrate with loose edematous granulation tissue and reactive vessels *(Fig. 2.18.7)*. 3. Necrosis and ulceration of the epidermis with dermal inflammation extending beyond area of ulceration. 4. Vessels may secondarily show fibrinoid mural change beneath the ulcer but no true vasculitis *(Fig. 2.18.8)*.
Special studies	Depending upon clinical history, histochemical stains to exclude infection.	Diagnosis of exclusion. Histochemical stains and microbiologic cultures to exclude bacterial, fungal, and mycobacterial infection.
Treatment	Oral corticosteroids are first-line therapy. Alternative treatments include colchicine, dapsone, and potassium iodide, but these are generally reserved for cases where systemic corticosteroids are contraindicated due to comorbidities.	Wound care, with limited manipulation of lesions, and analgesia. Topical corticosteroids and tacrolimus for mild forms. Systemic corticosteroids, cyclosporine, infliximab, and other biologic agents for more severe cases.
Prognosis	Highly steroid responsive in most cases with complete resolution with use of systemic corticosteroids. Recurrences may be seen in cases associated with underlying chronic disease or malignancy.	Unpredictable course that may be rapidly resolving, chronic, or relapsing. Typically, lesions resolve slowly over months. Risk for relapse variable and dependent upon comorbidities.

2.18 Sweet Syndrome vs Pyoderma Gangrenosum

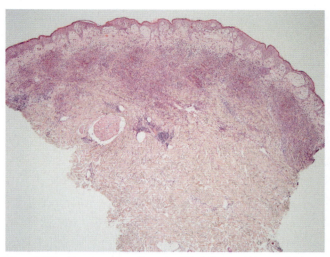

Figure 2.18.1 Sweet syndrome. Dense band-like infiltrate within superficial dermis with marked papillary dermal edema.

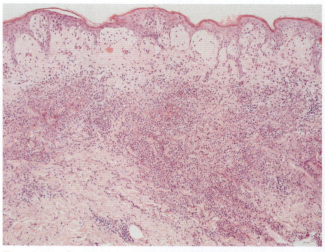

Figure 2.18.2 Sweet syndrome. Diffuse band of neutrophils with marked papillary dermal edema and mild neutrophilic exocytosis into epidermis.

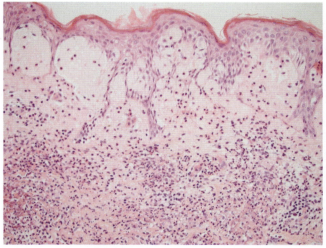

Figure 2.18.3 Sweet syndrome. Dense band of neutrophils with marked papillary dermal edema. Epidermis shows mild reactive changes but no significant hyperplasia.

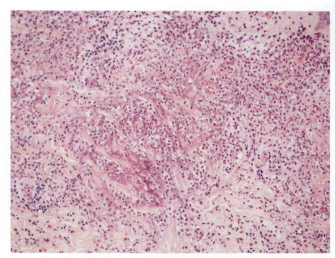

Figure 2.18.4 Sweet syndrome. Dense infiltrate of mature neutrophils with mild eosinophilic degeneration of collagen secondary to neutrophil degranulation.

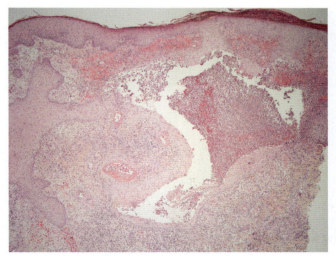

Figure 2.18.5 Pyoderma gangrenosum. Pseudoepitheliomatous epidermal hyperplasia with undermining of epidermis by reactive squamous epithelium. Dense neutrophilic infiltrate with erythrocyte extravasation.

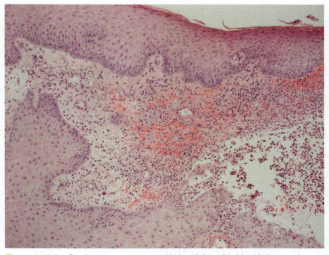

Figure 2.18.6 Pyoderma gangrenosum. Undermining of epidermis by reactive epidermis and dense neutrophilic infiltrate with hemorrhage.

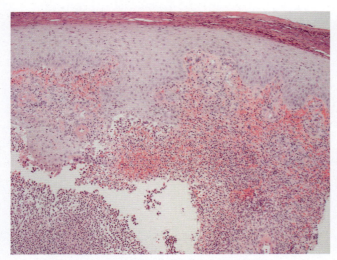

Figure 2.18.7 Pyoderma gangrenosum. Dermis is loose and edematous with dense neutrophilic inflammation, reactive vessels, and hemorrhage.

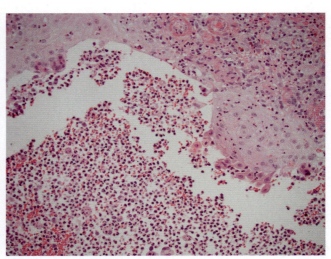

Figure 2.18.8 Pyoderma gangrenosum. Portions of pseudoepitheliomatous epidermis surrounded by sheets of neutrophils. Vessels show secondary fibrinous mural change near area of ulceration.

2.19 GRANULOMA FACIALE VS SWEET SYNDROME

	Granuloma Faciale	**Sweet Syndrome**
Age	Any age, but most commonly middle-aged individuals.	Any age, but typically between 30 and 60 years. Female predilection.
Location	Face including nose, cheeks, and forehead.	Most commonly on upper extremities and also head and neck region, trunk, and lower extremities. Rarely oral or genital mucosal lesions.
Etiology	Unknown. Thought to be a form of chronic vasculitis.	Most cases are idiopathic and may be associated with malignancy (most commonly myeloproliferative diseases), autoimmune disease, infection, and medications.
Presentation	Circumscribed, asymptomatic, red-brown to violaceous papules, plaques, or nodules with telangiectasia and follicular prominence.	Acute onset of multiple tender erythematous plaques or nodules that may be pustular or bullous. Fever generally accompanies lesions and may have other constitutional symptoms.
Histology	1. Unremarkable epidermis (Fig. 2.19.1). 2. Dermal infiltrate separated from epidermis and adnexal structures by grenz zone (Figs. 2.19.1 and 2.19.2). 3. Infiltrate is composed of neutrophils, eosinophils, lymphocytes, and plasma cells (Fig. 2.19.3). No granuloma formation (misnomer). 4. May have mild leukocytoclasis, erythrocyte extravasation, and hemosiderin deposition (Fig. 2.19.4).	1. Normal epidermis with marked subepidermal edema rather than grenz zone (Fig. 2.19.5). Formation of "gossamer fibers" in area of edema (Fig. 2.19.6). 2. Dense, diffuse superficial dermal infiltrate predominated by neutrophils (Fig. 2.19.7). Usually minimal component of other inflammatory cell types. 3. Leukocytoclasis but no fibrinoid necrosis of vessels walls (Fig. 2.19.7).
Special studies	None.	Depending upon clinical history, histochemical stains to exclude infection.
Treatment	Topical corticosteroids, tacrolimus, or dapsone to treat mild or moderate cases. Systemic corticosteroids and oral dapsone for more severe cases.	Oral corticosteroids are first-line therapy. Alternative treatments include colchicine, dapsone, and potassium iodide, but these are generally reserved for cases where systemic corticosteroids are contraindicated due to comorbidities.
Prognosis	Benign condition but with chronic, progressive course and recurrences. Frequently unresponsive to therapy.	Highly steroid responsive in most cases with complete resolution with corticosteroid therapy. Recurrences may be seen in cases associated with underlying chronic disease or malignancy.

2 Inflammatory Diseases of the Dermis

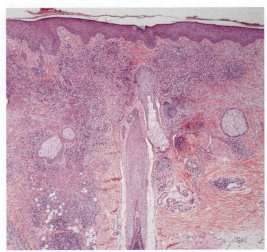

Figure 2.19.1 Granuloma faciale. Dense nodular inflammatory infiltrate within dermis that spares adnexal structures and is separated from epidermis by grenz zone.

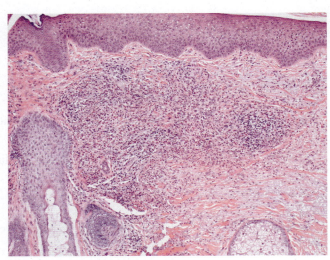

Figure 2.19.2 Granuloma faciale. Dense perivascular infiltrate of mixed composition. Vessels are swollen and have reactive endothelial cells.

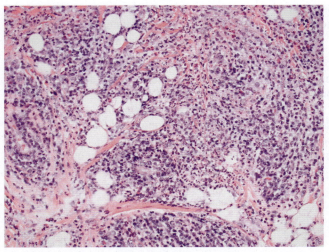

Figure 2.19.3 Granuloma faciale. Mixed perivascular infiltrate consisting of lymphocytes, neutrophils, eosinophils, and plasma cells. Note that there are no granulomas (misnomer).

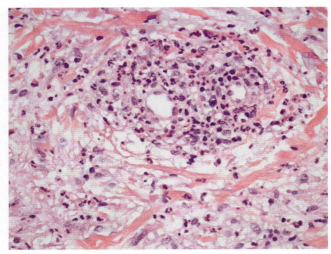

Figure 2.19.4 Granuloma faciale. Mild vasculitic change with invasion of small vessel walls by neutrophils and mild red blood cell extravasation.

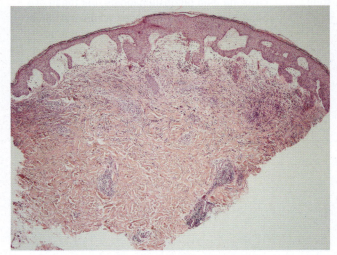

Figure 2.19.5 Sweet syndrome. Moderately dense band of inflammation within superficial reticular dermis and massive edema of papillary dermis.

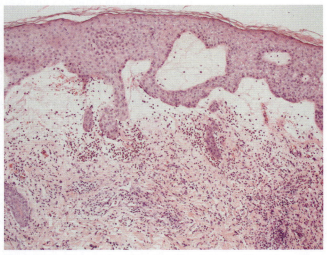

Figure 2.19.6 Sweet syndrome. Reactive epidermal changes with massive papillary dermal edema forming "gossamer fibers" and underlying neutrophilic infiltrate.

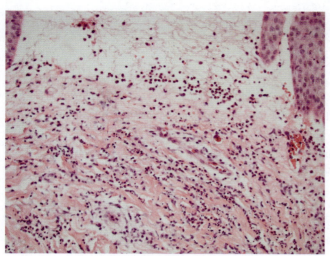

Figure 2.19.7 Sweet syndrome. Papillary dermal edema and neutrophilic dermal infiltrate with karyorrhectic debris. Note that eosinophils and plasma cells are not prominent and there is no vasculitis.

2.20 ERYTHEMA ELEVATUM DIUTINUM VS GRANULOMA FACIALE

	Erythema Elevatum Diutinum	**Granuloma Faciale**
Age	Any age. Most commonly fourth to sixth decades.	Any age, but most commonly middle age.
Location	Extensor surfaces of elbows, knees, hands, and feet. Other sites possible, but trunk and face usually spared.	Face including nose, cheeks, and forehead.
Etiology	Unknown. Postulated to be vasculitic process secondary to immune complex deposition induced by chronic antigen exposure.	Unknown. Thought to be a form of chronic vasculitis.
Presentation	Symmetric, asymptomatic, firm, red-brown or violaceous papules, plaques, or nodules.	Circumscribed, asymptomatic, red-brown to violaceous papules, plaques, or nodules with telangiectasia and follicular prominence.
Histology	1. Unremarkable epidermis (Fig. 2.20.1). 2. Dermal inflammatory infiltrate predominated by neutrophils and also including plasma cells and occasional eosinophils (Fig. 2.20.2). 3. Leukocytoclasis with vascular damage and erythrocyte extravasation (Fig. 2.20.4). 4. Nodular fibrosis with storiform pattern (late-stage lesions) (Fig. 2.20.3). 5. Histologic features overlap with granuloma faciale and correlation with anatomic site and history is essential.	1. Dermal infiltrate separated from epidermis and adnexal structures by grenz zone (Fig. 2.20.5). 2. Infiltrate is composed of neutrophils, eosinophils, lymphocytes, and plasma cells (Fig. 2.20.6). No granuloma formation (misnomer). 3. May have mild leukocytoclasis, erythrocyte extravasation, and hemosiderin deposition (Fig. 2.20.6). 4. Whorled fibrosis around vessels (late-stage lesions) (Fig. 2.20.7). 5. Histologic features overlap with erythema elevatum diutinum, and correlation with anatomic site and history is essential.
Special studies	None.	None.
Treatment	Dapsone is preferred therapy. Corticosteroids (high-potency topical, intralesional, systemic), colchicine, and niacinamide combined with tetracycline may be used in cases not responsive to dapsone.	Topical corticosteroids, tacrolimus, or dapsone to treat mild or moderate cases. Systemic corticosteroids and oral dapsone for more severe cases.
Prognosis	Chronic course with remittances and relapses. Most cases resolve over several years.	Benign condition but with chronic, progressive course with recurrences. Frequently unresponsive to therapy.

2.20 Erythema Elevatum Diutinum vs Granuloma Faciale

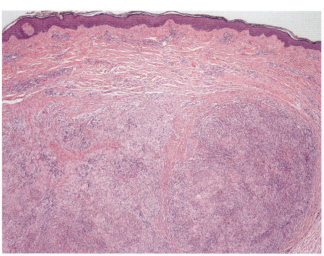

Figure 2.20.1 Erythema elevatum diutinum. Nodular dermal fibrosis ("onion-skinning") with dense inflammatory infiltrate sparing epidermis. Note location on extremity with moderately thick epidermis and stratum corneum.

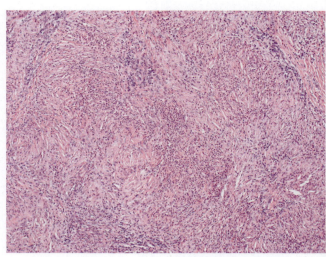

Figure 2.20.2 Erythema elevatum diutinum. Storiform fibrosis with dense infiltrate consisting of aggregates of neutrophils and clusters of plasma cells.

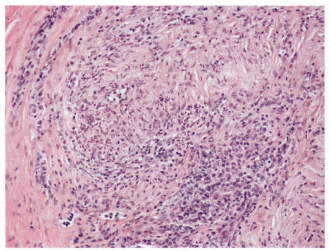

Figure 2.20.3 Erythema elevatum diutinum. "Onion-skinning" fibrosis surrounding vessels with neutrophils and plasma cells.

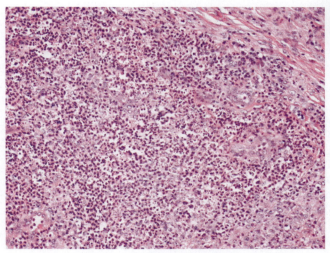

Figure 2.20.4 Erythema elevatum diutinum. Areas of dense neutrophilic inflammation with focal destruction of vessel walls.

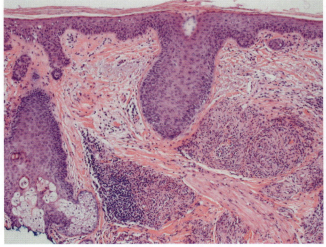

Figure 2.20.5 Granuloma faciale. Dense nodular perivascular infiltrate sparing the epidermis and adnexal structures. Note facial location with sebaceous hair follicles and solar elastosis.

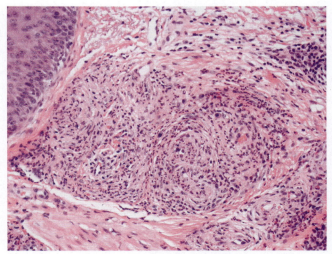

Figure 2.20.6 Granuloma faciale. Mixed infiltrate of neutrophils, eosinophils, and plasma cells involving small vessels. Vessels have reactive changes with mild erythrocyte extravasation.

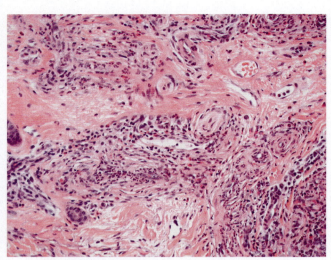

Figure 2.20.7 Granuloma faciale. Mild perivascular storiform fibrosis with mixed infiltrate of neutrophils, eosinophils, and plasma cells.

2.21 BEHCET DISEASE VS SWEET SYNDROME

	Behcet Disease	**Sweet Syndrome**
Age	Young adults, typically in third and fourth decades; infrequently seen in children.	Any age, but typically between 30 and 60 years. Female predilection.
Location	Mouth, eyes, and genital regions. Lower extremities (erythema nodosum-like lesions); head and neck, upper extremities, and trunk (papulopustular lesions).	Most commonly on upper extremities and also head and neck region, trunk, and lower extremities. Rarely oral or genital mucosal lesions.
Etiology	Unknown. Postulated to be dysfunctional immune activity, triggered by exposure to an antigen, in a genetically susceptible individual.	Most cases are idiopathic and may be associated with malignancy (most commonly myeloproliferative diseases), autoimmune disease, infection, and medications.
Presentation	Multiple, painful, "punched out" ulcers of oral and genital mucosa. Bilateral and recurrent uveitis. Skin lesions include eruption of multiple pustules and acneiform papules with pathergy.	Acute onset of multiple tender erythematous plaques or nodules that may be pustular or bullous. Fever generally accompanies lesions and may have other constitutional symptoms.
Histology	1. Intraepidermal pustule (follicular and nonfollicular) *(Fig. 2.21.1)*. 2. Neutrophilic infiltrate within dermis with nuclear debris *(Fig. 2.21.2)*. May have collagen degeneration but no massive edema. 3. Neutrophils within blood vessel walls and erythrocyte extravasation *(Figs. 2.21.3 and 2.21.4)*.	1. Reactive epidermis with marked subepidermal edema and formation of "gossamer fibers" *(Fig. 2.21.5)*. 2. Dense, diffuse superficial dermal infiltrate predominated by neutrophils *(Fig. 2.21.6)*. Not folliculocentric. 3. Leukocytoclasis but no fibrinoid necrosis of vessels walls *(Fig. 2.21.7)*.
Special studies	Depending upon history, histochemical stains to exclude infection.	Depending upon clinical history, histochemical stains to exclude infection.
Treatment	Colchicine is first-line therapy. Oral corticosteroids for refractory cases.	Oral corticosteroids are first-line therapy.
Prognosis	Chronic disease with relapsing and remitting course.	Highly steroid responsive in most cases with complete resolution. Recurrences may be seen in cases associated with underlying chronic disease or malignancy.

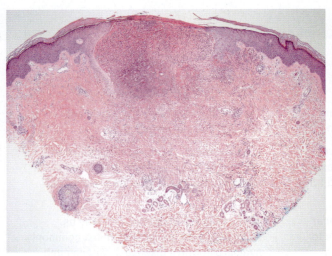

Figure 2.21.1 Behcet disease. Dermal neutrophilic inflammation with central pustule formation.

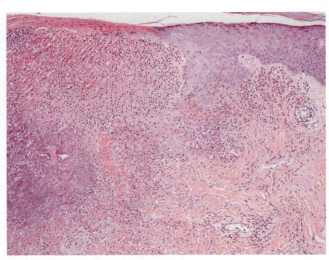

Figure 2.21.2 Behcet disease. Neutrophilic dermal inflammation with pustule formation and degeneration of the superficial dermal collagen beneath the pustule.

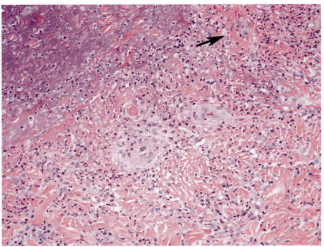

Figure 2.21.3 Behcet disease. Neutrophilic inflammation with karyorrhectic debris and focal vasculitic changes with extension of neutrophils into vessel walls and fibrinoid mural necrosis (arrow).

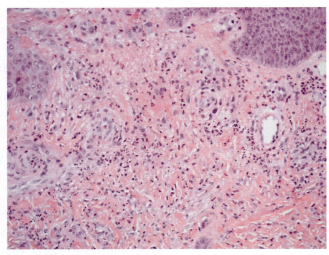

Figure 2.21.4 Behcet disease. Vasculitic changes with neutrophilic inflammation, leukocytoclasis, and destruction of vessels.

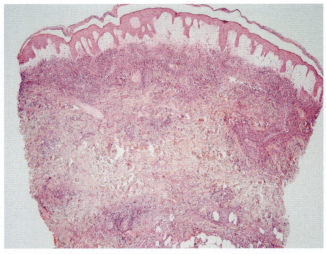

Figure 2.21.5 Sweet syndrome. Dense band-like dermal inflammatory infiltrate with massive papillary dermal edema.

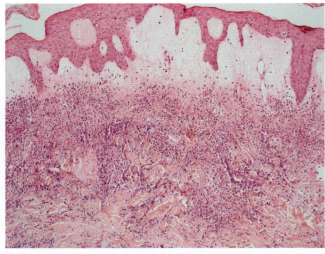

Figure 2.21.6 Sweet syndrome. Superficial band of neutrophils with massive papillary dermal edema creating "gossamer fibers."

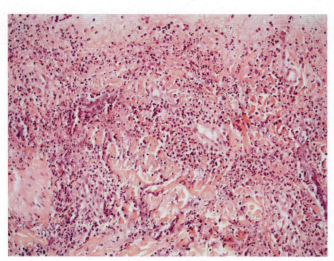

Figure 2.21.7 Sweet syndrome. Dermal infiltrate composed primarily of mature neutrophils with karyorrhectic debris. Note that vessels have reactive change but no vasculitis.

2.22 PERNIO VS TUMID LUPUS ERYTHEMATOSUS

	Pernio	**Tumid Lupus Erythematosus**
Age	Any age. Young and middle-aged women most commonly affected.	Any age.
Location	Hands and feet, particularly distal toes and fingers.	Sun-exposed areas including face, neck, chest, and upper back.
Etiology	Majority of cases are idiopathic with rare secondary cases associated with lupus erythematosus. Theorized to be caused by vasoconstriction or vasospasm due to cold exposure. Tissue hypoxemia induces the inflammatory reaction. Hyperviscosity and endothelial injury may also play a role.	Unknown. Thought to be a combination of factors including ultraviolet light exposure, immune system dysregulation, and medications.
Presentation	Symmetric, red-purple macules, papules, or nodules that develop within 24 hours after exposure to cold, damp conditions. May have associated burning, pain, or pruritus.	Annular, erythematous to violaceous, edematous plaques. Exacerbated by UV exposure.
Histology	1. Epidermis is normal or may have mild interface vacuolar alteration *(Fig. 2.22.1)*. Rare degenerated epidermal keratinocytes. 2. Superficial and deep perivascular and perieccrine lymphocytic infiltrate *(Fig. 2.22.1)*. Exocytosis of lymphocytes into eccrine units *(Fig. 2.22.3)*. 3. Fluffy papillary dermal edema *(Figs. 2.22.1 and 2.22.2)*. 4. Lymphocytic vasculopathy *(Fig. 2.22.3)*.	1. Normal epidermis without interface vacuolar change *(Figs. 2.22.4 and 2.22.5)*. No appreciable subepidermal edema. 2. Moderately dense superficial and deep perivascular and periadnexal lymphocytic infiltrate *(Figs. 2.22.5 and 2.22.6)* extending around eccrine unit *(Fig. 2.22.7)*. 3. Mucin deposition demonstrated with colloidal iron stain *(Fig. 2.22.8)*.
Special studies	None.	Colloidal iron or alcian blue stain to detect mucin in reticular dermis.
Treatment	Avoidance of cold, damp environments. Cessation of smoking to reduce vasoconstriction. Topical corticosteroids and nifedipine may also provide relief of symptoms.	Photoprotection. Topical or intralesional corticosteroids are first line of therapy. Antimalarials for refractory cases.
Prognosis	Excellent. Lesions generally resolve without sequelae.	Individual lesions resolve after days or few weeks but frequently recur. Rarely associated with systemic lupus erythematosus.

2.22 Pernio vs Tumid Lupus Erythematosus

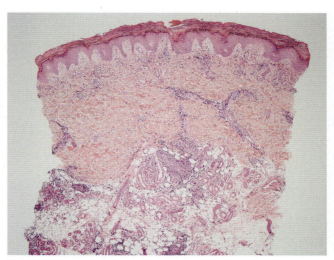

Figure 2.22.1 Pernio. Acral skin with superficial and deep perivascular and perieccrine lymphocytic infiltrate with papillary dermal edema.

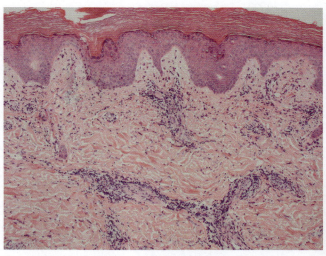

Figure 2.22.2 Pernio. Perivascular lymphocytic infiltrate with "fluffy" papillary dermal edema and mild erythrocyte extravasation. Epidermis has subtle interface vacuolar change.

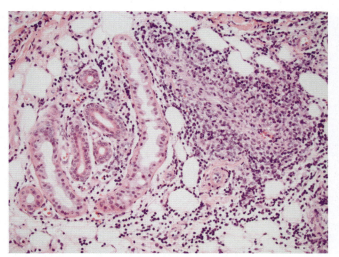

Figure 2.22.3 Pernio. Lymphocytic infiltrate extends around the eccrine unit (secretory and ductal components) and shows involvement of vessels of the deep dermis ("lymphocytic vasculopathy"). No true vasculitis.

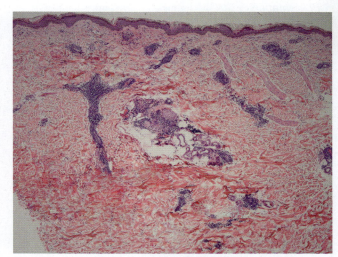

Figure 2.22.4 Tumid lupus erythematosus. Moderately dense superficial and deep perivascular and periadnexal lymphocytic infiltrate within dermis of truncal skin.

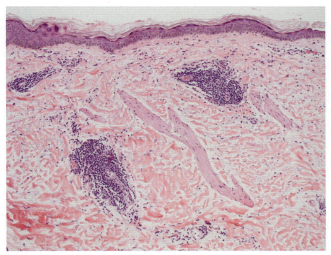

Figure 2.22.5 Tumid lupus erythematosus. Epidermis is thinned but does not show interface alteration (as opposed to other forms of lupus erythematosus). Moderately dense perivascular infiltrate of small lymphocytes. No appreciable subepidermal edema.

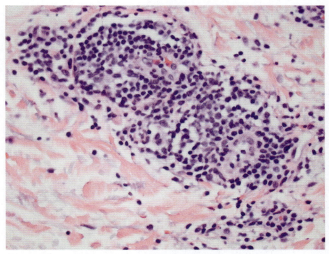

Figure 2.22.6 Tumid lupus erythematosus. Perivascular infiltrate of lymphocytes without vasculitis.

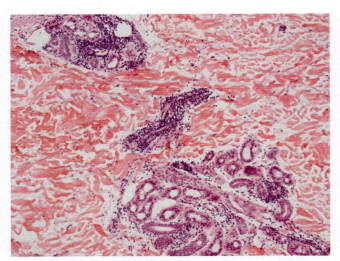

Figure 2.22.7 Tumid lupus erythematosus. Lymphocytic infiltrate extends around the deep vascular plexus and eccrine unit.

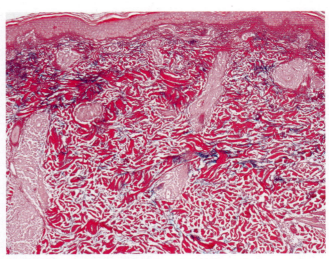

Figure 2.22.8 Tumid lupus erythematosus. Colloidal iron stain demonstrating mucin deposition within reticular dermis.

2.23 PLASMA CELL MUCOSITIS VS LICHEN SCLEROSUS

	Plasma Cell Mucositis	**Lichen Sclerosus**
Age	Adults, middle aged to elderly.	Any age; genital involvement primarily in postmenopausal women and older uncircumcised men.
Location	Genital mucosal surfaces including penis (Zoon balanitis) and vulva. May also affect oral sites including lips, tongue, gingiva, and buccal mucosa.	Most commonly involves genital skin but can be extragenital, particularly on trunk, often inframammary.
Etiology	Unknown. Inadequate hygiene and chronic irritation are suggested as potential causes due to the fact that Zoon balanitis occurs primarily in uncircumcised men.	Unknown. Possibly combination of immune dysfunction, genetic predisposition, and triggers including infection and trauma.
Presentation	Solitary or multiple, well-circumscribed, shiny, red-orange plaques.	Polygonal porcelain white patches and plaques with atrophy. Genital lesions may be associated with pruritus and tenderness; extragenital lesions are usually asymptomatic.
Histology	1. Epidermal hyperplasia (early) and thinning (late) with superficial erosion and exocytosis of neutrophils *(Fig. 2.23.1)*. 2. Mild spongiosis, especially in the lower half of epidermis. Keratinocytes in lower epidermis appear elongated and arranged parallel to the epidermis ("lozenge cells") *(Fig. 2.23.2)*. Notably, no interface vacuolar change. 3. Dense band of inflammation within dermis that is predominated by plasma cells and also including lymphocytes, neutrophils, and occasional eosinophils *(Fig. 2.23.3)*. 4. Vessels have reactive change with erythrocyte extravasation and hemosiderin deposition *(Fig. 2.23.3)*.	1. Epidermal atrophy with vacuolar interface alteration, occasional necrotic basal keratinocytes, and compact hyperkeratosis *(Fig. 2.23.4)*. 2. Edema and homogenization of papillary dermis with sclerotic collagen and telangiectatic vessels *(Figs. 2.23.5 and 2.23.6)*. 3. Moderately dense band of inflammatory cells including lymphocytes, histiocytes, and occasional eosinophils *(Figs. 2.23.4 and 2.23.5)*. No prominent plasma cell component.
Special studies	None.	None.
Treatment	Promotion of good hygiene. Topical corticosteroids, calcineurin inhibitors, and imiquimod are primary treatment options. Laser ablation has also been reported to be effective. Circumcision is recommended to reduce recurrences.	Potent to ultrapotent topical corticosteroids are first-line therapy. Topical calcineurin inhibitors are second-line treatment.
Prognosis	Benign condition with generally good response to therapy.	Chronic disease with unpredictable course. Genital lichen sclerosus associated with increased risk for squamous cell carcinoma.

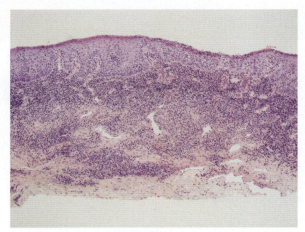

Figure 2.23.1 Plasma cell mucositis. Dense lichenoid band of lymphocytes and numerous plasma cells. Overlying epithelium is of variable thickness with mild spongiosis and exocytosis of lymphocytes and neutrophils.

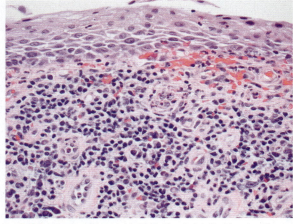

Figure 2.23.2 Plasma cell mucositis. Epithelium is focally thinned and has mild spongiosis with exocytosis of a few neutrophils. Some of the epithelial cells are flattened and assume a "lozenge" or "diamond" shape. Dermal infiltrate of plasma cells with red blood cell extravasation.

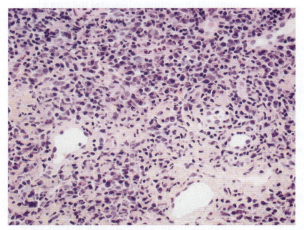

Figure 2.23.3 Plasma cell mucositis. Mature plasma cells predominate the dermal infiltrate and are associated with dilated, thin-walled blood vessels.

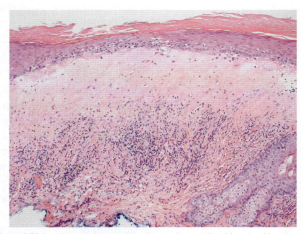

Figure 2.23.4 Lichen sclerosus. Hyperkeratosis overlying thinned epidermis with interface vacuolar change. Superficial dermis has a band of sclerotic collagen and underlying lichenoid infiltrate of lymphocytes.

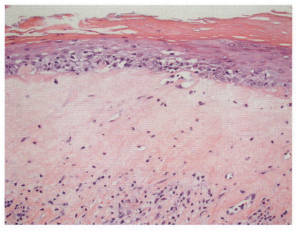

Figure 2.23.5 Lichen sclerosus. Interface vacuolar change with exocytosis of occasional lymphocytes and necrotic keratinocytes. Papillary dermis is sclerotic with telangiectasia and an infiltrate of lymphocytes, rather than plasma cells.

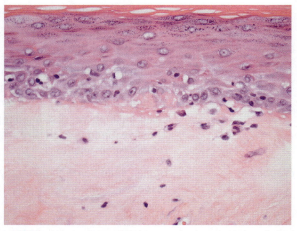

Figure 2.23.6 Lichen sclerosus. Interface vacuolar change with dermal sclerosis. Note that epidermis has reactive change with preserved granular layer and no lozenge- or diamond-shaped cells.

2.24 MORPHEA VS LICHEN SCLEROSUS

	Morphea	**Lichen Sclerosus**
Age	Any age, but majority of cases between the ages of 20 and 50 years. The linear form is the most common variant in children.	Any age; genital involvement primarily in postmenopausal women and older uncircumcised men.
Location	Any region of the body may be affected; however, rarely involves genital skin.	Most commonly involves genital skin, but can be extragenital, particularly on trunk, often inframammary.
Etiology	Not entirely known. Autoimmune, genetic, vascular, and environmental factors trigger production of cytokines that contribute to the development of sclerosis.	Unknown. Possibly combination of immune dysfunction, genetic predisposition, and triggers including infection and trauma.
Presentation	One or several well-delineated plaques of indurated skin that may be hyper- or hypopigmented. Early lesions have an erythematous to violaceous appearance and spread centrifugally. As lesions progress, they become more sclerotic and porcelain white. Lesions may be associated with pruritus, pain, and tightness.	Polygonal porcelain white patches and plaques with atrophy. Genital lesions may be associated with pruritus and tenderness; extragenital lesions usually asymptomatic.
Histology	1. Normal stratum corneum and epidermis; no appreciable hyperkeratosis or vacuolar interface change *(Fig. 2.24.1)*. Biopsy appears "squared off." 2. Reticular dermis expanded by thickened bundles of collagen arranged compactly with loss of usual fenestrated pattern *(Figs. 2.24.2 and 2.24.3)*. Papillary dermis generally unaffected. 3. Moderately dense mid and deep perivascular and interstitial infiltrate of lymphocytes, plasma cells and, sometimes, eosinophils *(Figs. 2.24.3 and 2.24.4)*. Infiltrate is accentuated in deep dermis. 4. Sclerotic collagen encroaches upon adnexal structures with loss of surrounding adipose tissue and eventual destruction of adnexae *(Fig. 2.24.3)*. 5. Some cases may have overlapping features of morphea and lichen sclerosus.	1. Epidermal atrophy with vacuolar interface alteration and occasional necrotic basal keratinocytes *(Figs. 2.24.5 and 2.24.7)*. Variable compact hyperkeratosis. 2. Edema and homogenization of papillary dermis with sclerotic collagen *(Figs. 2.24.5-2.24.7)*. 3. Sparse band of inflammatory cells including lymphocytes, histiocytes, and occasional eosinophils *(Fig. 2.24.6)*. Plasma cells not prominent. 4. Deep reticular dermis unremarkable *(Fig. 2.24.5)*. Adnexae generally preserved. 5. Some cases may have overlapping features of both morphea and lichen sclerosus.
Special studies	None.	None.
Treatment	Therapy is dependent upon the extent and level of activity of the disease as well as degree of functional impairment. Management options include observation, topical agents (corticosteroids, tacrolimus, vitamin D analogues), phototherapy, and systemic immunosuppressive agents.	Potent to ultrapotent topical corticosteroids are first-line therapy. Topical calcineurin inhibitors are second-line treatment.
Prognosis	Disease may persist for years with a remitting and relapsing course. Complications include functional impairment due to sclerosis and joint contractures depending upon the anatomic site and extent of disease.	Chronic disease with unpredictable course. Genital lichen sclerosus associated with increased risk for squamous cell carcinoma.

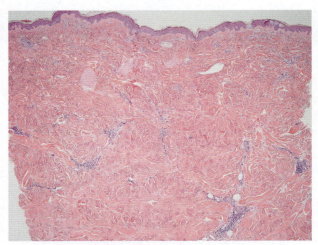

Figure 2.24.1 Morphea. "Squared off" punch biopsy showing expansion of the reticular dermis by thickened sclerotic collagen bundles and a moderately dense perivascular infiltrate within the mid and deep dermis.

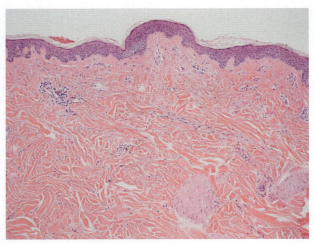

Figure 2.24.2 Morphea. Epidermis is unremarkable and notably does not show interface vacuolar change. The papillary dermis is normal. Slight thickening of the collagen bundles within the superficial reticular dermis.

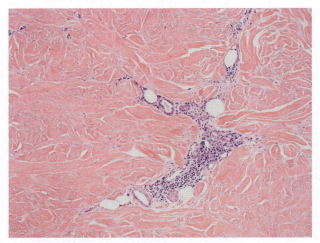

Figure 2.24.3 Morphea. Thick, sclerotic collagen bundles within the deep reticular dermis encroaching upon the eccrine unit. The fat surrounding the eccrine unit is replaced by sclerosis, and the gland is atrophic.

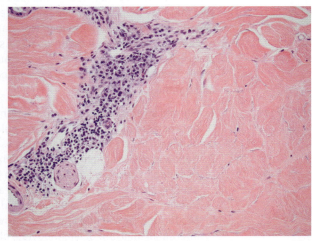

Figure 2.24.4 Morphea. Deep perivascular infiltrate of lymphocytes and plasma cells. Collagen bundles are sclerotic and have lost the normal fenestrated pattern.

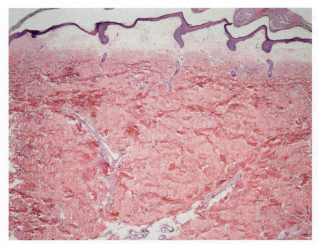

Figure 2.24.5 Lichen sclerosus. Epidermis is of variable thickness with areas of thinning and diminished rete ridge pattern. There is overlying compact hyperkeratosis, and the papillary dermis is expanded by edematous, homogenized collagen. Note that there is no significant deep dermal inflammation and the collagen of the reticular dermis appears normal with preserved eccrine unit.

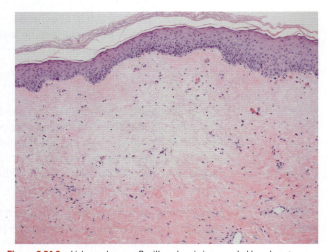

Figure 2.24.6 Lichen sclerosus. Papillary dermis is expanded by edematous, homogenized collagen with underlying sparse, patchy lymphocytic infiltrate.

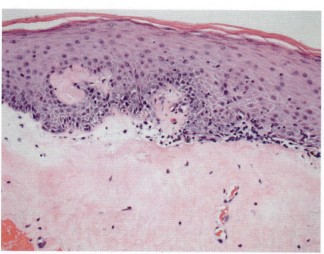

Figure 2.24.7 Lichen sclerosus. Interface vacuolar alteration with exocytosis of lymphocytes along the basal zone and rare degenerated keratinocytes. The papillary dermis has pale, sclerotic collagen with telangiectasia and erythrocyte extravasation.

SUGGESTED READING

Chapters 2.1-2.8

Abdelghany M, Massoud S. Eruptive xanthoma. *Cleve Clin J Med.* 2015;82(4):209-210.

Aldibane RT, Al Hawsawi K. Interstitial granulomatous drug reaction: a case report. *Cureus.* 2022;14(2):e21893.

Ball NJ, Kho GT, Martinka M. The histologic spectrum of cutaneous sarcoidosis: a study of twenty-eight cases. *J Cutan Pathol.* 2004;31(2):160-168.

Beuerlein KG, Martin ED, Strowd LC. Interstitial granulomatous dermatitis as an adverse reaction to vedolizumab. *Cutis.* 2022;109(3):167-169.

Caplan A, Rosenbach M, Imadojemu S. Cutaneous sarcoidosis. *Semin Respir Crit Care Med.* 2020;41(5):689-699.

Dodiuk-Gad RP, Shear NH. Granulomatous drug eruptions. *Dermatol Clin.* 2015;33(3):525-539.

Erfurt-Berge C, Dissemond J, Schwede K, et al. Updated results of 100 patients on clinical features and therapeutic options in necrobiosis lipoidica in a retrospective multicentre study. *Eur J Dermatol.* 2015;25(6):595-601.

Fernandez-Faith E, McDonnell J. Cutaneous sarcoidosis: differential diagnosis. *Clin Dermatol.* 2007;25(3):276-287.

Jacobson RK, Antia C, Sharaf MA. Disseminated interstitial granuloma annulare associated with hepatocellular carcinoma. *Clin Exp Dermatol.* 2019;44(1):110-112.

Johnson E, Patel MH, Brumfiel CM, et al. Histopathologic features of necrobiosis lipoidica. *J Cutan Pathol.* 2022;49(8):692-700.

Joshi TP, Duvic M. Granuloma annulare: an updated review of epidemiology, pathogenesis, and treatment options. *Am J Clin Dermatol.* 2022;23(1):37-50.

Khokhar O, Khachemoune A. A case of granulomatous rosacea: sorting granulomatous rosacea from other granulomatous diseases that affect the face. *Dermatol Online J.* 2004;10(1):6.

Kim YC, Triffet MK, Gibson LE. Foreign bodies in sarcoidosis. *Am J Dermatopathol.* 2000;22(5):408-412.

Kim SM, Lee H, Kim YC. Eruptive xanthoma with dermal mucin deposition. *Am J Dermatopathol.* 2021;43(8):583-584.

Lynch JM, Barrett TL. Collagenolytic (necrobiotic) granulomas: part II--the 'red' granulomas. *J Cutan Pathol.* 2004;31(6):409-418.

Magro CM, Crowson AN. The spectrum of cutaneous lesions in rheumatoid arthritis: a clinical and pathological study of 43 patients. *J Cutan Pathol.* 2003;30:1-10.

Mangas C, Fernández-Figueras MT, Fité E, Fernández-Chico N, Sàbat M, Ferrándiz C. Clinical spectrum and histological analysis of 32 cases of specific cutaneous sarcoidosis. *J Cutan Pathol.* 2006;33(12):772-777.

Molina-Ruiz AM, Requena L. Foreign body granulomas. *Dermatol Clin.* 2015;33(3):497-523.

Patterson JW. Rheumatoid nodule and subcutaneous granuloma annulare. A comparative histologic study. *Am J Dermatopathol.* 1988;10:1-8.

Pierce J, Patel T, Scott C. Eruptive xanthomas. *Mayo Clin Proc.* 2021;96(12):3097-3098.

Piette EW, Rosenbach M. Granuloma annulare: pathogenesis, disease associations and triggers, and therapeutic options. *J Am Acad Dermatol.* 2016;75(3):467-479.

Requena L, Fernández-Figueras MT. Subcutaneous granuloma annulare. *Semin Cutan Med Surg.* 2007;26(2):96-99.

Requena L, Cerroni L, Kutzner H. Histopathologic patterns associated with external agents. *Dermatol Clin.* 2012;30(4):731-748, vii.

Rodríguez-Garijo N, Bielsa I, Mascaró JM, Jr, et al. Reactive granulomatous dermatitis as a histological pattern including manifestations of interstitial granulomatous dermatitis and palisaded neutrophilic and granulomatous dermatitis: a study of 52 patients. *J Eur Acad Dermatol Venereol.* 2021;35(4):988-994.

Rosenbach M, English JC III. Reactive granulomatous dermatitis: a review of palisaded neutrophilic and granulomatous dermatitis, interstitial granulomatous dermatitis, interstitial granulomatous drug reaction, and a proposed reclassification. *Dermatol Clin.* 2015;33(3):373-387.

Sánchez JL, Berlingeri-Ramos AC, Dueño DV. Granulomatous rosacea. *Am J Dermatopathol.* 2008;30(1):6-9.

Shah N, Shah M, Drucker AM, Shear NH, Ziv M, Dodiuk-Gad RP. Granulomatous cutaneous drug eruptions: a systematic review. *Am J Clin Dermatol.* 2021;22(1):39-53.

Sibbald C, Reid S, Alavi A. Necrobiosis lipoidica. *Dermatol Clin.* 2015;33(3):343-360.

Teran VA, Belote KG, Cropley TG, Zlotoff BJ, Gru AA. Granulomatous facial dermatoses. *Cutis.* 2021;108(4):E5-E10.

Tilstra JS, Lienesch DW. Rheumatoid nodules. *Dermatol Clin.* 2015;33(3):361-371.

Two AM, Wu W, Gallo RL, Hata TR. Rosacea: part I. Introduction, categorization, histology, pathogenesis, and risk factors. *J Am Acad Dermatol.* 2015;72(5):749-758; quiz 759-60.

Yang C, Tang S, Li S, Ying S, Zhu D, Liu T, Chu Y, Fang H, Qiao J. Underlying systemic diseases in interstitial granulomatous dermatitis and palisaded neutrophilic granulomatous dermatitis: a systematic review. *Dermatology.* 2022;239:1-12.

Chapters 2.9-2.12

Batista M, Calado R, Gil F, Cardoso JC, Tellechea O, Gonçalo M. Histopathology of chronic spontaneous urticaria with occasional bruising lesions is not significantly different from urticaria with typical wheals. *J Cutan Pathol.* 2021;48(8):1020-1026.

Bhate C, Schwartz RA. Lyme disease: part I. Advances and perspectives. *J Am Acad Dermatol.* 2011;64(4):619-636; quiz 637-8.

Bhate C, Schwartz RA. Lyme disease: part II. Management and prevention. *J Am Acad Dermatol.* 2011;64(4):639-653; quiz 654, 653.

Brar KK. A review of contact dermatitis. *Ann Allergy Asthma Immunol.* 2021;126(1):32-39.

Gu SL, Jorizzo JL. Urticarial vasculitis. *Int J Womens Dermatol.* 2021;7(3):290-297.

Hannon GR, Wetter DA, Gibson LE. Urticarial dermatitis: clinical features, diagnostic evaluation, and etiologic associations in a series of 146 patients at Mayo Clinic (2006-2012). *J Am Acad Dermatol.* 2014;70(2):263-268.

Krahl D, Sellheyer K. A scanning microscopic clue to the diagnosis of arthropod assault reaction: alteration of interstitial tissue is more common than a wedge-shaped inflammatory infiltrate. *J Cutan Pathol.* 2009;36(3):308-313.

Marzano AV, Tavecchio S, Venturini M, Sala R, Calzavara-Pinton P, Gattorno M. Urticarial vasculitis and urticarial autoinflammatory syndromes. *G Ital Dermatol Venereol.* 2015;150(1):41-50.

Marzano AV, Maronese CA, Genovese G, et al, Urticarial vasculitis: clinical and laboratory findings with a particular emphasis on differential diagnosis. *J Allergy Clin Immunol.* 2022;149(4):1137-1149.

Müllegger RR, Glatz M. Skin manifestations of lyme borreliosis: diagnosis and management. *Am J Clin Dermatol.* 2008;9(6):355-368.

Nassau S, Fonacier L. Allergic contact dermatitis. *Med Clin North Am.* 2020;104(1):61-76.

Peroni A, Colato C, Schena D, Girolomoni G. Urticarial lesions: if not urticaria, what else? The differential diagnosis of urticaria – part I. Cutaneous diseases. *J Am Acad Dermatol.* 2010;62(4):541-555; quiz 555-6.

Peroni A, Colato C, Zanoni G, Girolomoni G. Urticarial lesions: if not urticaria, what else? The differential diagnosis of urticaria – part II. Systemic diseases. *J Am Acad Dermatol.* 2010;62(4):557-570; quiz 571-2.

Rosa G, Fernandez AP, Vij A, et al. Langerhans cell collections, but not eosinophils, are clues to a diagnosis of allergic contact dermatitis in appropriate skin biopsies. *J Cutan Pathol.* 2016;43(6):498-504.

Singh S, Mann BK. Insect bite reactions. *Indian J Dermatol Venereol Leprol.* 2013;79(2):151-164.

Steen CJ, Carbonaro PA, Schwartz RA. Arthropods in dermatology. *J Am Acad Dermatol.* 2004;50(6):819-842, quiz 842-4.

Chapters 2.13-2.17

Audemard-Verger A, Pillebout E, Guillevin L, Thervet E, Terrier B. IgA vasculitis (Henoch-Shönlein purpura) in adults: diagnostic and therapeutic aspects. *Autoimmun Rev.* 2015;14(7):579-585.

Barron GS, Jacob SE, Kirsner RS. Dermatologic complications of chronic venous disease: medical management and beyond. *Ann Vasc Surg.* 2007;21(5):652-662.

Bosco L, Peroni A, Schena D, Colato C, Girolomoni G. Cutaneous manifestations of Churg-Strauss syndrome: report of two cases and review of the literature. *Clin Rheumatol.* 2011;30(4):573-580.

Carlson JA, Chen KR. Cutaneous vasculitis update: small vessel neutrophilic vasculitis syndromes. *Am J Dermatopathol.* 2006;28(6):486-506.

Çaytemel C, Baykut B, Ağırgöl Ş, et al. Pigmented purpuric dermatosis: ten years of experience in a tertiary hospital and awareness of mycosis fungoides in differential diagnosis. *J Cutan Pathol.* 2021;48(5):611-616.

Comfere NI, Macaron NC, Gibson LE. Cutaneous manifestations of Wegener's granulomatosis: a clinicopathologic study of 17 patients and correlation to antineutrophil cytoplasmic antibody status. *J Cutan Pathol.* 2007;34(10):739-747.

Daoud MS, Gibson LE, DeRemee RA, Specks U, el-Azhary RA, Su WP. Cutaneous Wegener's granulomatosis: clinical, histopathologic, and immunopathologic features of thirty patients. *J Am Acad Dermatol.* 1994;31(4):605-612.

Davis MD, Su WP. Cryoglobulinemia: recent findings in cutaneous and extracutaneous manifestations. *Int J Dermatol.* 1996;35(4):240-248.

Demirkesen C. Approach to cutaneous vasculitides with special emphasis on small vessel vasculitis: histopathology and direct immunofluorescence. *Curr Opin Rheumatol.* 2017;29(1):39-44.

Frumholtz L, Laurent-Roussel S, Lipsker D, Terrier B. Cutaneous vasculitis: review on diagnosis and clinicopathologic correlations. *Clin Rev Allergy Immunol.* 2021;61(2):181-193.

Gajic-Veljic M, Nikolic M, Peco-Antic A, Bogdanovic R, Andrejevic S, Bonaci-Nikolic B. Granulomatosis with polyangiitis (Wegener's granulomatosis) in children: report of three cases with cutaneous manifestations and literature review. *Pediatr Dermatol.* 2013;30(4):e37-e42.

Goeser MR, Laniosz V, Wetter DA. A practical approach to the diagnosis, evaluation, and management of cutaneous small-vessel vasculitis. *Am J Clin Dermatol.* 2014;15(4):299-306.

Ishibashi M, Kawahara Y, Chen KR. Spectrum of cutaneous vasculitis in eosinophilic granulomatosis with polyangiitis (Churg-Strauss): a case series. *Am J Dermatopathol.* 2015;37(3):214-221.

Kim KE, Moon HR, Ryu HJ. Dermoscopic findings and the clinicopathologic correlation of pigmented purpuric dermatosis: a retrospective review of 60 cases. *Ann Dermatol.* 2021;33(3):214-221.

Kolopp-Sarda MN, Miossec P. Cryoglobulinemic vasculitis: pathophysiological mechanisms and diagnosis. *Curr Opin Rheumatol.* 2021;33:1-7.

Krishnaram AS, Geetha T, Pratheepa, Saigal A. Primary cryoglobulinemia with cutaneous features. *Indian J Dermatol Venereol Leprol.* 2013;79(3):427-430.

Linskey KR, Kroshinsky D, Mihm MC Jr, Hoang MP. Immunoglobulin-A--associated small-vessel vasculitis: a 10-year experience at the Massachusetts General Hospital. *J Am Acad Dermatol.* 2012;66(5):813-822.

Marques CC, Fernandes EL, Miquelin GM, Colferai MMT. Cutaneous manifestations of Churg-Strauss syndrome: key to diagnosis. *An Bras Dermatol.* 2017;92(5 suppl 1):56-58.

Marzano AV, Raimondo MG, Berti E, Meroni PL, Ingegnoli F. Cutaneous manifestations of ANCA-associated small vessels vasculitis. *Clin Rev Allergy Immunol.* 2017;53(3):428-438.

Pillebout E, Sunderkötter C. IgA vasculitis. *Semin Immunopathol.* 2021;43(5):729-738.

Ramos-Casals M, Stone JH, Cid MC, Bosch X. The cryoglobulinaemias. *Lancet.* 2012;379(9813):348-360.

Runge JS, Nakamura M, Sullivan AN, Harms PW, Chan MP. Pigmented purpuric dermatosis of the hand: clinicopathologic analysis of six cases with review of the literature. *Am J Dermatopathol.* 2022;44(8):553-558.

Sardana K, Sarkar R, Sehgal VN. Pigmented purpuric dermatoses: an overview. *Int J Dermatol.* 2004;43(7):482-488.

Spigariolo CB, Giacalone S, Nazzaro G. Pigmented purpuric dermatoses: a complete narrative review. *J Clin Med*. 2021;10(11):2283.

Sundaresan S, Migden MR, Silapunt S. Stasis dermatitis: pathophysiology, evaluation, and management. *Am J Clin Dermatol*. 2017;18(3):383-390.

Tabb ES, Duncan LM, Nazarian RM. Eosinophilic granulomatosis with polyangiitis: cutaneous clinical and histopathologic differential diagnosis. *J Cutan Pathol*. 2021;48(11):1379-1386.

Tolaymat L, Hall MR. Pigmented purpuric dermatitis. In: *StatPearls*. StatPearls Publishing; 2022.

Weaver J, Billings SD. Initial presentation of stasis dermatitis mimicking solitary lesions: a previously unrecognized clinical scenario. *J Am Acad Dermatol*. 2009;61(6):1028-1032.

Chapters 2.18-2.21

Alavi A, Sajic D, Cerci FB, Ghazarian D, Rosenbach M, Jorizzo J. Neutrophilic dermatoses: an update. *Am J Clin Dermatol*. 2014;15(5):413-423.

Alpsoy E, Bozca BC, Bilgic A. Behçet disease: an update for dermatologists. *Am J Clin Dermatol*. 2021;22(4):477-502.

Alpsoy E. Behçet's disease: a comprehensive review with a focus on epidemiology, etiology and clinical features, and management of mucocutaneous lesions. *J Dermatol*. 2016;43(6):620-632.

Baldessari EM, Garcia N, Mendez Villarroel A. Sweet's syndrome. *Intern Med J*. 2012;42(1):103-104.

Chen J, Yao X. A contemporary review of Behcet's syndrome. *Clin Rev Allergy Immunol*. 2021;61(3):363-376.

Chen KR, Kawahara Y, Miyakawa S, Nishikawa T. Cutaneous vasculitis in Behçet's disease: a clinical and histopathologic study of 20 patients. *J Am Acad Dermatol*. 1997;36(5 pt 1):689-696.

Cohen PR, Kurzrock R. Sweet's syndrome revisited: a review of disease concepts. *Int J Dermatol*. 2003;42(10):761-778.

Crowson AN, Mihm MC Jr, Magro C. Pyoderma gangrenosum: a review. *J Cutan Pathol*. 2003;30(2):97-107.

Doktor V, Hadi A, Hadi A, Phelps R, Goodheart H. Erythema elevatum diutinum: a case report and review of literature. *Int J Dermatol*. 2019;58(4):408-415.

Filosa A, Filosa G. Neutrophilic dermatoses: a broad spectrum of disease. *G Ital Dermatol Venereol*. 2018;153(2):265-272.

Frantz R, Chukwuma O, Sokumbi O, et al. Identifying histopathologic features of erythema elevatum diutinum and granuloma faciale. *J Cutan Pathol*. 2022;49(3):323-326.

Gibson LE, el-Azhary RA. Erythema elevatum diutinum. *Clin Dermatol*. 2000;18(3):295-299.

Joshi TP, Friske SK, Hsiou DA, Duvic M. New practical aspects of sweet syndrome. *Am J Clin Dermatol*. 2022;23(3):301-318.

Kaur M, Singh A, Ramesh V. Granuloma faciale. *Indian Dermatol Online J*. 2016;7:130-132.

LeBoit PE. Granuloma faciale: a diagnosis deserving of dignity. *Am J Dermatopathol*. 2002;24(5):440-443.

Mançano VS, Dinato SLME, Almeida JRP, Romiti N. Erythema elevatum diutinum. *An Bras Dermatol*. 2018;93(5):614-615.

Marcoval J, Moreno A, Peyr J. Granuloma faciale: a clinicopathological study of 11 cases. *J Am Acad Dermatol*. 2004;51(2):269-273.

Mat MC, Sevim A, Fresko I, Tüzün Y. Behçet's disease as a systemic disease. *Clin Dermatol*. 2014;32(3):435-442.

Nelson CA, Stephen S, Ashchyan HJ, James WD, Micheletti RG, Rosenbach M. Neutrophilic dermatoses: pathogenesis, sweet syndrome, neutrophilic eccrine hidradenitis, and Behçet disease. *J Am Acad Dermatol*. 2018;79(6):987-1006.

Okhovat JP, Shinkai K. Pyoderma gangrenosum. *JAMA Dermatol*. 2014;150(9):1032.

Rochet NM, Chavan RN, Cappel MA, Wada DA, Gibson LE. Sweet syndrome: clinical presentation, associations, and response to treatment in 77 patients. *J Am Acad Dermatol*. 2013;69(4):557-564.

Ruocco E, Sangiuliano S, Gravina AG, Miranda A, Nicoletti G. Pyoderma gangrenosum: an updated review. *J Eur Acad Dermatol Venereol*. 2009;23(9):1008-1017.

Wallach D, Vignon-Pennamen MD. Pyoderma gangrenosum and Sweet syndrome: the prototypic neutrophilic dermatoses. *Br J Dermatol*. 2018;178(3):595-602.

Ye MJ, Ye JM. Pyoderma gangrenosum: a review of clinical features and outcomes of 23 cases requiring inpatient management. *Dermatol Res Pract*. 2014;2014:461467.

Chapter 2.22

Alexiades-Armenakas MR, Baldassano M, Bince B, et al. Tumid lupus erythematosus: criteria for classification with immunohistochemical analysis. *Arthritis Rheum*. 2003;49(4):494-500.

Baker JS, Miranpuri S. Perniosis a case report with literature review. *J Am Podiatr Med Assoc*. 2016;106(2):138-140.

Boada A, Bielsa I, Fernández-Figueras MT, Ferrándiz C. Perniosis: clinical and histopathological analysis. *Am J Dermatopathol*. 2010;32(1):19-23.

Crowson AN, Magro CM. Idiopathic perniosis and its mimics: a clinical and histological study of 38 cases. *Hum Pathol*. 1997;28(4):478-484.

Hsu S, Hwang LY, Ruiz H. Tumid lupus erythematosus. *Cutis*. 2002;69(3):227-230.

Patsinakidis N, Kautz O, Gibbs BF, Raap U. Lupus erythematosus tumidus: clinical perspectives. *Clin Cosmet Investig Dermatol*. 2019;12:707-719.

Ruiz H, Sánchez JL. Tumid lupus erythematosus. *Am J Dermatopathol*. 1999;21(4):356-360.

Saleh D, Grubbs H, Koritala T, Crane JS. Tumid lupus erythematosus. In: *StatPearls*. StatPearls Publishing; 2022.

Chapters 2.23-2.24

Arif T, Fatima R, Sami M. Extragenital lichen sclerosus: a comprehensive review. *Australas J Dermatol*. 2022;63(4):452-462.

Brix WK, Nassau SR, Patterson JW, Cousar JB, Wick MR. Idiopathic lymphoplasmacellular mucositis-dermatitis. *J Cutan Pathol*. 2010;37(4):426-431.

Careta MF, Romiti R. Localized scleroderma: clinical spectrum and therapeutic update. *An Bras Dermatol.* 2015;90(1):62-73.

Chan MP, Zimarowski MJ. Vulvar dermatoses: a histopathologic review and classification of 183 cases. *J Cutan Pathol.* 2015;42:510-518.

Chiu YE, Abban CY, Konicke K, Segura A, Sokumbi O. Histopathologic spectrum of morphea. *Am J Dermatopathol.* 2021;43:1-8.

Damiani L, Quadros MD, Posser V, Minotto R, Boff AL. Zoon vulvitis. *An Bras Dermatol.* 2017;92(5 suppl 1):166-168.

Fistarol SK, Itin PH. Diagnosis and treatment of lichen sclerosus: an update. *Am J Clin Dermatol.* 2013;14(1):27-47.

Jindal R, Shirazi N, Chauhan P. Histopathology of morphea: sensitivity of various named signs, a retrospective study. *Indian J Pathol Microbiol.* 2020;63(4):600-603.

Keith PJ, Wolz MM, Peters MS. Eosinophils in lichen sclerosus et atrophicus. *J Cutan Pathol.* 2015;42(10):693-698.

Kowalewski C, Kozłowska A, Górska M, et al. Alterations of basement membrane zone and cutaneous microvasculature in morphea and extragenital lichen sclerosus. *Am J Dermatopathol.* 2005;27(6):489-496.

Sattler S, Elsensohn AN, Mauskar MM, Kraus CN. Plasma cell vulvitis: a systematic review. *Int J Womens Dermatol.* 2021;7(5 pt B):489-496.

3
Vesiculobullous Diseases

3.1 Bullous Pemphigoid vs Pemphigus Vulgaris
3.2 Bullous Pemphigoid vs Epidermolysis Bullosa Acquisita
3.3 Linear IgA Dermatosis vs Bullous Pemphigoid
3.4 Bullous Pemphigoid vs Dermatitis Herpetiformis
3.5 Pemphigoid (Herpes) Gestationis vs Polymorphic Eruption of Pregnancy
3.6 Dermatitis Herpetiformis vs Linear IgA Dermatosis
3.7 Porphyria Cutanea Tarda vs Bullous Pemphigoid
3.8 Mucous Membrane (Cicatricial) Pemphigoid vs Bullous Pemphigoid
3.9 Porphyria Cutanea Tarda vs Epidermolysis Bullosa Acquisita
3.10 Epidermolysis Bullosa vs Porphyria Cutanea Tarda
3.11 Pemphigus Vulgaris vs Darier Disease
3.12 Darier Disease vs Transient Acantholytic Dermatosis (Grover Disease)
3.13 Pemphigus Vulgaris vs Pemphigus Foliaceus
3.14 Pemphigus Foliaceus vs Bullous Impetigo
3.15 Pemphigus Vulgaris vs Transient Acantholytic Dermatosis (Grover Disease)
3.16 Pemphigus Vulgaris vs Benign Familial Pemphigus (Hailey-Hailey Disease)
3.17 Benign Familial Pemphigus (Hailey-Hailey Disease) vs Transient Acantholytic Dermatosis (Grover Disease)
3.18 Darier Disease vs Benign Familial Pemphigus (Hailey-Hailey Disease)

3.1 BULLOUS PEMPHIGOID VS PEMPHIGUS VULGARIS

	Bullous Pemphigoid	**Pemphigus Vulgaris**
Age	Elderly adults, typically between ages of 60 and 80 y.	Adults, generally between ages of 45 and 65 y.
Location	Trunk and extremities, especially intertriginous areas of axilla, lower abdomen, inguinal crease, and inner thighs. Mucosal involvement rare.	Typically begins in oral mucosa. Skin lesions can develop at any site with a predilection for head and neck region, axillae, and upper trunk.
Etiology	Autoantibodies against antigens at the basement membrane zone. The antigens are BP180 (BPAG2) and BP230 (BPAG1), which are key proteins within the hemidesmosome. The binding of the autoantibodies activates complement followed by mast cell degranulation, attraction and activation of neutrophils and eosinophils, degradation of BP180, and subsequent subepidermal vesicle formation. Some cases are drug-induced.	Autoantibodies targeted at the Ca^{2+}-dependent cadherin desmoglein 3 and, to a lesser degree, desmoglein 1. Binding of the antibodies disrupts the integrity of the desmosomes responsible for cell-cell adhesion with resultant vesicle formation.
Presentation	Pruritic, tense vesicles and bulla on an erythematous base. May have a prebullous phase of pruritic, urticarial plaques. Negative Nikolsky sign (induction of vesicle when mechanical pressure is applied to perilesional skin).	Flaccid vesicles and bullae that are fragile and become eroded and crusted. Nikolsky sign (induction of vesicle when mechanical pressure is applied to perilesional skin) present.
Histology	1. Subepidermal vesicle filled with serum, fibrin, and eosinophils *(Fig. 3.1.1)*. 2. Intact epidermis forming roof of vesicle *(Fig. 3.1.2)*. 3. Eosinophil-rich infiltrate within superficial dermis *(Figs. 3.1.2 and 3.1.3)*.	1. Suprabasal acantholysis with formation of an intraepidermal (suprabasal) vesicle *(Figs. 3.1.5 and 3.1.6)*. 2. Superficial epidermis forming roof of vesicle is intact. Basal keratinocytes retained along basement membrane zone resembling "tombstones" *(Fig. 3.1.7)*. 3. Sparse superficial perivascular inflammatory infiltrate that includes eosinophils *(Fig. 3.1.7)*.
Special studies	Direct immunofluorescence shows linear IgG and C3 deposition at the dermal-epidermal junction *(Fig. 3.1.4)*. Serology detecting serum antibodies to BP180 and BP230.	Direct immunofluorescence shows intercellular deposition of IgG and/or C3 *(Fig. 3.1.8)*. Serology detecting serum antibodies to desmoglein 3.
Treatment	Treatment depends upon extent of disease and comorbidities. For limited disease, potent topical steroids are used. Systemic corticosteroids are used for extensive disease. Immunosuppressive agents such as azathioprine, mycophenolate mofetil, methotrexate, and cyclophosphamide may be necessary for disease unresponsive to steroids or in patients with contraindications to systemic steroid use.	Systemic corticosteroids to rapidly slow disease progression. Other immunosuppressive agents, such as rituximab, azathioprine, mycophenolate mofetil, and cyclophosphamide, typically utilized for steroid-sparing effect.

	Bullous Pemphigoid	**Pemphigus Vulgaris**
Prognosis	Very good. Disease typically resolves within months but can occasionally persist for few years.	Severe disease with potential for significant morbidity and mortality. Without treatment, often fatal within 5 y of onset of disease. Morbidity from infection, fluid and electrolyte disturbances, and medication-related complications.

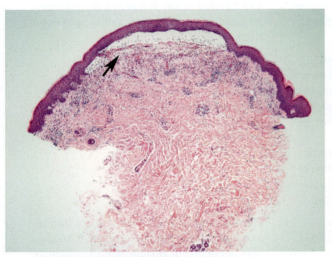

Figure 3.1.1 Bullous pemphigoid. Subepidermal fluid-filled vesicle (arrow) with a moderately dense superficial dermal inflammatory infiltrate.

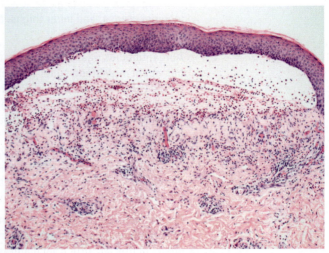

Figure 3.1.2 Bullous pemphigoid. The roof of the vesicle is formed by epidermis with mild degenerative changes. The subepidermal vesicle contains fibrin and is associated with an eosinophil-rich infiltrate.

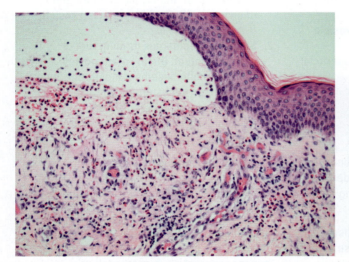

Figure 3.1.3 Bullous pemphigoid. Subepidermal vesicle containing fibrin, erythrocytes, and eosinophils.

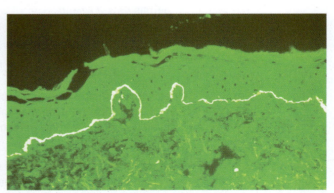

Figure 3.1.4 Bullous pemphigoid. Direct immunofluorescence for C3 showing linear fluorescence along the dermal-epidermal junction. IgG would show a similar pattern.

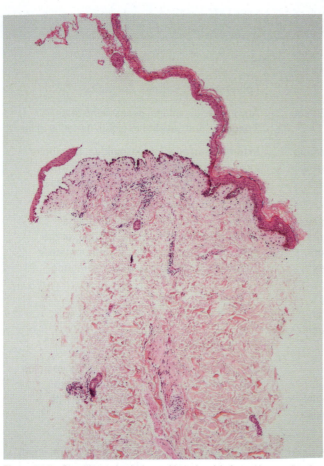

Figure 3.1.5 Pemphigus vulgaris. Intraepidermal vesicle formed by suprabasal acantholysis. The epidermis forming the roof of the vesicle is intact. There is a sparse superficial dermal infiltrate.

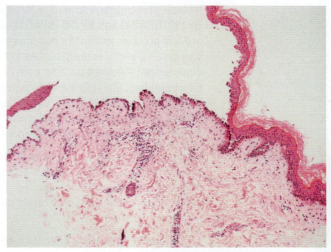

Figure 3.1.6 Pemphigus vulgaris. Suprabasal acantholysis forming an intraepidermal vesicle. No vesicle contents present due to disruption of vesicle by biopsy procedure.

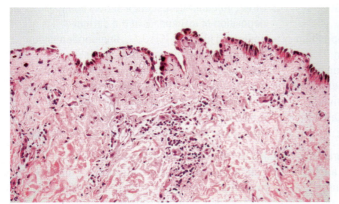

Figure 3.1.7 Pemphigus vulgaris. Intact basal epidermal layer at floor of vesicle with a "tombstone" appearance of basal keratinocytes.

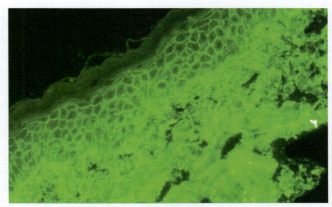

Figure 3.1.8 Pemphigus vulgaris. Intercellular deposition of IgG in a "chicken wire" pattern on direct immunofluorescence.

3.2 BULLOUS PEMPHIGOID VS EPIDERMOLYSIS BULLOSA ACQUISITA

	Bullous Pemphigoid	**Epidermolysis Bullosa Acquisita**
Age	Elderly adults, typically between ages of 60 and 80 y.	Any age, with bimodal peaks in the first 3 decades and seventh to eighth decades of life.
Location	Trunk and extremities, especially intertriginous areas of axilla, lower abdomen, inguinal crease, and inner thighs. Mucosal involvement rare.	Extensor surfaces of extremities. May have more widespread disease involving trunk, flexural regions, and intertriginous areas.
Etiology	Autoantibodies against antigens at the basement membrane zone. The antigens are BP180 (BPAG2) and BP230 (BPAG1), which are key proteins within the hemidesmosome. The binding of the autoantibodies activates complement followed by mast cell degranulation, attraction and activation of neutrophils and eosinophils, degradation of BP180, and subsequent subepidermal vesicle formation. Some cases are drug-induced.	Autoantibodies against collagen VII in the anchoring fibrils of the sublamina densa of skin and mucosa. Binding of the autoantibodies promotes an inflammatory pathway that leads to vesicle formation.
Presentation	Pruritic, tense vesicles and bulla on an erythematous base. May have a prebullous phase of pruritic, urticarial plaques. Typically, no associated scarring but may rarely have milia formation.	Skin fragility with formation of tense vesicles and bullae on a nonerythematous base. Vesicles rupture easily and resolve with scarring and milia formation.
Histology	1. Subepidermal vesicle filled with serum, fibrin, and eosinophils (Figs. 3.2.1 and 3.2.3). 2. Intact epidermis forming roof of vesicle (Fig. 3.2.2). 3. Eosinophil-rich infiltrate within superficial dermis (Figs. 3.2.2 and 3.2.3). 4. Mild dermal edema but no dermal fibrosis (Fig. 3.2.3).	1. Subepidermal vesicle formation with small amount of serum within vesicle (Figs. 3.2.5 and 3.2.6). 2. Sparse superficial perivascular mixed dermal inflammatory infiltrate (Fig. 3.2.7). 3. Mild superficial dermal fibrosis. May have milia formation (Figs. 3.2.5 and 3.2.6).
Special studies	Direct immunofluorescence shows linear deposition of IgG and C3 at the dermal-epidermal junction (Fig. 3.2.4). Immunodeposition has an n-serrated pattern. Salt-split-skin technique shows immunofluorescence on the epidermal (roof) side of the basement membrane zone. Immunohistochemistry for collagen IV (component of lamina densa) exhibits staining on the floor of the subepidermal vesicle.	Direct immunofluorescence shows linear deposition of IgG and C3 at the dermal-epidermal junction (Fig. 3.2.8). Immunodeposition has a u-serrated pattern. Salt-split-skin technique shows immunofluorescence on the dermal (floor) side of the basement membrane zone. Immunohistochemistry for collagen IV (component of lamina densa) demonstrates staining on the roof of the subepidermal vesicle.
Treatment	Depends upon extent of disease and comorbidities. For limited disease, potent topical steroids are used. Systemic corticosteroids are used for extensive disease. Immunosuppressive agents such as azathioprine, mycophenolate mofetil, methotrexate, and cyclophosphamide may be necessary for disease unresponsive to steroids or in patients with contraindications to systemic steroid use.	Initial treatment generally consists of colchicine and dapsone. Refractory disease may require systemic immunosuppressants, intravenous immunoglobulin, or rituximab.

(continued)

	Bullous Pemphigoid	**Epidermolysis Bullosa Acquisita**
Prognosis	Very good. Disease typically resolves within months but can occasionally persist for few years.	Chronic disease with a prolonged course. Disease is often recalcitrant to multiple therapies. Complications include joint contractures due to scarring.

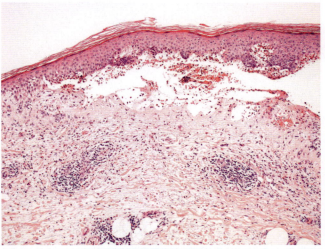

Figure 3.2.1 Bullous pemphigoid. Subepidermal vesicle formation with moderately dense superficial dermal infiltrate. Vesicle contains fibrin, erythrocytes, and inflammatory cells.

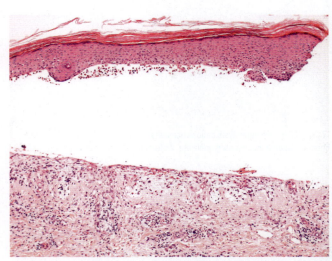

Figure 3.2.2 Bullous pemphigoid. Subepidermal vesicle with inflammatory cell contents. Overlying epidermis forming roof has degenerative changes.

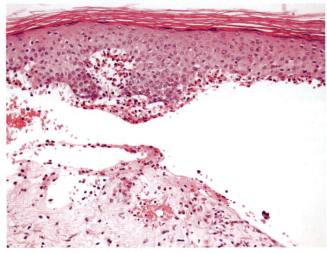

Figure 3.2.3 Bullous pemphigoid. Subepidermal vesicle containing fibrin, erythrocytes, and eosinophils.

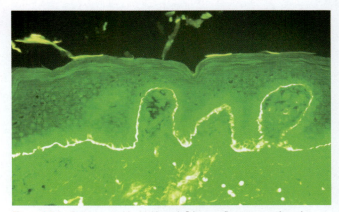

Figure 3.2.4 Bullous pemphigoid. Linear IgG immunofluorescence along the dermal-epidermal junction. Note that epidermolysis bullosa acquisita may show identical light microscopic and direct immunofluorescence findings necessitating salt-split-skin study or immunohistochemistry for collagen IV to differentiate.

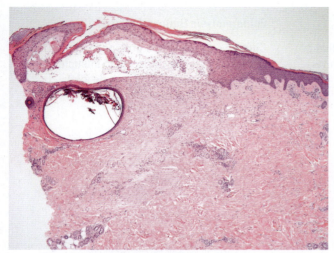

Figure 3.2.5 Epidermolysis bullosa acquisita. Subepidermal vesicle filled with fibrin and sparse inflammatory infiltrate. Note milia beneath the vesicle.

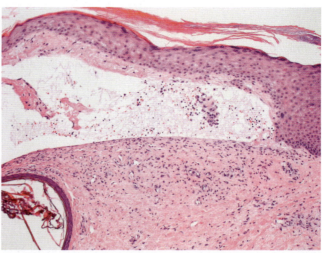

Figure 3.2.6 Epidermolysis bullosa acquisita. Subepidermal vesicle with fibrin, blood, and few inflammatory cells. The underlying dermis has reparative changes.

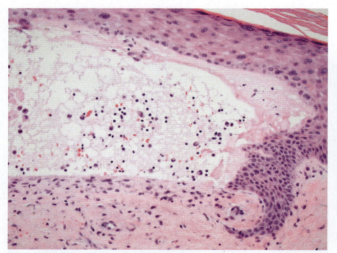

Figure 3.2.7 Epidermolysis bullosa acquisita. Subepidermal vesicle filled with fibrin, red blood cells, and scant lymphomononuclear inflammation.

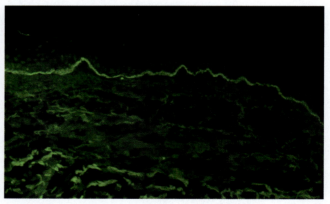

Figure 3.2.8 Epidermolysis bullosa acquisita. Direct immunofluorescence revealing linear IgG deposition along the dermal-epidermal junction. Note that a similar pattern is seen with bullous pemphigoid, and additional studies, such as salt-split-skin indirect immunofluorescence or immunohistochemistry for collagen IV, may be necessary to differentiate between the two entities.

3.3 LINEAR IgA DERMATOSIS VS BULLOUS PEMPHIGOID

	Linear IgA Dermatosis	**Bullous Pemphigoid**
Age	Adult form has bimodal age distribution with peaks in the third and sixth decades of life.	Elderly adults, typically between ages of 60 and 80 y.
Location	Trunk and extremities primarily but may involve face and genital regions. May have mucous membrane involvement.	Trunk and extremities, especially intertriginous areas of axilla, lower abdomen, inguinal crease, and inner thighs. Mucosal involvement rare.
Etiology	Circulating IgA autoantibodies directed against the 97- and 120-kDa portions of the bullous pemphigoid antigen 2 (BPAG2) in the lamina lucida of the basement membrane zone. Some cases involve autoantibodies against type VII collagen, laminin-332, or laminin gamma 1. The adult form may be idiopathic but is most frequently drug-induced with vancomycin being the most commonly associated drug.	Autoantibodies against antigens at the basement membrane zone. The antigens are BP180 (BPAG2) and BP230 (BPAG1), which are key proteins within the hemidesmosome. The binding of the autoantibodies activates complement followed by mast cell degranulation, attraction and activation of neutrophils and eosinophils, degradation of BP180, and subsequent subepidermal vesicle formation. Some cases are drug-induced, but vancomycin not a common culprit.
Presentation	Abrupt onset of tense vesicles and bullae on nonerythematous or erythematous base. Some lesions may consist of annular, erythematous plaques with peripheral vesicles.	Pruritic, tense vesicles and bulla on an erythematous base. May have a prebullous phase of pruritic, urticarial plaques.
Histology	1. Subepidermal vesicle formation (Fig. 3.3.1). 2. Vesicle contains neutrophils and fibrin (Figs. 3.3.2 and 3.3.3). 3. Dermal infiltrate predominated by neutrophils with few eosinophils (Figs. 3.3.2 and 3.3.3).	1. Subepidermal vesicle filled with serum, fibrin, and eosinophils (Fig. 3.3.5). 2. Intact epidermis forming roof of vesicle (Fig. 3.3.6). 3. Eosinophil-rich infiltrate within superficial dermis (Figs. 3.3.6 and 3.3.7). 4. Dermal edema (Fig. 3.3.6).
Special studies	Direct immunofluorescence shows linear deposition of IgA along the dermal-epidermal junction (Fig. 3.3.4).	Direct immunofluorescence shows linear IgG and C3 deposition at the dermal-epidermal junction (Fig. 3.3.8). Serology detecting serum antibodies to BP180 and BP230.
Treatment	Dapsone is first-line therapy. Colchicine and sulfonamides are also effective. Systemic corticosteroids or other immunosuppressants may be necessary for severe or refractory disease.	Depends upon extent of disease and comorbidities. For limited disease, potent topical steroids are used. Systemic corticosteroids are used for extensive disease. Immunosuppressive agents such as azathioprine, mycophenolate mofetil, methotrexate, and cyclophosphamide may be necessary for disease unresponsive to steroids or in patients with contraindications to systemic steroid use.

	Linear IgA Dermatosis	**Bullous Pemphigoid**
Prognosis	Idiopathic cases have a variable course but generally spontaneously resolve after months to years. Drug-induced cases generally resolve within a few weeks of cessation of the offending agent.	Very good. Disease typically resolves within months but can occasionally persist for few years.

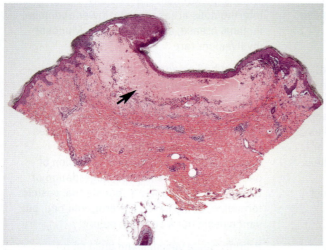

Figure 3.3.1 Linear IgA dermatosis. Fluid-filled subepidermal vesicle formation (arrow) associated with a moderately dense inflammatory infiltrate.

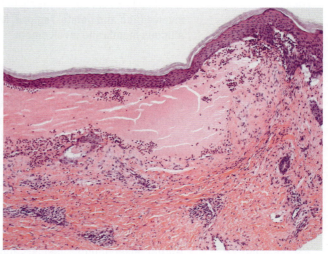

Figure 3.3.2 Linear IgA dermatosis. Subepidermal vesicle filled with serum and neutrophil-rich inflammation.

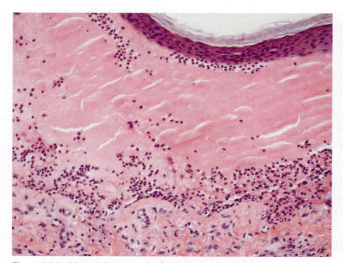

Figure 3.3.3 Linear IgA dermatosis. Subepidermal vesicle filled with serum and numerous neutrophils.

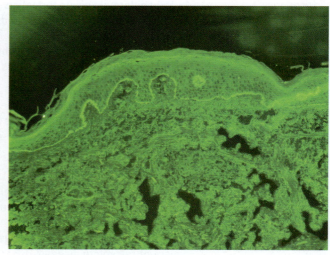

Figure 3.3.4 Linear IgA dermatosis. Direct immunofluorescence demonstrating linear staining along the dermal-epidermal junction with IgA immunoreactant.

3.3 Linear IgA Dermatosis vs Bullous Pemphigoid

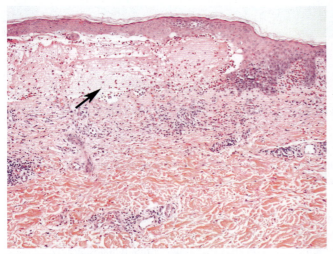

Figure 3.3.5 Bullous pemphigoid. Subepidermal vesicle (arrow) associated with a moderately dense eosinophil-rich inflammatory infiltrate.

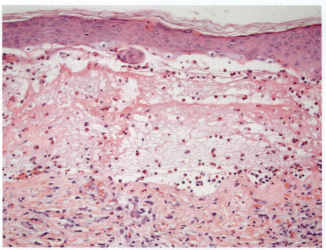

Figure 3.3.6 Bullous pemphigoid. Infiltrate associated with the subepidermal vesicle is predominated by eosinophils, rather than neutrophils, in the classic presentation of bullous pemphigoid.

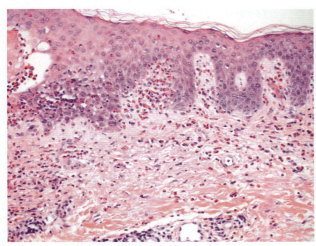

Figure 3.3.7 Bullous pemphigoid. Eosinophilic spongiosis adjacent to the subepidermal vesicle with a few eosinophils tagging along the basal zone.

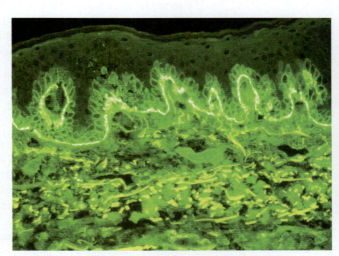

Figure 3.3.8 Bullous pemphigoid. Linear IgG along the dermal-epidermal junction. There is a similar fluorescence pattern with C3.

3.4 BULLOUS PEMPHIGOID VS DERMATITIS HERPETIFORMIS

	Bullous Pemphigoid	**Dermatitis Herpetiformis**
Age	Elderly adults, typically between ages of 60 and 80 y.	Any age but typically presents in adults in the fourth and fifth decades of life.
Location	Trunk and extremities, especially intertriginous areas of axilla, lower abdomen, inguinal crease, and inner thighs. Mucosal involvement rare.	Extensor surfaces of elbows, knees, scalp, and buttocks. Involvement of mucosal surfaces is rare.
Etiology	Autoantibodies against antigens at the basement membrane zone. The antigens are BP180 (BPAG2) and BP230 (BPAG1), which are key proteins within the hemidesmosome. The binding of the autoantibodies activates complement followed by mast cell degranulation, attraction and activation of neutrophils and eosinophils, degradation of BP180, and subsequent subepidermal vesicle formation. Some cases are drug-induced.	Autoimmune disease with underlying genetic predisposition in individuals with HLA DQ2 and HLA DQ8 haplotypes. It is caused by development of IgA autoantibodies against transglutaminases. The immune complexes are deposited in the papillary dermis and initiate neutrophil chemotaxis and proteolytic degradation of the lamina lucida with resultant blister formation.
Presentation	Pruritic, tense vesicles and bulla on an erythematous base. May have a prebullous phase of pruritic, urticarial plaques.	Grouped, intensely pruritic papules and vesicles with crusted erosions due to scratching. Majority of patients have associated gluten-sensitive enteropathy.
Histology	1. Subepidermal vesicle filled with serum, fibrin, and eosinophils (*Figs. 3.4.1* and *3.4.2*). 2. Adjacent epidermis may have variable spongiosis with eosinophilic exocytosis. 3. Dermal papillae adjacent to vesicle are preserved (*Fig. 3.4.2*). 4. Eosinophil-rich infiltrate within superficial dermis; neutrophils uncommon (*Figs. 3.4.2* and *3.4.3*).	1. Collections of neutrophils and fibrin at the top of flattened dermal papillae (*Figs. 3.4.5* and *3.4.6*). 2. Epidermal rete ridges preserved with no appreciable spongiosis (*Fig. 3.4.6*). 3. Papillary dermal edema with subepidermal vesicle formation (*Fig. 3.4.7*). 4. Superficial perivascular infiltrate of lymphocytes, neutrophils, and a small number of eosinophils (*Figs. 3.4.6* and *3.4.7*).
Special studies	Direct immunofluorescence shows linear IgG and C3 deposition at the dermal-epidermal junction (*Fig. 3.4.4*). Serology detecting serum antibodies to BP180 and BP230.	Direct immunofluorescence shows granular deposition of IgA within the dermal papillae (*Fig. 3.4.8*). Serology for anti-endomysial, anti–epidermal transglutaminase, and anti–tissue transglutaminase IgA antibodies.
Treatment	Depends upon extent of disease and comorbidities. For limited disease, potent topical steroids are used. Systemic corticosteroids are used for extensive disease. Immunosuppressive agents such as azathioprine, mycophenolate mofetil, methotrexate, and cyclophosphamide may be necessary for disease unresponsive to steroids or in patients with contraindications to systemic steroid use.	Dapsone and life-long adherence to gluten-free diet.

(continued)

3.4 Bullous Pemphigoid vs Dermatitis Herpetiformis

	Bullous Pemphigoid	**Dermatitis Herpetiformis**
Prognosis	Very good. Disease typically resolves within months but can occasionally persist for few years.	Life-long condition with remittances and exacerbations. Strongly associated with gluten-sensitive enteropathy with a concomitant risk of lymphoma of the small bowel.

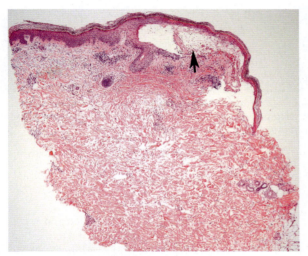

Figure 3.4.1 Bullous pemphigoid. Subepidermal vesicle formation (arrow) with detachment of the epidermis from the dermis. There is a moderately dense inflammatory infiltrate in the superficial dermis.

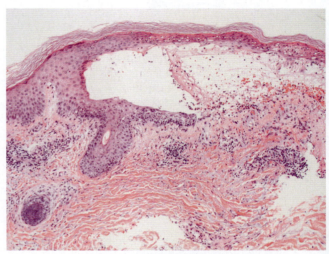

Figure 3.4.2 Bullous pemphigoid. Subepidermal vesicle containing fibrin, erythrocytes, and inflammatory cells predominated by eosinophils.

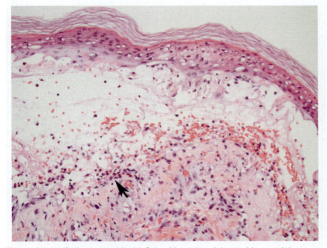

Figure 3.4.3 Bullous pemphigoid. Subepidermal vesicle notably containing eosinophils (arrow).

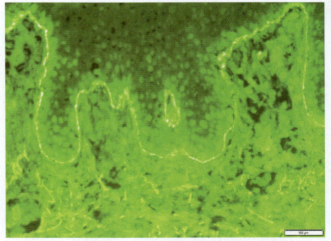

Figure 3.4.4 Bullous pemphigoid. Linear IgG along the dermal-epidermal junction on direct immunofluorescence. C3 conjugate has similar pattern. Note that there is no IgA deposition.

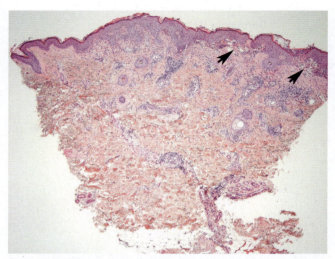

Figure 3.4.5 Dermatitis herpetiformis. Superficial dermal inflammatory infiltrate with subepidermal vesicle formation (arrows).

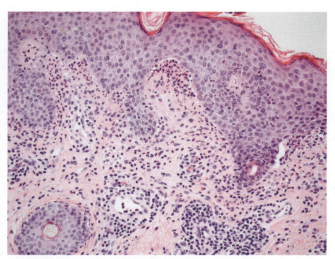

Figure 3.4.6 Dermatitis herpetiformis. Early lesions show papillary dermal microabscesses with collections of neutrophils associated with a small amount of fibrin and neutrophilic nuclear debris at the tips of papillae.

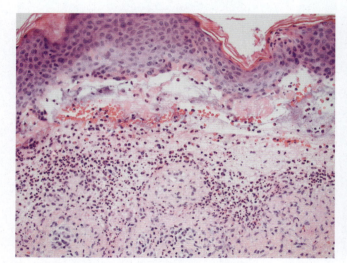

Figure 3.4.7 Dermatitis herpetiformis. Established lesions have subepidermal vesicle formation. The vesicle is filled with fibrin, erythrocytes, and neutrophils with only rare eosinophils.

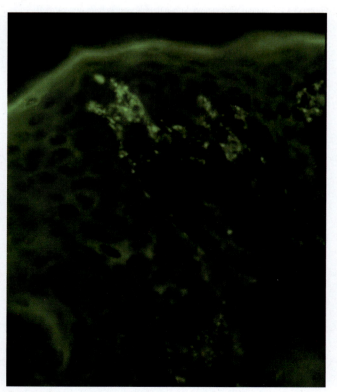

Figure 3.4.8 Dermatitis herpetiformis. Immune complexes deposit in dermal papillae resulting in a granular pattern on direct immunofluorescence with IgA immunoreactant.

3.5 PEMPHIGOID (HERPES) GESTATIONIS VS POLYMORPHIC ERUPTION OF PREGNANCY

	Pemphigoid (Herpes) Gestationis	**Polymorphic Eruption of Pregnancy**
Age	Women of child-bearing years.	Women of childbearing age; predominately primigravidas.
Location	Periumbilical region initially, then extends to remainder of the abdomen and extremities. Face and mucous membranes generally spared.	Abdomen, particularly within striae, sparing periumbilical area. Spreads to trunk and extremities; spares face, mucosa, and acral skin.
Etiology	Autoimmune vesiculobullous process with autoantibodies directed toward the basement membrane autoantigen BP180 (BPAG2, collagen XVII).	Unknown. Stretching of the skin of the gravid abdomen causing connective tissue damage that reveals antigens activating an inflammatory reaction is postulated. Other hypotheses include hormonal flux and fetal antigens as having a role.
Presentation	Erythematous urticarial papules and plaques that progress to vesicles and tense bullae. Lesions accompanied by intense pruritus that is often the first symptom. Majority of cases present in the third trimester, between the 28th and 32nd w of gestation.	Intensely pruritic erythematous, edematous wheals, papules, and plaques. May have small vesicles or scale. Develops late in pregnancy, usually in the last week of the third trimester and, sometimes, postpartum.
Histology	1. Subepidermal vesicle formation *(Figs. 3.5.1-3.5.3)*. 2. Vesicle contains serum, fibrin, and eosinophils *(Figs. 3.5.2 and 3.5.3)*. 3. Superficial dermal infiltrate with eosinophils and lymphocytes *(Fig. 3.5.3)*.	1. Epidermis may be normal or have mild spongiosis with exocytosis of a small number of lymphocytes *(Figs. 3.5.5, 3.5.6, and 3.5.8)*. 2. Perivascular and interstitial infiltrate of eosinophils, lymphocytes, and occasional neutrophils *(Figs. 3.5.6 and 3.5.7)*. 3. Dermal edema but no subepidermal vesicle formation *(Figs. 3.5.5 and 3.5.7)*.
Special studies	Direct immunofluorescence demonstrates linear deposition of IgG and C3 along the dermal-epidermal junction *(Fig. 3.5.4)*. Enzyme-linked immunosorbent assay (ELISA)-BP180 for diagnosis and monitoring of disease activity.	Negative direct immunofluorescence.
Treatment	Topical steroids and antihistamines in early or mild forms of disease. Systemic corticosteroids or other immunosuppressant agents in severe or recalcitrant cases.	Symptomatic relief of pruritus with topical corticosteroids and antihistamines.
Prognosis	Generally responsive to therapy and typically resolves completely within 2 m of delivery. Recurrence may be seen in subsequent pregnancies. May have effects on fetus include prematurity, low birth weight, and transitory skin lesions.	Self-limiting with no maternal or fetal risk. Eruption typically resolves spontaneously within 4 w or at the time of delivery. Generally does not recur with subsequent pregnancies.

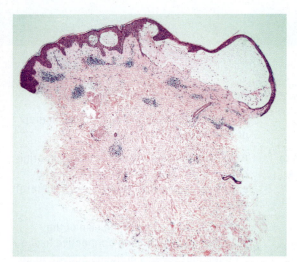

Figure 3.5.1 Pemphigoid (herpes) gestationis. Subepidermal vesicle formation with moderately dense superficial dermal inflammatory infiltrate.

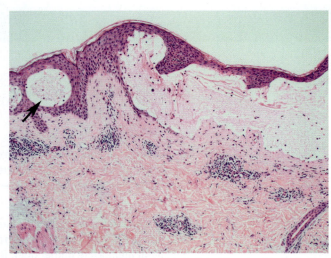

Figure 3.5.2 Pemphigoid (herpes) gestationis. Subepidermal vesicle filled with fibrin and inflammatory cells including eosinophils. Note that there is eosinophilic spongiosis adjacent to the vesicle (arrow).

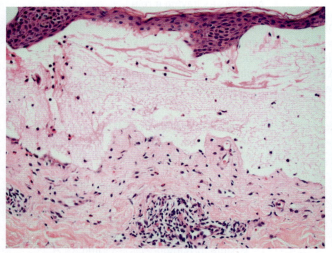

Figure 3.5.3 Pemphigoid (herpes) gestationis. Subepidermal vesicle containing fibrin, eosinophils, and lymphocytes.

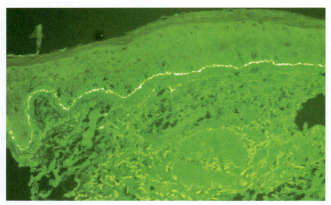

Figure 3.5.4 Pemphigoid (herpes) gestationis. Direct immunofluorescence has pattern identical to classic bullous pemphigoid with linear deposition of C3 along the dermal-epidermal junction. IgG has a similar pattern of fluorescence. This is a distinguishing feature from polymorphic eruption of pregnancy, which would have negative immunofluorescence.

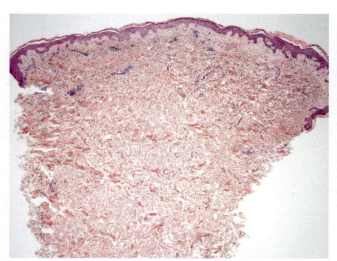

Figure 3.5.5 Polymorphic eruption of pregnancy. Superficial to mid dermal perivascular inflammatory infiltrate with mild papillary dermal edema. Note that there is no subepidermal vesicle formation.

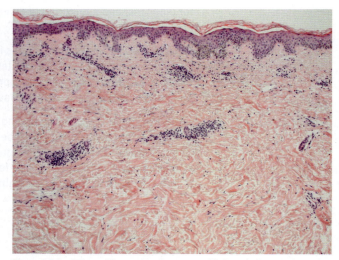

Figure 3.5.6 Polymorphic eruption of pregnancy. Moderately dense perivascular and interstitial infiltrate with minimal epidermal change.

3.5 Pemphigoid (Herpes) Gestationis vs Polymorphic Eruption of Pregnancy

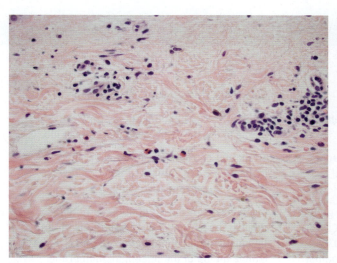

Figure 3.5.7 Polymorphic eruption of pregnancy. Dermal infiltrate is composed primarily of lymphocytes but includes a small number of eosinophils.

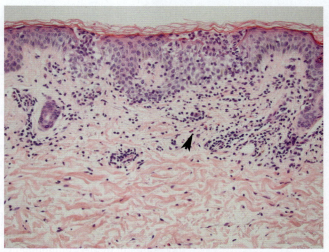

Figure 3.5.8 Polymorphic eruption of pregnancy. Some cases have foci of epidermal spongiosis with lymphocytic exocytosis. Notably, no subepidermal vesiculation despite the density of the inflammatory infiltrate that includes eosinophils (arrow).

3.6 DERMATITIS HERPETIFORMIS VS LINEAR IgA DERMATOSIS

	Dermatitis Herpetiformis	**Linear IgA Dermatosis**
Age	Any age, but typically presents in adults in the fourth and fifth decades of life.	Adult form has bimodal age distribution with peaks in the third and sixth decades of life.
Location	Extensor surfaces of elbows, knees, scalp, and buttocks. Involvement of mucosal surfaces is rare.	Trunk and extremities primarily but may involve face and genital regions. May have mucous membrane involvement.
Etiology	Autoimmune disease with underlying genetic predisposition in individuals with HLA DQ2 and HLA DQ8 haplotypes. It is caused by development of IgA autoantibodies against transglutaminases. The immune complexes are deposited in the papillary dermis and initiate neutrophil chemotaxis and proteolytic degradation of the lamina lucida with resultant blister formation.	Circulating IgA autoantibodies directed against the 97- and 120-kDa portions of the bullous pemphigoid antigen 2 (BPAG2) in the lamina lucida of the basement membrane zone. Some cases involve autoantibodies against type VII collagen, laminin-332, or laminin gamma 1. The adult form may be idiopathic but is most frequently drug-induced with vancomycin being the most commonly associated drug.
Presentation	Grouped, intensely pruritic papules and vesicles with crusted erosions due to scratching. Majority of patients have associated gluten-sensitive enteropathy.	Abrupt onset of tense vesicles and bullae on nonerythematous or erythematous base. Some lesions may consist of annular, erythematous plaques with peripheral vesicles.
Histology	1. Collections of neutrophils and fibrin at the top of slightly flattened dermal papillae (Figs. 3.6.2 and 3.6.3). Often karyorrhexis in dermis. 2. Epidermal rete ridges preserved with minimal spongiosis (Figs. 3.6.2 and 3.6.3). 3. Papillary dermal edema with subepidermal vesicle formation (Fig. 3.6.1). 4. Superficial perivascular infiltrate of lymphocytes, neutrophils, and a small number of eosinophils (Figs. 3.6.2 and 3.6.3).	1. Subepidermal vesicle formation with flattened epidermal rete ridges (Figs. 3.6.5 and 3.6.6). 2. Vesicle contains neutrophils and fibrin (Fig. 3.6.6). 3. Neutrophils align along the dermal-epidermal junction, rather than forming microabscesses (Fig. 3.6.7). 4. Dermal infiltrate predominated by neutrophils with few eosinophils (Figs. 3.6.6 and 3.6.7).
Special studies	Direct immunofluorescence shows granular deposition of IgA within the dermal papillae (Fig. 3.6.4). Serology for anti-endomysial, anti–epidermal transglutaminase, and anti–tissue transglutaminase IgA antibodies.	Direct immunofluorescence shows homogeneous linear, rather than granular, deposition of IgA along the dermal-epidermal junction (Fig. 3.6.8).
Treatment	Dapsone and life-long adherence to gluten-free diet.	Dapsone is first-line therapy. Colchicine and sulfonamides are also effective. Systemic corticosteroids or other immunosuppressants may be necessary for severe or refractory disease.
Prognosis	Life-long condition with remittances and exacerbations. Strongly associated with gluten-sensitive enteropathy with a concomitant risk of lymphoma of the small bowel.	Idiopathic cases have a variable course but generally spontaneously resolve after months to years. Drug-induced cases generally resolve within a few weeks of cessation of the offending agent.

3.6 Dermatitis Herpetiformis vs Linear IgA Dermatosis

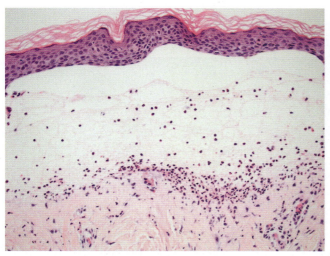

Figure 3.6.1 Dermatitis herpetiformis. Subepidermal vesicle filled with fibrin and neutrophils. Note that identical features may be seen in linear IgA dermatosis.

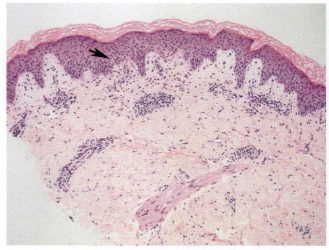

Figure 3.6.2 Dermatitis herpetiformis. Examination of the dermal-epidermal junction adjacent to the vesicle is helpful in making the distinction from linear IgA dermatosis. In dermatitis herpetiformis, the neutrophils form discrete aggregates (microabscesses) within the dermal papillae (arrow).

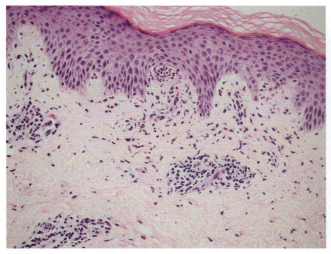

Figure 3.6.3 Dermatitis herpetiformis. Discrete papillary dermal microabscess associated with small amount of fibrin and nuclear debris.

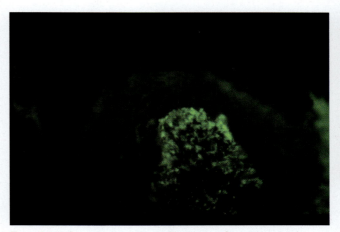

Figure 3.6.4 Dermatitis herpetiformis. Direct immunofluorescence reveals granular deposition of IgA within the dermal papillae due to immune complex deposition.

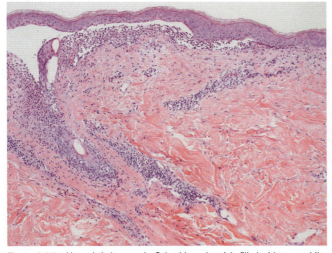

Figure 3.6.5 Linear IgA dermatosis. Subepidermal vesicle filled with neutrophils. Note that identical features may be seen in dermatitis herpetiformis.

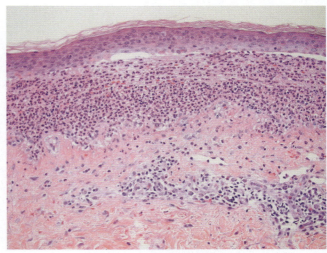

Figure 3.6.6 Linear IgA dermatosis. Subepidermal vesicle filled with numerous neutrophils and fibrin.

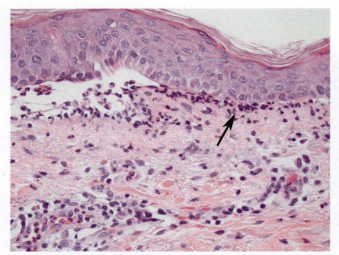

Figure 3.6.7 Linear IgA dermatosis. Adjacent to the vesicle, neutrophils are aligned along the dermal-epidermal junction (arrow) rather than forming discrete microabscesses.

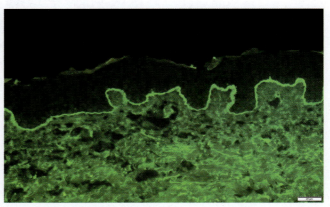

Figure 3.6.8 Linear IgA dermatosis. Continuous linear IgA deposition along the dermal-epidermal junction.

3.7 PORPHYRIA CUTANEA TARDA VS BULLOUS PEMPHIGOID

	Porphyria Cutanea Tarda	**Bullous Pemphigoid**
Age	Adults, typically middle age.	Elderly adults, typically between ages of 60 and 80 y.
Location	Sun-exposed areas of skin including face, ears, neck, dorsum of hands, forearms, and feet.	Trunk and extremities, especially intertriginous areas of axilla, lower abdomen, inguinal crease, and inner thighs. Mucosal involvement rare.
Etiology	Deficiency in uroporphyrinogen decarboxylase enzyme in the heme biosynthesis pathway. This results in excess porphyrins, including uroporphyrinogen, that deposit in the skin. Interaction with light causes excitation of porphyrins and release of energy that creates singlet-excited oxygen that leads to tissue damage.	Autoantibodies against antigens at the basement membrane zone. The antigens are BP180 (BPAG2) and BP230 (BPAG1), which are key proteins within the hemidesmosome. The binding of the autoantibodies activates complement followed by mast cell degranulation, attraction and activation of neutrophils and eosinophils, degradation of BP180, and subsequent subepidermal vesicle formation. Some cases are drug-induced.
Presentation	Skin fragility and formation of tense vesicles and bullae containing serous or bloody fluid. Vesicles are accompanied by crusted erosions and heal with scars. Mottled pigmentation and milia formation are commonly associated with the scars.	Pruritic, tense vesicles and bulla on an erythematous base. May have a prebullous phase of pruritic, urticarial plaques.
Histology	1. Subepidermal vesicle formation with small amount of blood or serum within the vesicle cavity *(Figs. 3.7.1* and *3.7.2)*. 2. Vesicle is associated with minimal inflammation ("pauci-inflammatory") *(Figs. 3.7.1* and *3.7.2)*. 3. Epidermis forming roof of vesicle has degenerative change with linear, eosinophilic, globules ("caterpillar bodies") along the base *(Fig. 3.7.1)*. 4. Preservation of dermal papillae ("festooning") *(Figs. 3.7.2* and *3.7.3)*. 5. Hyalinized thickening of the walls of superficial dermal vessels highlighted with PAS stain *(Fig. 3.7.4)*.	1. Subepidermal vesicle filled with serum, fibrin, and eosinophils *(Fig. 3.7.6)*. 2. Intact epidermis forming roof of vesicle; papillae are flattened *(Fig. 3.7.7)*. 3. Eosinophil-rich infiltrate within superficial dermis *(Figs. 3.7.7* and *3.7.8)*.
Special studies	PAS stain demonstrating thickening of the walls of blood vessels in superficial dermis and, in some cases, stacked globules ("caterpillar bodies") along the roof of the vesicle. Direct immunofluorescence shows nonspecific deposition of immunoglobulins in and around superficial dermal vessels *(Fig. 3.7.5)*. Confirmation with measurement of urine and/or plasma total porphyrins with fractionation if elevated.	Direct immunofluorescence shows linear IgG and C3 deposition at the dermal-epidermal junction *(Fig. 3.7.9)*. Serology detecting serum antibodies to BP180 and BP230.

	Porphyria Cutanea Tarda	**Bullous Pemphigoid**
Treatment	Avoidance of sun and other triggering factors. Therapies include phlebotomy, hydroxychloroquine, and iron chelation.	Depends upon extent of disease and comorbidities. For limited disease, potent topical steroids are used. Systemic corticosteroids are used for extensive disease. Immunosuppressive agents such as azathioprine, mycophenolate mofetil, methotrexate, and cyclophosphamide may be necessary for disease unresponsive to steroids or in patients with contraindications to systemic steroid use.
Prognosis	Treatable condition with a normal life expectancy. Relapses may occur especially if triggering factors are not removed.	Very good. Disease typically resolves within months but can occasionally persist for few years.

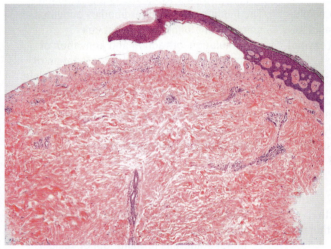

Figure 3.7.1 Porphyria cutanea tarda. Subepidermal vesicle with no appreciable inflammation. Note preservation of dermal papillae.

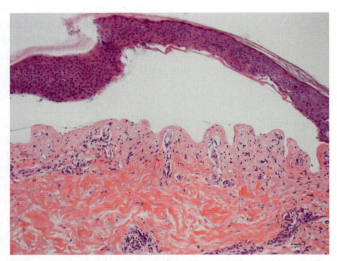

Figure 3.7.2 Porphyria cutanea tarda. Subepidermal vesicle containing a small amount of fibrin and red blood cells. Note that there is minimal inflammation associated with the vesicle.

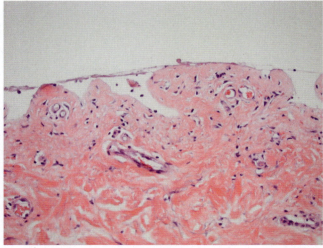

Figure 3.7.3 Porphyria cutanea tarda. Floor of subepidermal vesicle with preservation of the dermal papillae in a "festooning" fashion. Blood vessels within papillae have thickened walls.

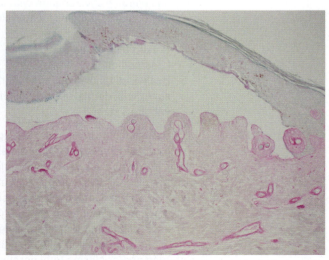

Figure 3.7.4 Porphyria cutanea tarda. PAS stain demonstrating thickening of the walls of the vessels in the dermal papillae.

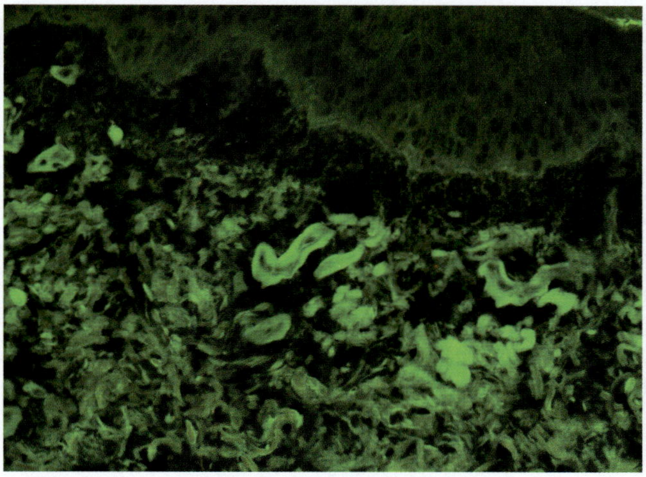

3.7 Porphyria Cutanea Tarda vs Bullous Pemphigoid

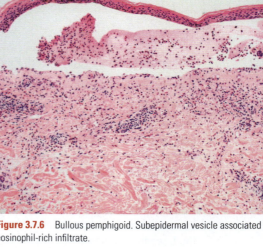

Figure 3.7.5 Porphyria cutanea tarda. Direct immunofluorescence showing vascular fluorescence with IgM representing nonspecific trapping of immunoglobulin due to abnormal vessel walls.

Figure 3.7.6 Bullous pemphigoid. Subepidermal vesicle associated with dense eosinophil-rich infiltrate.

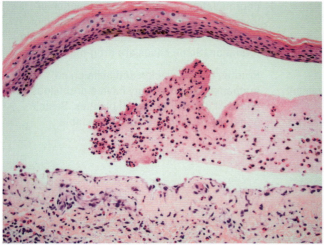

Figure 3.7.7 Bullous pemphigoid. Subepidermal vesicle filled with inflammation predominated by eosinophils. Note that floor of vesicle has flattened papillae.

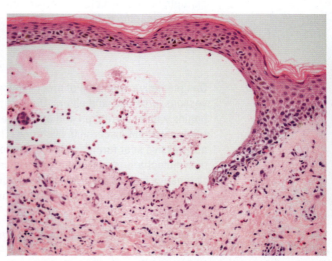

Figure 3.7.8 Bullous pemphigoid. Edge of subepidermal vesicle with eosinophilic infiltrate. Papillae are flattened and the vessels do not appear thickened.

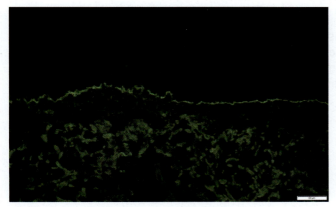

Figure 3.7.9 Bullous pemphigoid. Direct immunofluorescence revealing linear deposition of C3 along the dermal-epidermal junction. A similar pattern is seen with IgG.

3.8 MUCOUS MEMBRANE (CICATRICIAL) PEMPHIGOID VS BULLOUS PEMPHIGOID

	Mucous Membrane (Cicatricial) Pemphigoid	**Bullous Pemphigoid**
Age	Older adults with onset in the sixth to seventh decades of life.	Elderly adults, typically between ages of 60 and 80 y.
Location	May involve the skin only, mucous membranes only, or both skin and mucous membranes. Oral cavity and ocular mucosa are the most common locations. Skin lesions may be generalized or localized to head and neck region.	Trunk and extremities, especially intertriginous areas of axilla, lower abdomen, inguinal crease, and inner thighs. Mucosal involvement rare.
Etiology	Autoimmune disease with autoantibodies to components of the hemidesmosome region of the basement membrane zone including 180 kD bullous pemphigoid antigen (BP180), laminin 332, and beta-4-integrin. Binding of the antibodies disrupts normal structure of epidermal-dermal interface leading to blister formation.	Autoantibodies against antigens at the basement membrane zone. The antigens are BP180 (BPAG2) and BP230 (BPAG1), which are key proteins within the hemidesmosome. The binding of the autoantibodies activates complement followed by mast cell degranulation, attraction and activation of neutrophils and eosinophils, degradation of BP180, and subsequent subepidermal vesicle formation. Some cases are drug-induced.
Presentation	Desquamative mucositis of oral cavity with vesicles, erosions, and ulcers. Ocular involvement begins with eye irritation and excessive tearing without discernible blistering. There is progressive scar formation leading to formation of symblepharons, entropion, and trichiasis. Cutaneous lesions present with tense blisters on erythematous base with or without atrophy and scarring.	Pruritic, tense vesicles and bulla on an erythematous base. May have a prebullous phase of pruritic, urticarial plaques. Vesicle generally resolve without appreciable scarring.
Histology	1. Subepidermal vesicle formation *(Figs. 3.8.1 and 3.8.2)*. 2. Mixed inflammatory infiltrate in superficial dermis composed of lymphocytes, neutrophils, and eosinophils *(Figs. 3.8.1 and 3.8.2)*. 3. Fibrosis and milia formation in superficial dermis *(Fig. 3.8.3)*.	1. Subepidermal vesicle filled with serum, fibrin, and eosinophils *(Figs. 3.8.5 and 3.8.6)*. 2. Intact epidermis forming roof of vesicle *(Fig. 3.8.6)*. 3. Eosinophil-rich infiltrate within superficial dermis *(Fig. 3.8.7)*.
Special studies	Direct immunofluorescence demonstrates linear deposition of IgG, C3, and/or IgA along the dermal-epidermal junction *(Fig. 3.8.4)*. Indirect immunofluorescence may be performed but is generally of low sensitivity.	Direct immunofluorescence shows linear IgG and C3 deposition at the dermal-epidermal junction *(Fig. 3.8.8)*. Serology detecting serum antibodies to BP180 and BP230.

(continued)

	Mucous Membrane (Cicatricial) Pemphigoid	**Bullous Pemphigoid**
Treatment	Topical corticosteroids for mild or moderate disease. Systemic corticosteroids alone or combined with other immunosuppressant agents for severe or rapidly progressive disease.	Depends upon extent of disease and comorbidities. For limited disease, potent topical steroids are used. Systemic corticosteroids are used for extensive disease. Immunosuppressive agents such as azathioprine, mycophenolate mofetil, methotrexate, and cyclophosphamide may be necessary for disease unresponsive to steroids or in patients with contraindications to systemic steroid use.
Prognosis	Chronic disease that may have aggressive course. Complications due to scarring, particularly of the mucous membranes, may be debilitating and lead to blindness and tooth loss. Remission of disease is possible, but long-term treatment is often necessary to avoid relapses. Mucous membrane pemphigoid with antibodies against laminin 332 has been associated with increased risk for internal malignancy.	Very good. Disease typically resolves within months but can occasionally persist for few years.

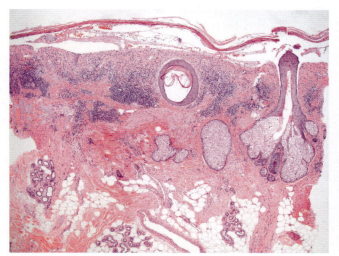

Figure 3.8.1 Mucous membrane (cicatricial) pemphigoid. Cutaneous subepidermal fluid-filled vesicle with dense mixed inflammation and milia formation.

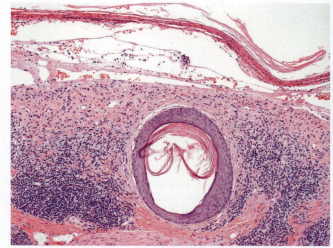

Figure 3.8.2 Mucous membrane (cicatricial) pemphigoid. Subepidermal vesicle containing fibrin, blood, and inflammatory cells. The dermis has dense mixed inflammation and fibrosis with milia formation.

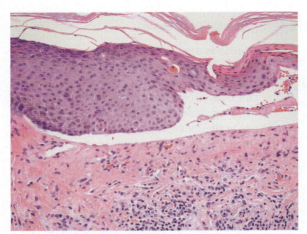

Figure 3.8.3 Mucous membrane (cicatricial) pemphigoid. Subepidermal vesicle with lymphomononuclear inflammation and fibrosis.

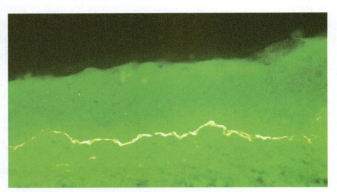

Figure 3.8.4 Mucous membrane (cicatricial) pemphigoid. Linear immunofluorescence with IgG immunoreactant. May also have similar immunofluorescence with IgA and C3 immunoreactants.

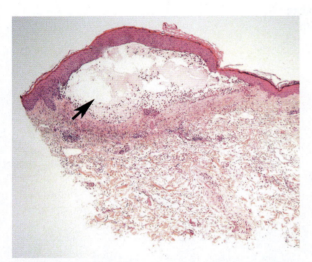

Figure 3.8.5 Bullous pemphigoid. Subepidermal vesicle filled with serum and eosinophil-rich inflammation (arrow).

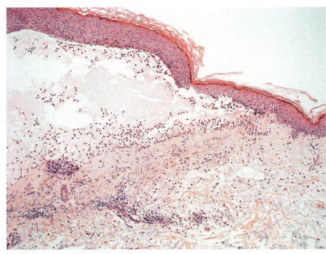

Figure 3.8.6 Bullous pemphigoid. Subepidermal vesicle with numerous eosinophils. Note that there is no appreciable fibrosis within the dermis.

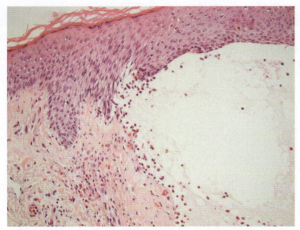

Figure 3.8.7 Bullous pemphigoid. Edge of subepidermal vesicle with eosinophilic infiltrate within the vesicle and the underlying dermis.

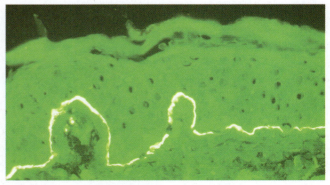

Figure 3.8.8 Bullous pemphigoid. Linear deposition of C3 along the dermal-epidermal junction. Similar pattern with IgG usually present but no appreciable deposition of IgA.

3.9 PORPHYRIA CUTANEA TARDA VS EPIDERMOLYSIS BULLOSA ACQUISITA

	Porphyria Cutanea Tarda	**Epidermolysis Bullosa Acquisita**
Age	Adults, typically middle age.	Any age, with bimodal peaks in the first 3 decades and seventh to eighth decades of life.
Location	Sun-exposed areas of skin including face, ears, neck, dorsum of hands, forearms, and feet.	Extensor surfaces of extremities. May have more widespread disease involving trunk, flexural regions, and intertriginous areas.
Etiology	Deficiency in uroporphyrinogen decarboxylase enzyme in the heme biosynthesis pathway. This results in excess porphyrins, including uroporphyrinogen, that deposit in the skin. Interaction with light causes excitation of porphyrins and release of energy that creates singlet-excited oxygen that leads to tissue damage.	Autoantibodies against collagen VII in the anchoring fibrils in the sublamina densa of skin and mucosa. Binding of the autoantibodies promotes an inflammatory pathway that leads to vesicle formation.
Presentation	Skin fragility and formation of tense vesicles and bullae containing serous or bloody fluid. Vesicles are accompanied by crusted erosions and heal with scars. Mottled pigmentation and milia formation are commonly associated with the scars.	Skin fragility with formation of tense vesicles and bullae on a nonerythematous base. Vesicles rupture easily and resolve with scarring and milia formation.
Histology	1. Subepidermal vesicle formation with small amount of blood or serum within the vesicle cavity *(Figs. 3.9.1 and 3.9.2)*. 2. Vesicle is associated with minimal inflammation ("pauci-inflammatory") *(Figs. 3.9.1 and 3.9.2)*. 3. Epidermal forming roof of vesicle has degenerative change with linear, eosinophilic, globules ("caterpillar bodies") along the base *(Fig. 3.9.3)*. 4. Preservation of dermal papillae ("festooning") *(Fig. 3.9.3)*. 5. Hyalinized thickening of the walls of superficial dermal vessels *(Fig. 3.9.3)*.	1. Subepidermal vesicle formation with small amount of serum within vesicle *(Figs. 3.9.5 and 3.9.6)*. Dermal papillae are flattened. 2. Sparse superficial perivascular mixed dermal inflammatory infiltrate *(Figs. 3.9.6 and 3.9.7)*. 3. Mild superficial dermal fibrosis *(Fig. 3.9.7)*.
Special studies	PAS stain demonstrating thickening of the walls of blood vessels in superficial dermis and, in some cases, stacked globules ("caterpillar bodies") along the roof of the vesicle. Direct immunofluorescence shows nonspecific deposition of immunoglobulins in and around superficial dermal vessels *(Fig. 3.9.4)*. Confirmation with measurement of urine and/or plasma total porphyrins with fractionation if elevated.	Direct immunofluorescence shows linear deposition of IgG and C3 at the dermal-epidermal junction *(Fig. 3.9.8)*. Immunodeposition has a u-serrated pattern. Salt-split-skin technique shows immunofluorescence on the dermal (floor) side of the basement membrane zone. ELISA testing for antibodies to type VII collagen.

	Porphyria Cutanea Tarda	**Epidermolysis Bullosa Acquisita**
Treatment	Avoidance of sun and other triggering factors. Therapies include phlebotomy, hydroxychloroquine, and iron chelation.	Initial treatment generally consists of colchicine and dapsone. Refractory disease may require systemic immunosuppressants, intravenous immunoglobulin, or rituximab.
Prognosis	Treatable condition with a normal life expectancy. Relapses may occur especially if triggering factors are not removed.	Chronic disease with a prolonged course. Disease is often recalcitrant to multiple therapies. Complications include joint contractures due to progressive scarring.

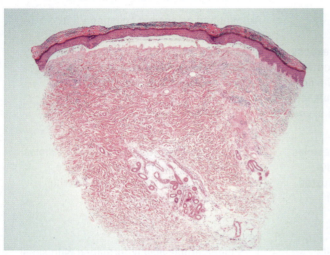

Figure 3.9.1 Porphyria cutanea tarda. Skin of distal extremity with subepidermal vesicle formation.

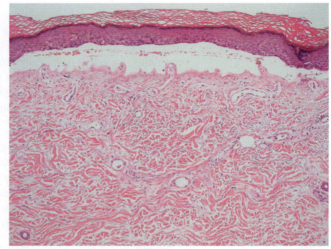

Figure 3.9.2 Porphyria cutanea tarda. Subepidermal vesicle with no appreciable inflammation. The floor of the vesicle has preserved papillae in a "festooning" fashion. Blood vessels within the superficial dermis are prominent and have mildly thickened walls.

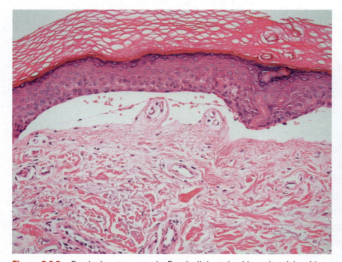

Figure 3.9.3 Porphyria cutanea tarda. Paucicellular subepidermal vesicle with "festooning" papillae.

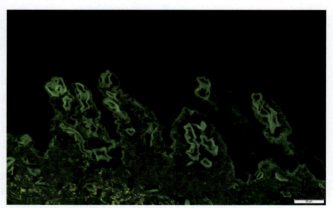

Figure 3.9.4 Porphyria cutanea tarda. Direct immunofluorescence showing vascular fluorescence with IgG representing nonspecific trapping of immunoglobulin due to abnormal vessel walls.

3.9 Porphyria Cutanea Tarda vs Epidermolysis Bullosa Acquisita

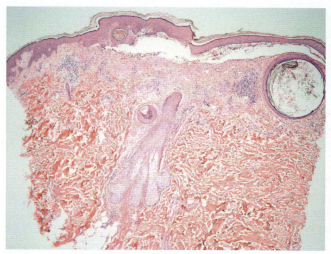

Figure 3.9.5 Epidermolysis bullosa acquisita. Subepidermal vesicle with patchy inflammatory infiltrate and milium.

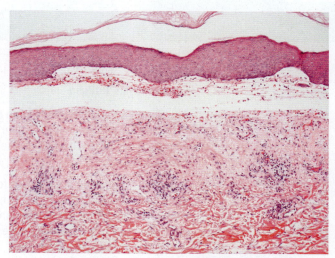

Figure 3.9.6 Epidermolysis bullosa acquisita. Subepidermal vesicle associated with moderate mixed inflammatory infiltrate including lymphocytes, neutrophils, and eosinophils. Note that the dermal papillae at the floor of the vesicle are generally flattened.

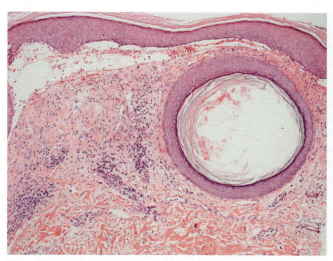

Figure 3.9.7 Epidermolysis bullosa acquisita. Milium formation associated with subepidermal vesicle, mixed inflammatory infiltrate, and fibrosis.

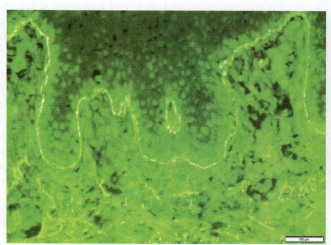

Figure 3.9.8 Epidermolysis bullosa acquisita. Linear deposition of IgG along the dermal-epidermal junction on direct immunofluorescence.

3.10 EPIDERMOLYSIS BULLOSA VS PORPHYRIA CUTANEA TARDA

	Epidermolysis Bullosa	**Porphyria Cutanea Tarda**
Age	Age of presentation depends upon subtype. Many individuals present at birth or early infancy, while others may not present until early adulthood.	Adults, typically middle age.
Location	Localized forms have predilection for distal acral surfaces. Generalized forms have more widespread involvement of trunk and neck, in addition to extremities. Mucosae may be involved in some subtypes.	Sun-exposed areas of skin including face, ears, neck, dorsum of hands, forearms, and feet.
Etiology	Variety of mutations involving genes encoding structural proteins involved in the epidermal-dermal anchoring complex forming the basement membrane zone in skin and mucosa. Dysfunction of the proteins leads to blister formation, erosions and ulcerations, and scarring. Four major groups are recognized including simplex, junctional, dystrophic, and Kindler epidermolysis bullosa.	Deficiency in uroporphyrinogen decarboxylase enzyme in the heme biosynthesis pathway. This results in excess porphyrins, including uroporphyrinogen, that deposit in the skin. Interaction with light causes excitation of porphyrins and release of energy that creates singlet-excited oxygen that leads to tissue damage.
Presentation	Skin fragility and blister formation is common to all subtypes. Depending upon the subtype, the blisters may be associated with scarring, milia, nail dystrophy, and contractures. Severe forms may have involvement of conjunctiva and noncutaneous mucosa of gastrointestinal, respiratory, and genitourinary tracts.	Skin fragility and formation of tense vesicles and bullae containing serous or bloody fluid. Vesicles are accompanied by crusted erosions and heal with scars. Mottled pigmentation and milia formation are commonly associated with the scars.
Histology	1. Epidermis of normal thickness with basket weave stratum corneum *(Fig. 3.10.1)*. 2. Subepidermal vesicle with no or minimal inflammatory infiltrate *(Fig. 3.10.2)*. 3. Dermal papillae are flattened and no appreciable thickening of the papillary dermal vessels *(Fig. 3.10.3)*.	1. Subepidermal vesicle formation with small amount of blood or serum within the vesicle cavity *(Figs. 3.10.4 and 3.10.6)* 2. Vesicle is associated with minimal inflammation ("pauci-inflammatory") *(Figs. 3.10.4 and 3.10.6)*. 3. Epidermal forming roof of vesicle has degenerative change with linear, eosinophilic, PAS-positive globules ("caterpillar bodies") along the base *(Figs. 3.10.4 and 3.10.5)*. 4. Preservation of dermal papillae ("festooning") *(Figs. 3.10.4 and 3.10.6)*. 5. Hyalinized thickening of the walls of superficial dermal vessels *(Fig. 3.10.6)*.

(continued)

	Epidermolysis Bullosa	**Porphyria Cutanea Tarda**
Special studies	Immunofluorescence mapping is generally performed to confirm the diagnosis as the light microscopic features are nonspecific. Alternatively, transmission electron microscopy may be used to identify the cleavage plane and structural abnormalities. Mutational analysis is often performed as confirmatory test.	PAS stain demonstrating thickening of the walls of blood vessels in superficial dermis *(Fig. 3.10.7)* and, in some cases, stacked globules ("caterpillar bodies") along the roof of the vesicle. Direct immunofluorescence shows nonspecific deposition of immunoglobulins in and around superficial dermal vessels *(Fig. 3.10.8)*. Confirmation with measurement of urine and/or plasma total porphyrins with fractionation if elevated.
Treatment	Treatment is primarily supportive and focused on wound care, prevention of infection, and management of complications. Treatment plans are individualized depending upon extent and severity of the blistering process and complications.	Avoidance of sun and other triggering factors. Therapies include phlebotomy, hydroxychloroquine, and iron chelation.
Prognosis	Prognosis is highly variable due to the heterogeneous nature of the underlying mutations. Prognosis is more favorable, in general, for the localized, autosomal dominant, and simplex forms. Some forms are associated with death in infancy. Substantial morbidity may be experienced from complications of scarring, contractures, infection, and secondary development of squamous cell carcinoma.	Treatable condition with a normal life expectancy. Relapses may occur especially if triggering factors are not removed.

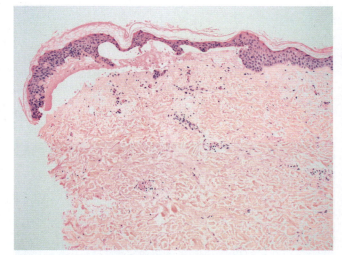

Figure 3.10.1 Epidermolysis bullosa. Paucicellular subepidermal vesicle containing fibrin and serum. Note that there is no appreciable inflammation and the dermis is unremarkable.

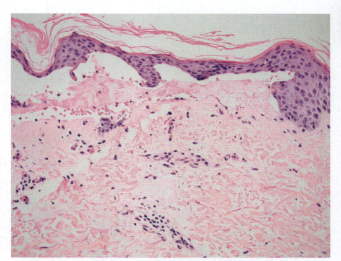

Figure 3.10.2 Epidermolysis bullosa. Subepidermal vesicle with rare inflammatory cells.

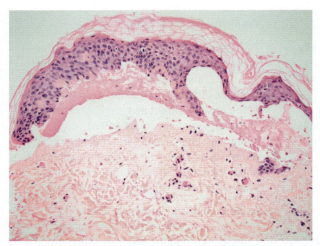

Figure 3.10.3 Epidermolysis bullosa. Subepidermal vesicle with fibrin and rare eosinophils. Epidermis forming roof of vesicle has degenerative changes. Note that dermal papillae are attenuated and the vessels are unremarkable.

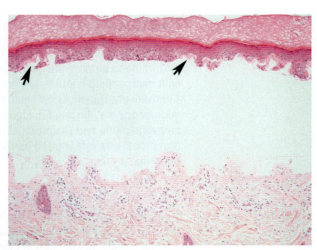

Figure 3.10.4 Porphyria cutanea tarda. Subepidermal vesicle with no appreciable inflammation. Dermal papillae extend into the vesicle cavity in a "festooning" fashion. Eosinophilic globules ("caterpillar bodies") are present along the base of the vesicle roof (arrows).

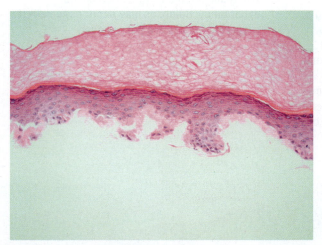

Figure 3.10.5 Porphyria cutanea tarda. Epidermal roof of subepidermal vesicle with eosinophilic globules ("caterpillar bodies").

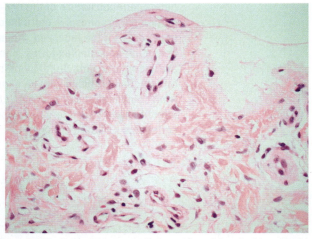

Figure 3.10.6 Porphyria cutanea tarda. Dermal floor of the subepidermal vesicle with preserved "festooning" papilla. Vessels have thick, hyalinized walls.

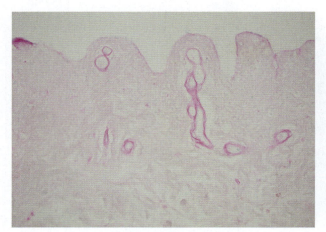

Figure 3.10.7 Porphyria cutanea tarda. PAS stain demonstrating thick vessel walls in superficial dermis beneath vesicle.

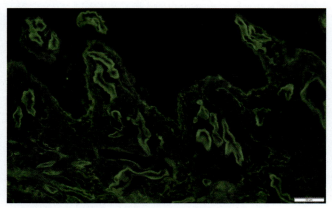

Figure 3.10.8 Porphyria cutanea tarda. Direct immunofluorescence showing vascular fluorescence with IgG representing nonspecific trapping of immunoglobulin due to abnormal vessel walls.

3.11 PEMPHIGUS VULGARIS VS DARIER DISEASE

	Pemphigus Vulgaris	**Darier Disease**
Age	Adults, generally between ages of 45 and 65 y.	Develops in childhood through adolescence with peak in teenage years.
Location	Typically begins in oral mucosa. Skin lesions can develop at any site with a predilection for head and neck region, axillae, and upper trunk.	Seborrheic areas particularly scalp, upper forehead along hairline, nasolabial folds, neck, and chest. Intertriginous regions may also be involved as well as hands and feet. May involve oral mucosa.
Etiology	Autoantibodies targeted at the Ca^{2+}-dependent cadherin desmoglein 3 and, to a lesser degree, desmoglein 1. Binding of the antibodies disrupts the integrity of the desmosomes responsible for cell-cell adhesion with resultant vesicle formation.	Autosomal dominant genodermatosis due to mutations in the *ATP2A2* gene on chromosome 12 that encodes a sarco/endoplasmic reticulum Ca^{2+}-ATPase pump (SERCA2). SERCA2 is responsible for transportation of calcium ions from the cytoplasm into the endoplasmic reticulum. Loss of function leads to acantholysis and dyskeratosis of epidermal keratinocytes.
Presentation	Flaccid vesicles and bullae that are fragile and become eroded and crusted. Nikolsky sign (induction of vesicle when mechanical pressure in applied to perilesional skin) present.	Symmetric, brown, keratotic papules that coalesce into verrucous plaques. Often associated with pruritus and malodor. Exacerbated by high temperature, sweating, mechanical irritation, and UV radiation. Punctate keratoses or pits on palms and soles. Nails are brittle and have subungual hyperkeratosis and alternating longitudinal bands. Cobblestone white papules in the oral mucosa.
Histology	1. Suprabasal acantholysis with formation of an intraepidermal (suprabasal) vesicle *(Figs. 3.11.1* and *3.11.2)*. 2. Superficial epidermis forming roof of vesicle intact. Basal keratinocytes retained along basement membrane zone resembling "tombstones" *(Figs. 3.11.2* and *3.11.3)*. 3. Superficial perivascular inflammatory infiltrate that includes eosinophils *(Fig. 3.11.3)*.	1. Hyperkeratosis and parakeratosis with entrapped neutrophils and bacteria *(Figs. 3.11.5* and *3.11.6)*. 2. Epidermal hyperplasia with papillomatosis *(Figs. 3.11.5* and *3.11.6)*. 3. Suprabasal acantholytic dyskeratosis with formation of corps ronds (dyskeratotic cells in superficial epidermis) and grains (dyskeratotic cells in stratum corneum) *(Fig. 3.11.7)*. 4. Superficial perivascular infiltrate of lymphocytes *(Figs. 3.11.6* and *3.11.7)*.
Special studies	Direct immunofluorescence shows intercellular deposition of IgG and/or C3 *(Fig. 3.11.4)*. Serology detecting serum antibodies to desmoglein 3.	None.

	Pemphigus Vulgaris	**Darier Disease**
Treatment	Systemic corticosteroids to rapidly slow disease progression. Other immunosuppressive agents, such as rituximab, azathioprine, mycophenolate mofetil, and cyclophosphamide, typically utilized for steroid-sparing effect.	Reduction of exacerbating factors combined with keratolytics and antiseptic washes. Topical corticosteroids to reduce inflammation. Topical or oral retinoids to decrease hyperkeratosis.
Prognosis	Severe disease with potential for significant morbidity and mortality. Without treatment, often fatal within 5 y of onset of disease. Morbidity from infection, fluid and electrolyte disturbances, and medication-related complications.	Chronic disease that may be recalcitrant to treatment or relapse when therapy is stopped. Most individuals have significant impairment in quality of life.

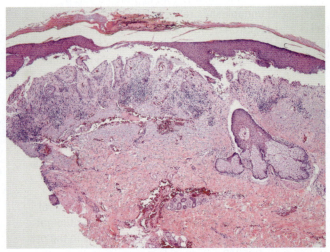

Figure 3.11.1 Pemphigus vulgaris. Suprabasal vesicle formation with overlying crust and moderate superficial dermal inflammatory infiltrate.

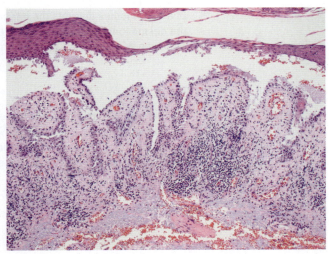

Figure 3.11.2 Pemphigus vulgaris. Intraepidermal vesicle formation resulting from suprabasilar acantholysis. The basal keratinocytes are intact creating a "tombstone" appearance along the junction. Note that the epidermis forming the roof of the vesicle is intact and does not show any appreciable dyskeratosis.

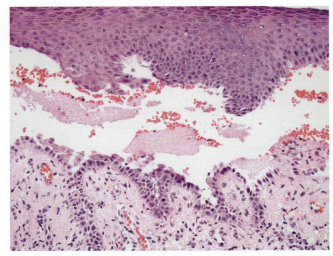

Figure 3.11.3 Pemphigus vulgaris. Suprabasilar acantholysis, without dyskeratosis, forming intraepidermal vesicle. Basal cells form "tombstones" along the papillae.

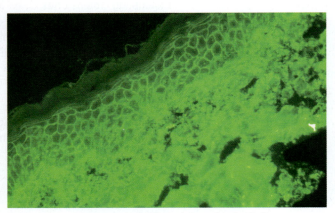

Figure 3.11.4 Pemphigus vulgaris. Diagnosis is confirmed with direct immunofluorescence showing intercellular deposition of IgG and C3.

3.11 Pemphigus Vulgaris vs Darier Disease

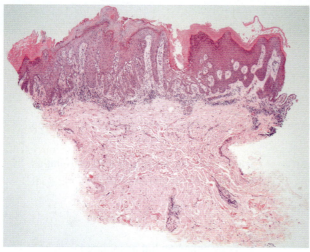

Figure 3.11.5 Darier disease. Epidermal hyperplasia with hyperkeratosis and parakeratosis. The epidermis has suprabasilar acantholysis with cleft formation and acantholytic dyskeratosis.

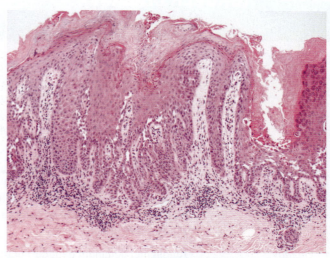

Figure 3.11.6 Darier disease. Hyperplastic epidermis with suprabasilar acantholysis and acantholytic dyskeratosis forming corps ronds and grains.

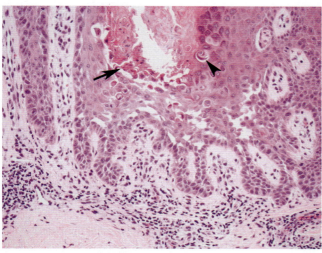

Figure 3.11.7 Darier disease. Acantholytic dyskeratosis with formation of corps ronds (arrowhead) and grains (arrow).

3.12 DARIER DISEASE VS TRANSIENT ACANTHOLYTIC DERMATOSIS (GROVER DISEASE)

	Darier Disease	**Transient Acantholytic Dermatosis (Grover Disease)**
Age	Develops in childhood through adolescence with peak in teenage years.	Typically older adults, male predominance.
Location	Seborrheic areas particularly scalp, upper forehead along hairline, nasolabial folds, neck, and chest. Intertriginous regions may also be involved as well as hands and feet. May involve oral mucosa.	Trunk, predominately, and also extremities and rarely head and neck region.
Etiology	Autosomal dominant genodermatosis due to mutations in the *ATP2A2* gene on chromosome 12 that encodes a sarco/endoplasmic reticulum Ca^{2+}-ATPase pump (SERCA2). SERCA2 is responsible for transportation of calcium ions from the cytoplasm into the endoplasmic reticulum. Loss of function leads to acantholysis and dyskeratosis of epidermal keratinocytes.	Etiology unknown but associated with heat and sweating.
Presentation	Symmetric, brown, keratotic papules that coalesce into verrucous plaques. Often associated with pruritus and malodor. Exacerbated by high temperature, sweating, mechanical irritation, and UV radiation. Punctate keratoses or pits on palms and soles. Nails are brittle and have subungual hyperkeratosis and alternating longitudinal bands. Cobblestone white papules in the oral mucosa.	Pruritic, 1-3 mm, pink papules and tiny vesicles.
Histology	1. Hyperkeratosis and parakeratosis with entrapped neutrophils and bacteria (Figs. 3.12.1 and 3.12.2). 2. Epidermal hyperplasia with papillomatosis (Figs. 3.12.1 and 3.12.2). 3. Suprabasal acantholytic dyskeratosis with formation of corps ronds (dyskeratotic cells in superficial epidermis) and grains (dyskeratotic cells in stratum corneum) (Fig. 3.12.3). Acantholytic dyskeratosis involves much of the epidermis. 4. Superficial perivascular infiltrate of lymphocytes (Figs. 3.12.2 and 3.12.3).	1. Epidermis of relatively normal thickness and rete architecture (Fig. 3.12.4). 2. Subtle small foci of suprabasal acantholysis and dyskeratosis (Figs. 3.12.4 and 3.12.5). May have multiple minute foci of acantholysis with different patterns and/or spongiosis in same biopsy (Fig. 3.12.6). 3. Sparse superficial perivascular lymphocytic infiltrate with occasional eosinophils (Figs. 3.12.5 and 3.12.6). 4. Examination of multiple levels of biopsy tissue may be necessary to reveal minute foci of acantholysis.

(continued)

3.12 Darier Disease vs Transient Acantholytic Dermatosis (Grover Disease)

	Darier Disease	Transient Acantholytic Dermatosis (Grover Disease)
Special studies	None.	None.
Treatment	Reduction of exacerbating factors combined with keratolytics and antiseptic washes. Topical corticosteroids to reduce inflammation. Topical or oral retinoids to decrease hyperkeratosis.	Topical corticosteroids and moisturizers are first-line therapy. Oral antihistamines for pruritus. Topical vitamin D analogues, systemic retinoids, and phototherapy for persistent disease.
Prognosis	Chronic disease that may be recalcitrant to treatment or relapse when therapy is stopped. Most individuals have significant impairment in quality of life.	Self-limited disease that typically resolves within a few weeks to months.

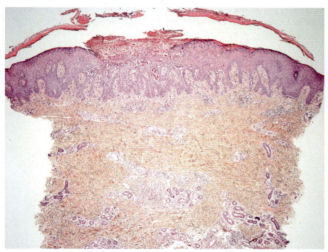

Figure 3.12.1 Darier disease. The epidermis is irregularly acanthotic and has overlying hyperkeratosis and parakeratosis. There is suprabasal acantholysis with prominent acantholytic dyskeratosis.

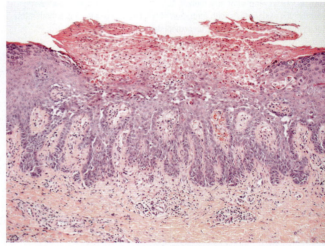

Figure 3.12.2 Darier disease. Epidermal hyperplasia with acantholysis forming a suprabasal cleft and superficial keratinocytes showing acantholytic dyskeratosis with corps ronds and grains.

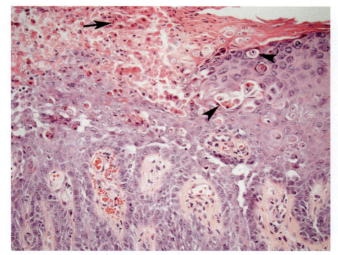

Figure 3.12.3 Darier disease. Suprabasilar acantholysis with dyskeratosis forming numerous corps ronds (arrowheads) and grains (arrow) in superficial epidermis and stratum corneum, respectively.

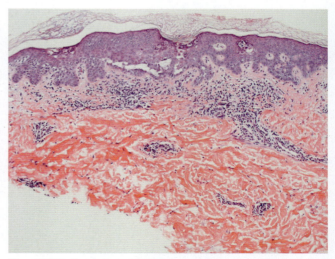

Figure 3.12.4 Transient acantholytic dermatosis (Grover disease). Focal, subtle epidermal acantholysis and spongiosis with moderately dense superficial dermal inflammatory infiltrate. Note that there is only mild epidermal hyperplasia and no parakeratosis (scale).

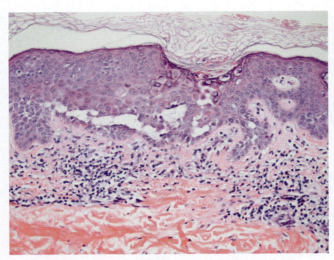

Figure 3.12.5 Transient acantholytic dermatosis (Grover disease). Subtle acantholytic dyskeratosis with formation of corps ronds. Dermis has a moderately dense infiltrate that includes rare eosinophils.

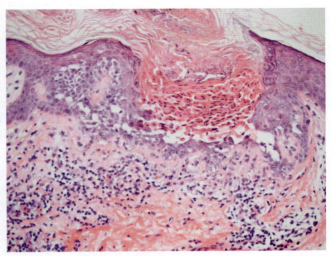

Figure 3.12.6 Transient acantholytic dermatosis (Grover disease). Small focus of acantholytic dyskeratosis with focal formation of dyskeratotic cells in the stratum corneum (grains).

3.13 PEMPHIGUS VULGARIS VS PEMPHIGUS FOLIACEUS

	Pemphigus Vulgaris	**Pemphigus Foliaceus**
Age	Adults, generally between ages of 45 and 65 y.	Adults between the ages of 45 and 65 y.
Location	Typically begins in oral mucosa. Skin lesions can develop at any site with a predilection for head and neck region, axillae, and upper trunk.	Face, scalp, and seborrheic areas of trunk. No mucosal lesions as opposed to pemphigus vulgaris.
Etiology	Autoantibodies targeted at the Ca^{2+}-dependent cadherin desmoglein 3 and, to a lesser degree, desmoglein 1. Binding of the antibodies disrupts the integrity of the desmosomes responsible for cell-cell adhesion with resultant vesicle formation.	Autoimmune disease with autoantibodies against desmoglein 1, a Ca^{2+}-dependent transmembrane adhesion molecule present in the epidermal desmosomes.
Presentation	Flaccid vesicles and bullae that are fragile and become eroded and crusted. Nikolsky sign (induction of vesicle when mechanical pressure is applied to perilesional skin) present.	Erythematous eroded plaques with "cornflake" scales and crusts. May have superficial fragile vesicles. Erosions heal without scarring.
Histology	1. Suprabasal acantholysis with formation of an intraepidermal (suprabasal) vesicle *(Figs. 3.13.1* and *3.13.2)*. 2. Superficial epidermis forming roof of vesicle intact. Basal keratinocytes retained along basement membrane zone resembling "tombstones" *(Figs. 3.13.2* and *3.13.3)*. 3. Sparse superficial perivascular inflammatory infiltrate that includes eosinophils *(Fig. 3.13.3)*.	1. Stratum corneum is detached and partially absent *(Figs. 3.13.5* and *3.13.6)*. 2. Subcorneal acantholysis with rounding up of keratinocytes along the surface of the epidermis *(Figs. 3.13.6* and *3.13.7)*. 3. Aggregates of neutrophils in areas of acantholysis and crust formation *(Fig. 3.13.5)*. 4. Sparse superficial perivascular lymphomononuclear infiltrate.
Special studies	Direct immunofluorescence shows intercellular deposition of IgG and/or C3 *(Fig. 3.13.4)*. May be accentuated in lower half of epidermis. Note that pemphigus foliaceus may have identical direct immunofluorescence findings so imperative to correlate with level of cleavage plane on light microscopy. Serology detecting serum antibodies to desmoglein 3 by ELISA.	Direct immunofluorescence demonstrates intercellular "netlike" deposition of IgG and C3 within the epidermis *(Fig. 3.13.8)*. May be accentuated in upper half of epidermis. Note that pemphigus vulgaris may have identical direct immunofluorescence findings so imperative to correlate with level of cleavage plane on light microscopy. Detection of serum antibodies against desmoglein 1 by ELISA.
Treatment	Systemic corticosteroids to rapidly slow disease progression. Other immunosuppressive agents, such as rituximab, azathioprine, mycophenolate mofetil, and cyclophosphamide, typically utilized for steroid-sparing effect.	Initial course of systemic corticosteroids with addition of steroid-sparing immunomodulators such as rituximab, azathioprine, cyclophosphamide, and mycophenolate mofetil.

	Pemphigus Vulgaris	**Pemphigus Foliaceus**
Prognosis	Severe disease with potential for significant morbidity and mortality. Without treatment, often fatal within 5 y of onset of disease. Morbidity from infection, fluid and electrolyte disturbances, and medication-related complications.	Chronic disease with unpredictable course. May be associated with considerable morbidity including infections, concurrent autoimmune diseases, and medication-related complications. Mortality is estimated to be two- to three-fold higher than in the general population.

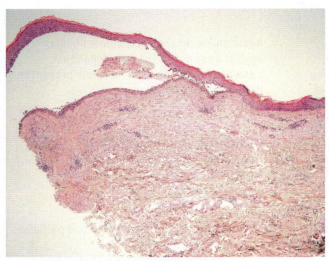

Figure 3.13.1 Pemphigus vulgaris. Large intraepidermal vesicle formed by suprabasal acantholysis.

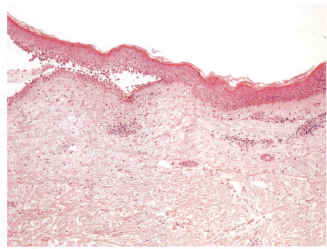

Figure 3.13.2 Pemphigus vulgaris. Suprabasal acantholysis forming intraepidermal vesicle associated with sparse dermal inflammatory infiltrate. Note the intact stratum corneum and lack of parakeratosis.

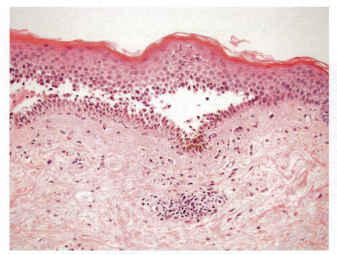

Figure 3.13.3 Pemphigus vulgaris. Acantholysis involving the lower, suprabasal region of the epidermis resulting in an intraepidermal vesicle. Basal keratinocytes along the floor of the vesicle have a "tombstone" appearance.

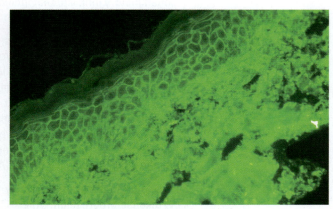

Figure 3.13.4 Pemphigus vulgaris. Direct immunofluorescence reveals an intercellular network with IgG and C3 immunoreactants. The fluorescence is most intense in the lower half of the epidermis.

3.13 Pemphigus Vulgaris vs Pemphigus Foliaceus

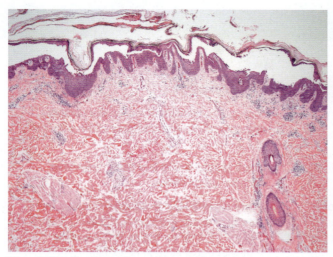

Figure 3.13.5 Pemphigus foliaceus. Subcorneal/intragranular acantholysis with partial detachment of the stratum corneum from the epidermis. The acantholysis forms a cleft in the upper third of the epidermis.

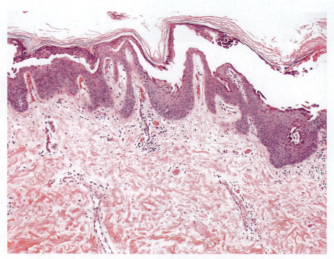

Figure 3.13.6 Pemphigus foliaceus. Superficial epidermal acantholysis within the granular layer. Note that the lower portion of the epidermis is intact.

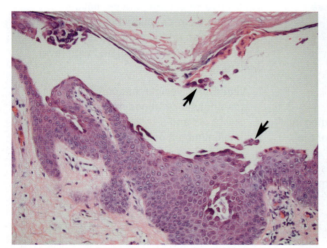

Figure 3.13.7 Pemphigus foliaceus. Acantholysis within the granular layer of the epidermis with dissociated, rounded keratinocytes (arrows) within the superficial epidermal cleft.

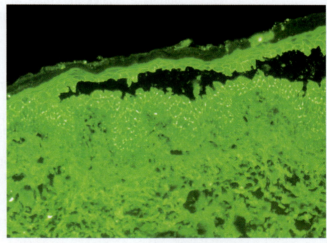

Figure 3.13.8 Pemphigus foliaceus. Direct immunofluorescence of lesional tissue demonstrates intercellular deposition of IgG and C3 in a "chicken wire" pattern. The intensity of the fluorescence is somewhat accentuated in the upper half of the epidermis.

3.14 PEMPHIGUS FOLIACEUS VS BULLOUS IMPETIGO

	Pemphigus Foliaceus	**Bullous Impetigo**
Age	Adults between the ages of 45 and 65 y.	Any age, but most common in the pediatric population, especially infants under the age of 2 y.
Location	Face, scalp, and seborrheic areas of trunk. No mucosal lesions.	Intertriginous areas and trunk; may have mucosal involvement.
Etiology	Autoimmune disease with autoantibodies against desmoglein 1, a Ca^{2+}-dependent transmembrane adhesion molecule present in the epidermal desmosomes.	Acute superficial skin infection caused by *Staphylococcus aureus* (coagulase-positive, group II). Blister formation is induced by staphylococcal exotoxins (exfoliatin A-D) that target desmoglein 1, a Ca^{2+}-dependent transmembrane adhesion molecule present in the epidermal desmosomes.
Presentation	Erythematous eroded plaques with "cornflake" scales and crusts. May have fragile vesicles. Erosions heal without scarring.	Solitary or small number of vesicles that rapidly evolve to large, flaccid bullae containing clear or yellow fluid. Ruptured bullae have an erythematous base with rim of scale. May be associated with fever, weakness, and diarrhea.
Histology	1. Stratum corneum is detached and partially absent *(Fig. 3.14.1)*. 2. Subcorneal acantholysis with rounding up of keratinocytes along the surface of the epidermis *(Figs. 3.14.2 and 3.14.3)*. 3. May have aggregates of neutrophils in areas of acantholysis and crust formation *(Fig. 3.14.1)*. 4. Sparse superficial perivascular lymphomononuclear infiltrate *(Fig. 3.14.3)*.	1. Subcorneal vesicle that contains acantholytic keratinocytes and neutrophils *(Figs. 3.14.5 and 3.14.6)*. 2. Small numbers of cocci within vesicle *(Fig. 3.14.7)*. 3. Sparse superficial perivascular infiltrate of lymphocytes and neutrophils *(Fig. 3.14.5)*.
Special studies	Direct immunofluorescence demonstrates intercellular "netlike" deposition of IgG and C3 within the epidermis *(Fig. 3.14.4)*. Detection of serum antibodies against desmoglein 1 by ELISA. Tissue Gram and PAS stains negative for bacterial and fungal organisms.	Tissue Gram stain to detect possible bacteria in vesicle. Direct immunofluorescence is negative.
Treatment	Initial course of systemic corticosteroids with addition of steroid-sparing immunomodulators such as rituximab, azathioprine, cyclophosphamide, and mycophenolate mofetil.	Topical and oral antibiotics.

(continued)

3.14 Pemphigus Foliaceus vs Bullous Impetigo

	Pemphigus Foliaceus	**Bullous Impetigo**
Prognosis	Chronic disease with unpredictable course. May be associated with considerable morbidity including infections, concurrent autoimmune diseases, and medication-related complications. Mortality is estimated to be two- to three-fold higher than in the general population.	Lesions generally resolve, with treatment, within 10-14 d. Approximately 20% spontaneously resolve without treatment.

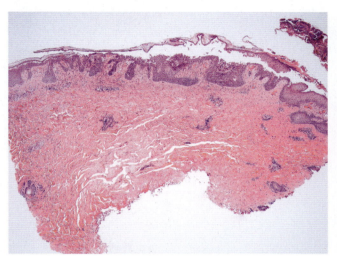

Figure 3.14.1 Pemphigus foliaceus. Subcorneal and intragranular acantholysis with partial detachment of the stratum corneum from superficial epidermis. There is serum crust in the upper right corner of image.

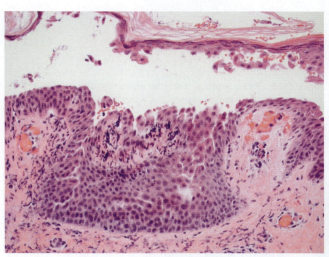

Figure 3.14.2 Pemphigus foliaceus. Acantholysis within granular layer with loss of cohesion and rounding up of superficial keratinocytes.

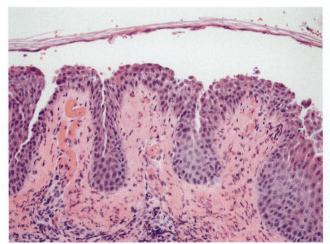

Figure 3.14.3 Pemphigus foliaceus. Acantholysis involving the granular layer of the epidermis with rounded keratinocytes along the surface of the intact lower epidermis. Note that there is no significant neutrophilic inflammation and no bacteria.

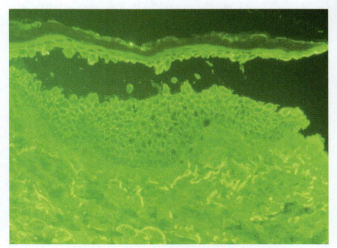

Figure 3.14.4 Pemphigus foliaceus. Diagnosis is confirmed with direct immunofluorescence showing intercellular deposition of IgG and C3 within the epidermis.

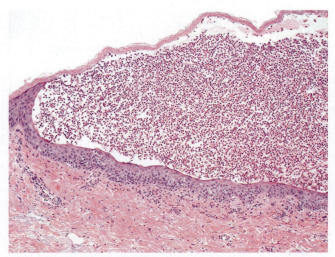

Figure 3.14.5 Bullous impetigo. Subcorneal vesicle filled with neutrophils. There are rare acantholytic superficial keratinocytes within the vesicle.

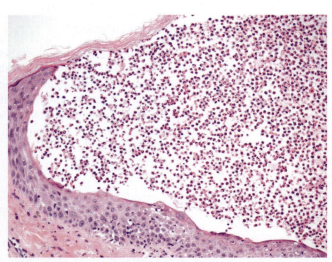

Figure 3.14.6 Bullous impetigo. Discrete subcorneal vesicle filled with neutrophils and rare acantholytic cells.

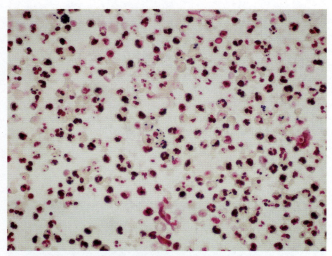

Figure 3.14.7 Bullous impetigo. Brown and Brenn tissue Gram stain demonstrates gram-positive cocci within the vesicle, including intracellular organisms.

3.15 PEMPHIGUS VULGARIS VS TRANSIENT ACANTHOLYTIC DERMATOSIS (GROVER DISEASE)

	Pemphigus Vulgaris	**Transient Acantholytic Dermatosis (Grover Disease)**
Age	Adults, generally between ages of 45 and 65 y.	Typically older adults, male predominance.
Location	Typically begins in oral mucosa. Skin lesions can develop at any site with a predilection for head and neck region, axillae, and upper trunk.	Trunk predominately, and also extremities and rarely head and neck region.
Etiology	Autoantibodies targeted at the Ca^{2+}-dependent cadherin desmoglein 3 and, to a lesser degree, desmoglein 1. Binding of the antibodies disrupts the integrity of the desmosomes responsible for cell-cell adhesion with resultant vesicle formation.	Etiology unknown but associated with heat and sweating.
Presentation	Flaccid vesicles and bullae that are fragile and become eroded and crusted. Nikolsky sign (induction of vesicle when mechanical pressure is applied to perilesional skin) present.	Pruritic, 1-3 mm, pink papules and tiny vesicles.
Histology	1. Suprabasal acantholysis with formation of an intraepidermal (suprabasal) vesicle/bulla *(Fig. 3.15.1)*. 2. Superficial epidermis forming roof of vesicle intact. Basal keratinocytes retained along basement membrane zone resembling "tombstones" *(Figs. 3.15.2 and 3.15.3)*. 3. Sparse superficial perivascular inflammatory infiltrate composed of lymphocytes with occasional eosinophils *(Figs. 3.15.2 and 3.15.3)*.	1. Epidermis of normal thickness and rete architecture *(Fig. 3.15.5)*. 2. Subtle small foci of suprabasal acantholysis. May have multiple minute foci of acantholysis with different patterns (acantholytic dyskeratosis, superficial acantholysis) and/or spongiosis in same biopsy *(Figs. 3.15.5-3.15.7)*. 3. Sparse superficial perivascular lymphocytic infiltrate with occasional eosinophils *(Fig. 3.15.6)*. 4. Examination of multiple levels of biopsy tissue may be necessary to reveal minute foci of acantholysis.
Special studies	Direct immunofluorescence shows intercellular deposition of IgG and/or C3 *(Fig. 3.15.4)*. Serology detecting serum antibodies to desmoglein 3 by ELISA.	None.
Treatment	Systemic corticosteroids to rapidly slow disease progression. Other immunosuppressive agents, such as rituximab, azathioprine, mycophenolate mofetil, and cyclophosphamide, typically utilized for steroid-sparing effect.	Topical corticosteroids and moisturizers are first-line therapy. Oral antihistamines for pruritus. Topical vitamin D analogues, systemic retinoids, and phototherapy for persistent disease.

	Pemphigus Vulgaris	**Transient Acantholytic Dermatosis (Grover Disease)**
Prognosis	Severe disease with potential for significant morbidity and mortality. Without treatment, often fatal within 5 y of onset of disease. Morbidity from infection, fluid and electrolyte disturbances, and medication-related complications.	Self-limited disease that typically resolves within a few weeks to months.

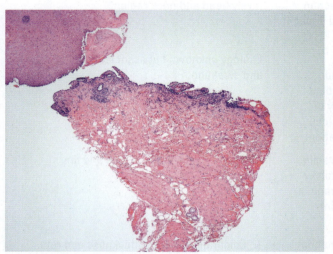

Figure 3.15.1 Pemphigus vulgaris. Suprabasilar acantholysis across the breadth of the oral mucosal biopsy forming an intraepithelial vesicle. The entire mucosa is detached from underlying tissues.

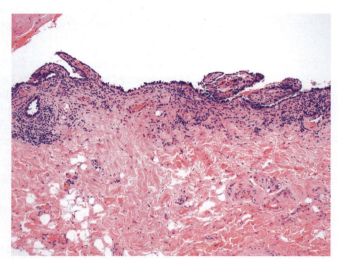

Figure 3.15.2 Pemphigus vulgaris. Retention of basal layer forming a "tombstone" pattern along the floor of the vesicle. There is a moderate inflammatory infiltrate.

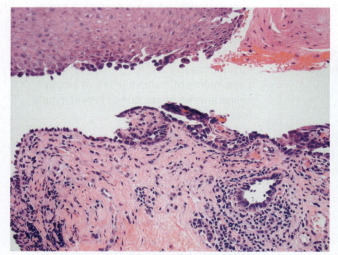

Figure 3.15.3 Pemphigus vulgaris. Suprabasal vesicle with "tombstone" pattern of intact basal cells along floor. Detached epithelium forming roof of vesicle has detached rounded acantholytic cells.

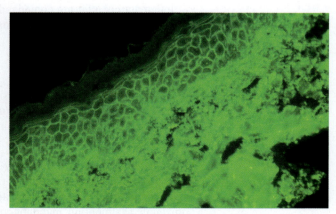

Figure 3.15.4 Pemphigus vulgaris. Direct immunofluorescence demonstrates intercellular deposition of IgG and C3 within perilesional epithelium.

3.15 Pemphigus Vulgaris vs Transient Acantholytic Dermatosis (Grover Disease)

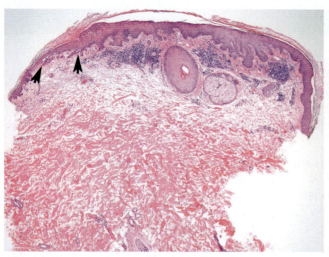

Figure 3.15.5 Transient acantholytic dermatosis (Grover disease). Superficial perivascular inflammatory infiltrate with mild epidermal hyperplasia and subtle suprabasal acantholysis (arrows).

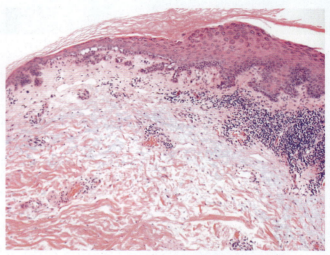

Figure 3.15.6 Transient acantholytic dermatosis (Grover disease). Subtle suprabasal acantholysis with mild epidermal hyperplasia and moderately dense lymphomononuclear infiltrate.

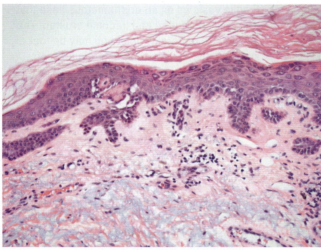

Figure 3.15.7 Transient acantholytic dermatosis (Grover disease). Subtlety of acantholysis differentiates Grover disease from pemphigus vulgaris. Examination of multiple levels of the biopsy is often necessary to find the acantholysis in cases of Grover disease.

3.16 PEMPHIGUS VULGARIS VS BENIGN FAMILIAL PEMPHIGUS (HAILEY-HAILEY DISEASE)

	Pemphigus Vulgaris	**Benign Familial Pemphigus (Hailey-Hailey Disease)**
Age	Adults, typically between ages of 45 and 65 y.	Adults, typically between 20 and 40 y of age.
Location	Typically begins in oral mucosa. Skin lesions can develop at any site with a predilection for head and neck region, axillae, and upper trunk.	Intertriginous regions including axillae, groin, perianal region, and lateral neck. Oral mucosa generally not involved.
Etiology	Autoantibodies targeted at the Ca^{2+}-dependent cadherin desmoglein 3 and, to a lesser degree, desmoglein 1. Binding of the antibodies disrupts the integrity of the desmosomes responsible for cell-cell adhesion with resultant vesicle formation.	Mutation of the *ATP2C1* gene on chromosome 3 that encodes proteins of calcium ATPase on the Golgi apparatus. This results in failure of calcium transport leading to loss of desmosomal integrity and acantholysis.
Presentation	Flaccid vesicles and bullae that are fragile and become eroded and crusted. Nikolsky sign (induction of vesicle when mechanical pressure is applied to perilesional skin) present.	Fragile vesicles on an erythematous base that are easily disrupted and become crusted. The lesions are generally moist and may be foul smelling due to secondary impetiginization. Nikolsky sign is negative.
Histology	1. Suprabasal acantholysis with formation of an intraepidermal (suprabasal) vesicle *(Figs. 3.16.1* and *3.16.2)*. 2. Superficial epidermis forming roof of vesicle intact. Basal keratinocytes retained along basement membrane zone resembling "tombstones" *(Fig. 3.16.3)*. 3. Involvement of follicular epithelium by acantholysis in pemphigus vulgaris aids in distinguishing from benign familial pemphigus (Hailey-Hailey disease) *(Fig. 3.16.4)*. 4. Sparse superficial perivascular inflammatory infiltrate that includes eosinophils *(Figs. 3.16.2* and *3.16.3)*.	1. Epidermal hyperplasia with hyperkeratosis and parakeratosis with crust formation *(Fig. 3.16.6)*. 2. Suprabasal acantholysis with florid acantholysis throughout upper levels of the epidermis ("dilapidated brick wall") *(Figs. 3.16.6-3.16.8)*. 3. Rare foci of acantholytic dyskeratosis with corps ronds formation. 4. Sparse superficial perivascular lymphocytic infiltrate *(Fig. 3.16.7)*.
Special studies	Direct immunofluorescence shows intercellular deposition of IgG and/or C3 *(Fig. 3.16.5)*. Serology detecting serum antibodies to desmoglein 3 by ELISA.	Direct immunofluorescence, to exclude other autoimmune bullous disorders, is negative.
Treatment	Systemic corticosteroids to rapidly slow disease progression. Other immunosuppressive agents, such as rituximab, azathioprine, mycophenolate mofetil, and cyclophosphamide, typically utilized for steroid-sparing effect.	Reduction of exacerbating factors such as friction from clothing, sweating, and secondary infection is key to control of the disease. First-line therapies include combination of topical antibiotics and intermittent topical corticosteroids or topical calcineurin inhibitors. Botulinum toxin injections efficacious in some cases to reduce sweating.

(continued)

3.16 Pemphigus Vulgaris vs Benign Familial Pemphigus (Hailey-Hailey Disease)

	Pemphigus Vulgaris	Benign Familial Pemphigus (Hailey-Hailey Disease)
Prognosis	Severe disease with potential for significant morbidity and mortality. Without treatment, often fatal within 5 y of onset of disease. Morbidity from infection, fluid and electrolyte disturbances, and medication-related complications.	Chronic disease with relapsing and remitting course.

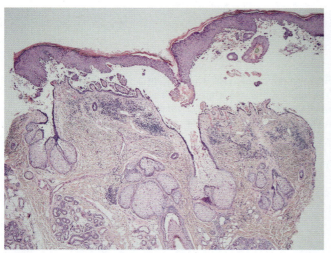

Figure 3.16.1 Pemphigus vulgaris. Intraepidermal vesicle formed by suprabasilar acantholysis.

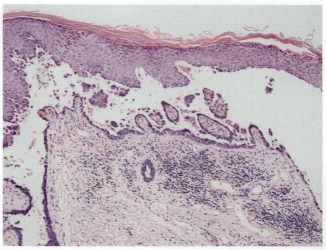

Figure 3.16.2 Pemphigus vulgaris. Intraepidermal vesicle formed by suprabasilar acantholysis with preservation of dermal papillae creating a "villous" appearance. Note that the epidermis forming the roof of the vesicle is generally intact.

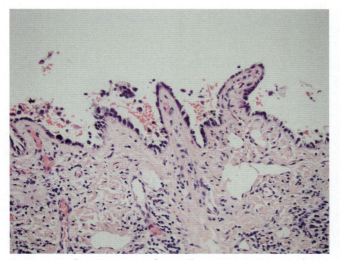

Figure 3.16.3 Pemphigus vulgaris. Suprabasilar acantholysis with retained basal keratinocytes with a characteristic "tombstone" pattern.

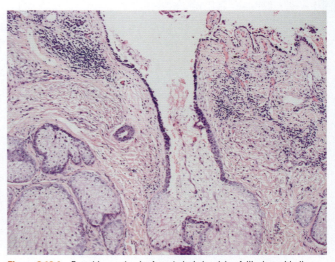

Figure 3.16.4 Pemphigus vulgaris. Acantholysis involving follicular epithelium aids in distinguishing from Hailey-Hailey disease.

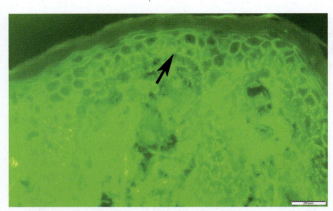

Figure 3.16.5 Pemphigus vulgaris. Direct immunofluorescence demonstrating intercellular network of IgG and C3 immunoreactants (arrow).

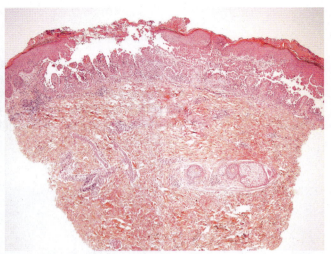

Figure 3.16.6 Benign familial pemphigus (Hailey-Hailey disease). Epidermal hyperplasia with prominent hyperkeratosis and parakeratosis. There is suprabasal cleft formation, and the epidermis shows prominent acantholysis creating a "dilapidated brick wall" appearance.

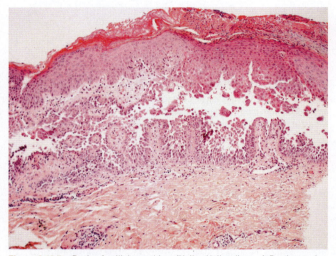

Figure 3.16.7 Benign familial pemphigus (Hailey-Hailey disease). Parakeratosis and crust with prominent epidermal acantholysis involving much of the mid epidermis. The epidermis has the appearance of a "dilapidated brick wall."

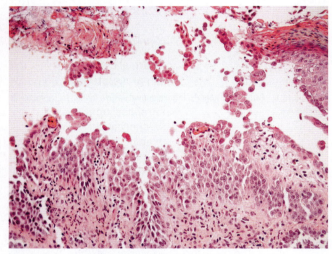

Figure 3.16.8 Benign familial pemphigus (Hailey-Hailey disease). The acantholytic keratinocytes are disassociated from each other and have a rounded-up appearance within the vesicle cavity.

3.17 BENIGN FAMILIAL PEMPHIGUS (HAILEY-HAILEY DISEASE) VS TRANSIENT ACANTHOLYTIC DERMATOSIS (GROVER DISEASE)

	Benign Familial Pemphigus (Hailey-Hailey Disease)	**Transient Acantholytic Dermatosis (Grover Disease)**
Age	Adults, typically between 20 and 40 y of age.	Typically older adults, male predominance.
Location	Intertriginous regions including axillae, groin, perianal region, and lateral neck. Oral mucosa generally not involved.	Trunk predominately, and also extremities and, rarely, head and neck region.
Etiology	Mutation of the *ATP2C1* gene on chromosome 3 that encodes proteins of calcium ATPase on the Golgi apparatus. This results in failure of calcium transport leading to loss of desmosomal integrity and acantholysis.	Etiology unknown but associated with heat and sweating.
Presentation	Fragile vesicles on an erythematous base that are easily disrupted and become crusted. The lesions are generally moist and may be foul smelling due to secondary impetiginization. Nikolsky sign is negative.	Pruritic, 1-3 mm, pink papules and tiny vesicles.
Histology	1. Epidermal hyperplasia with hyperkeratosis and parakeratosis with crust formation *(Fig. 3.17.1)*. 2. Suprabasal acantholysis with florid acantholysis throughout upper levels of the epidermis ("dilapidated brick wall") *(Figs. 3.17.1-3.17.3)*. 3. Rare foci of acantholytic dyskeratosis with corps ronds formation. 4. Sparse superficial perivascular lymphocytic infiltrate *(Figs. 3.17.1* and *3.17.2)*.	1. Epidermis of normal thickness and rete architecture *(Fig. 3.17.4)*. 2. Subtle small foci of suprabasal acantholysis. May have multiple minute foci of acantholysis with different patterns (acantholytic dyskeratosis, superficial acantholysis) and/or spongiosis in the same biopsy *(Figs. 3.17.5* and *3.17.6)*. 3. Sparse superficial perivascular lymphocytic infiltrate with occasional eosinophils *(Figs. 3.17.5* and *3.17.6)*. 4. Examination of multiple levels of biopsy tissue may be necessary to reveal minute foci of acantholysis.
Special studies	Direct immunofluorescence, to exclude other autoimmune bullous disorders, is negative.	None.
Treatment	Reduction of exacerbating factors such as friction from clothing, sweating, and secondary infection is key to control of the disease. First-line therapies include combination of topical antibiotics and intermittent topical corticosteroids or topical calcineurin inhibitors. Botulinum toxin injections efficacious in some cases to reduce sweating.	Topical corticosteroids and moisturizers are first-line therapy. Oral antihistamines for pruritus. Topical vitamin D analogues, systemic retinoids, and phototherapy for persistent disease.
Prognosis	Chronic disease with relapsing and remitting course.	Self-limited disease that typically resolves within a few weeks to months.

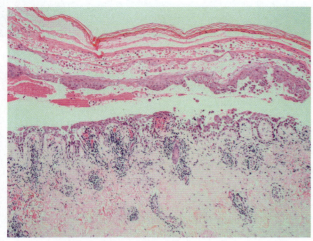

Figure 3.17.1 Benign familial pemphigus (Hailey-Hailey disease). Prominent epidermal acantholysis involving the entire biopsy. Epidermis is hyperplastic, and there is overlying hyperkeratosis and parakeratosis.

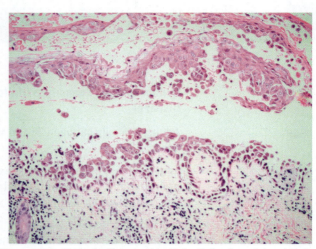

Figure 3.17.2 Benign familial pemphigus (Hailey-Hailey disease). Acantholysis involves much of the thickness of the epidermis creating a "dilapidated brick wall" appearance.

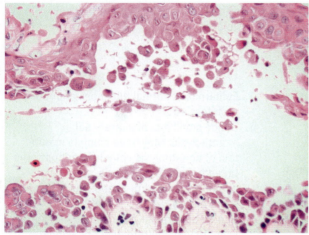

Figure 3.17.3 Benign familial pemphigus (Hailey-Hailey disease). The acantholytic keratinocytes are rounded and float within the vesicle cavity.

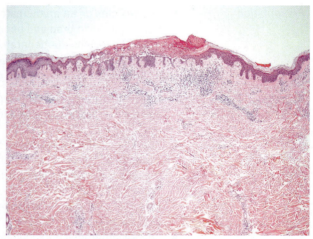

Figure 3.17.4 Transient acantholytic dermatosis (Grover disease). Small focus of epidermal acantholysis associated with a superficial dermal inflammatory infiltrate. Note that there is no significant epidermal hyperplasia.

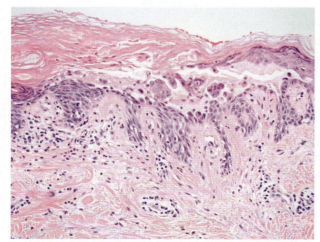

Figure 3.17.5 Transient acantholytic dermatosis (Grover disease). The pattern of acantholysis mimics Hailey-Hailey disease with involvement of much of the mid and upper levels of the epidermis with "dilapidated brick wall" appearance. However, the focus is small and subtle.

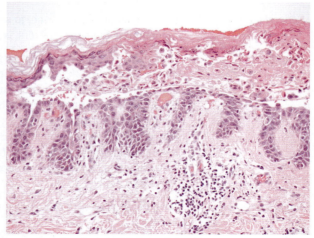

Figure 3.17.6 Transient acantholytic dermatosis (Grover disease). Small focus of epidermal acantholysis. Given that the histologic features may mimic those of Hailey-Hailey disease, correlation with the clinical history is essential.

3.18 DARIER DISEASE VS BENIGN FAMILIAL PEMPHIGUS (HAILEY-HAILEY DISEASE)

	Darier Disease	**Benign Familial Pemphigus (Hailey-Hailey Disease)**
Age	Develops in childhood through adolescence with peak in teenage years.	Adults, typically between 20 and 40 y of age.
Location	Seborrheic areas particularly scalp, upper forehead along hairline, nasolabial folds, neck, and chest. Intertriginous regions may also be involved as well as hands and feet. May involve oral mucosa.	Intertriginous regions including axillae, groin, perianal region, and lateral neck. Oral mucosa generally not involved.
Etiology	Autosomal dominant genodermatosis due to mutations in the *ATP2A2* gene on chromosome 12 that encodes a sarco/endoplasmic reticulum Ca^{2+}-ATPase pump (SERCA2). SERCA2 is responsible for transportation of calcium ions from the cytoplasm into the endoplasmic reticulum. Loss of function leads to acantholysis and dyskeratosis of epidermal keratinocytes.	Mutation of the *ATP2C1* gene on chromosome 3 that encodes proteins of calcium ATPase on the Golgi apparatus. This results in failure of calcium transport leading to loss of desmosomal integrity and acantholysis.
Presentation	Symmetric, brown, keratotic papules that coalesce into verrucous plaques. Often associated with pruritus and malodor. Exacerbated by high temperature, sweating, mechanical irritation, and UV radiation. Punctate keratoses or pits on palms and soles. Nails are brittle and have subungual hyperkeratosis and alternating longitudinal bands. Cobblestone white papules in the oral mucosa.	Fragile vesicles on an erythematous base that are easily disrupted and become crusted. The lesions are generally moist and may be foul smelling due to secondary impetiginization. Nikolsky sign is negative.
Histology	1. Hyperkeratosis and parakeratosis that may have entrapped neutrophils and bacteria *(Fig. 3.18.1)*. 2. Epidermal hyperplasia with papillomatosis *(Figs. 3.18.1 and 3.18.2)*. 3. Suprabasal acantholytic dyskeratosis with formation of corps ronds and grains *(Figs. 3.18.2 and 3.18.3)*. 4. Superficial perivascular infiltrate of lymphocytes *(Fig. 3.18.3)*.	1. Epidermal hyperplasia with hyperkeratosis and parakeratosis with crust formation *(Figs. 3.18.4 and 3.18.5)*. 2. Suprabasal acantholysis with florid acantholysis throughout upper levels of the epidermis ("dilapidated brick wall") *(Figs. 3.18.5 and 3.18.6)*. 3. Little or no dyskeratosis. 4. Sparse superficial perivascular lymphocytic infiltrate *(Fig. 3.18.5)*.
Special studies	None.	Direct immunofluorescence, to exclude other autoimmune bullous disorders, is negative.
Treatment	Reduction of exacerbating factors combined with keratolytics and antiseptic washes. Topical corticosteroids to reduce inflammation. Topical or oral retinoids to decrease hyperkeratosis.	Reduction of exacerbating factors such as friction from clothing, sweating, and secondary infection is key to control of the disease. First-line therapies include combination of topical antibiotics and intermittent topical corticosteroids or topical calcineurin inhibitors. Botulinum toxin injections efficacious in some cases to reduce sweating.

	Darier Disease	**Benign Familial Pemphigus (Hailey-Hailey Disease)**
Prognosis	Chronic disease that may be recalcitrant to treatment or relapse when therapy is stopped. Most individuals have significant impairment in quality of life.	Chronic disease with relapsing and remitting course.

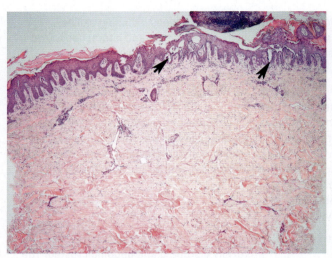

Figure 3.18.1 Darier disease. Hyperkeratosis and crust overlying an acanthotic epidermis with acantholysis (arrows).

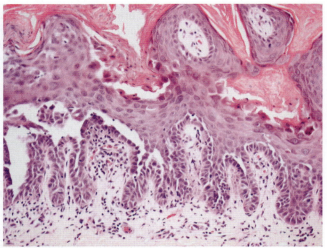

Figure 3.18.2 Darier disease. Suprabasal acantholysis with formation of a cleft. Note that the mid epidermis is generally intact and lacks a dilapidated look.

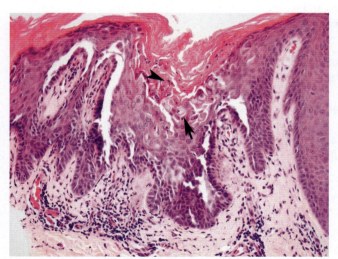

Figure 3.18.3 Darier disease. Suprabasal acantholysis with dyskeratosis and formation of corps ronds (arrow) and grains (arrowhead). Although Hailey-Hailey disease may have occasional dyskeratotic cells, the dyskeratosis is more prominent in Darier disease.

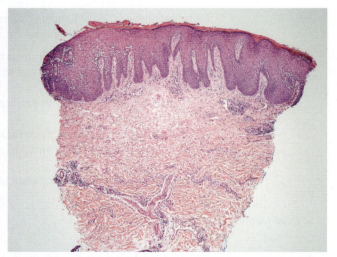

Figure 3.18.4 Benign familial pemphigus (Hailey-Hailey disease). Hyperplastic epidermis with hyperkeratosis and parakeratosis. Areas of the epidermis have a clefted appearance due to acantholysis.

3.18 Darier Disease vs Benign Familial Pemphigus (Hailey-Hailey Disease)

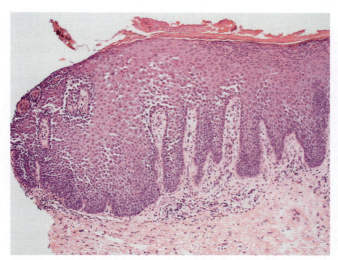

Figure 3.18.5 Benign familial pemphigus (Hailey-Hailey disease). Acantholysis involving the mid epidermis creating a "dilapidated brick wall" appearance. Note that there is no dyskeratosis (no formation of corps ronds or grains).

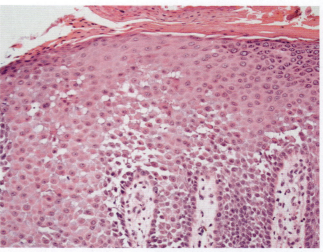

Figure 3.18.6 Benign familial pemphigus (Hailey-Hailey disease). Acantholysis of the epidermis with rounding up of dissociated keratinocytes throughout the epidermis. No corps ronds or grains are present.

SUGGESTED READINGS

Chapters 3.1-3.10

Agostinis P, Antonello RM. Pemphigoid gestationis. *N Engl J Med*. 2020;383(9):e61.

Al-Fouzan A W S, Galadari I, Oumeish I, Oumeish OY. Herpes gestationis (Pemphigoid gestationis). *Clin Dermatol*. 2006;24(2):109-112.

Bernard P, Antonicelli F. Bullous pemphigoid: a review of its diagnosis, associations and treatment. *Am J Clin Dermatol*. 2017;18(4):513-528.

Bolotin D, Petronic-Rosic V. Dermatitis herpetiformis. Part I. Epidemiology, pathogenesis, and clinical presentation. *J Am Acad Dermatol*. 2011;64(6):1017-1024; quiz 1025-1026.

Bolotin D, Petronic-Rosic V. Dermatitis herpetiformis. Part II. Diagnosis, management, and prognosis. *J Am Acad Dermatol*. 2011;64(6):1027-1033; quiz 1033-1034.

Buonavoglia A, Leone P, Dammacco R, et al. Pemphigus and mucous membrane pemphigoid: An update from diagnosis to therapy. *Autoimmun Rev*. 2019;18(4):349-358.

Caux F. Diagnosis and clinical features of epidermolysis bullosa acquisita. *Dermatol Clin*. 2011;29(3):485-491, x.

Chanal J, Ingen-Housz-Oro S, Ortonne N, et al. Linear IgA bullous dermatosis: comparison between the drug-induced and spontaneous forms. *Br J Dermatol*. 2013;169(5):1041-1048.

Du G, Patzelt S, van Beek N, Schmidt E. Mucous membrane pemphigoid. *Autoimmun Rev*. 2022;21(4):103036.

Fleming TE, Korman NJ. Cicatricial pemphigoid. *J Am Acad Dermatol*. 2000;43(4):571-591; quiz 591-594.

Gupta R, Woodley DT, Chen M. Epidermolysis bullosa acquisita. *Clin Dermatol*. 2012;30(1):60-69.

Hammers CM, Stanley JR. Mechanisms of disease: pemphigus and bullous pemphigoid. *Annu Rev Pathol*. 2016;11:175-197.

Jin MF, Wieland CN. Porphyria cutanea tarda. *Mayo Clin Proc*. 2021;96(5):1248-1249.

Junkins-Hopkins JM. Dermatitis herpetiformis: pearls and pitfalls in diagnosis and management. *J Am Acad Dermatol*. 2010;63(3):526-528.

Kanda N, Nakadaira N, Otsuka Y, Ishii N, Hoashi T, Saeki H. Linear IgA bullous dermatosis associated with ulcerative colitis: a case report and literature review. *Australas J Dermatol*. 2020;61(1):e82-e86.

Kershenovich R, Hodak E, Mimouni D. Diagnosis and classification of pemphigus and bullous pemphigoid. *Autoimmun Rev*. 2014;13(4-5):477-481.

Lammer J, Hein R, Roenneberg S, Biedermann T, Volz T. Drug-induced linear IgA bullous dermatosis: a case report and review of the literature. *Acta Derm Venereol*. 2019;99(6):508-515.

Long H, Zhang G, Wang L, Lu Q. Eosinophilic skin diseases: a comprehensive review. *Clin Rev Allergy Immunol*. 2016;50(2):189-213.

Massone C, Cerroni L, Heidrun N, Brunasso AMG, Nunzi E, Gulia A, Ambros-Rudolph CM. Histopathological diagnosis of atopic eruption of pregnancy and polymorphic eruption of pregnancy: a study on 41 cases. *Am J Dermatopathol*. 2014;36(10):812-821.

Montagnon CM, Lehman JS, Murrell DF, Camilleri MJ, Tolkachjov SN. Subepithelial autoimmune bullous dermatoses disease activity assessment and therapy. *J Am Acad Dermatol*. 2021;85(1):18-27.

Montagnon CM, Tolkachjov SN, Murrell DF, Camilleri MJ, Lehman JS. Subepithelial autoimmune blistering dermatoses: clinical features and diagnosis. *J Am Acad Dermatol*. 2021;85:1-14.

Onodera H, Mihm MC Jr, Yoshida A, Akasaka T. Drug-induced linear IgA bullous dermatosis. *J Dermatol*. 2005;32(9):759-764.

Patel PM, Jones VA, Murray TN, Amber KT. A review comparing international guidelines for the management of bullous pemphigoid, pemphigoid gestationis, mucous membrane pemphigoid, and epidermolysis bullosa acquisita. *Am J Clin Dermatol*. 2020;21(4):557-565.

Poblete-Gutiérrez P, Wiederholt T, Merk HF, Frank J. The porphyrias: clinical presentation, diagnosis and treatment. *Eur J Dermatol*. 2006;16(3):230-240.

Reunala T, Hervonen K, Salmi T. Dermatitis herpetiformis: an update on diagnosis and management. *Am J Clin Dermatol*. 2021;22(3):329-338.

Sarkany RP. The management of porphyria cutanea tarda. *Clin Exp Dermatol*. 2001;26(3):225-232.

Taylor D, Pappo E, Aronson IK. Polymorphic eruption of pregnancy. *Clin Dermatol*. 2016;34(3):383-391.

Tekin B, Johnson EF, Wieland CN, et al. Histopathology of autoimmune bullous dermatoses: what's new? *Hum Pathol*. 2022;128:69-89.

Ujiie H, Nishie W, Shimizu H. Pathogenesis of bullous pemphigoid. *Dermatol Clin*. 2011;29(3):439-446, ix.

Venning VA. Linear IgA disease: clinical presentation, diagnosis, and pathogenesis. *Dermatol Clin*. 2011;29(3):453-458, ix.

Vorobyev A, Ludwig RJ, Schmidt E. Clinical features and diagnosis of epidermolysis bullosa acquisita. *Expert Rev Clin Immunol*. 2017;13(2):157-169.

Chapters 3.10-3.18

Aldana PC, Khachemoune A. Grover disease: review of subtypes with a focus on management options. *Int J Dermatol*. 2020;59(5):543-550.

Ben Lagha I, Ashack K, Khachemoune A. Hailey-Hailey disease: an update review with a focus on treatment data. *Am J Clin Dermatol*. 2020;21(1):49-68.

Cooper SM, Burge SM. Darier's disease: epidemiology, pathophysiology, and management. *Am J Clin Dermatol*. 2003;4(2):97-105.

Davis MD, Dinneen AM, Landa N, Gibson LE. Grover's disease: clinicopathologic review of 72 cases. *Mayo Clin Proc*. 1999;74(3):229-234.

Engin B, Kutlubay Z, Çelik U, Serdaroğlu S, Tüzün Y. Hailey-Hailey disease: a fold (intertriginous) dermatosis. *Clin Dermatol*. 2015;33(4):452-455.

Grekin SJ, Fox MC, Gudjonsson JE, Fullen DR. Psoriasiform pemphigus foliaceus: a report of two cases. *J Cutan Pathol*. 2012;39(5):549-553.

Kassar S, Tounsi-Kettiti H, Charfeddine C, et al. Histological characterization of Darier's disease in Tunisian families. *J Eur Acad Dermatol Venereol.* 2009;23(10):1178-1183.

Korman AM, Milani-Nejad N. Darier disease. *JAMA Dermatol.* 2020;156(10):1125.

Lacarrubba F, Verzì AE, Errichetti E, Stinco G, Micali G. Darier disease: dermoscopy, confocal microscopy, and histologic correlations. *J Am Acad Dermatol.* 2015;73(3):e97-e99.

Lacarrubba F, Boscaglia S, Nasca MR, Caltabiano R, Micali G. Grover's disease: dermoscopy, reflectance confocal microscopy and histopathological correlation. *Dermatol Pract Concept.* 2017;7(3):51-54.

Maghfour J, Ly S, Haidari W, Taylor SL, Feldman SR. Treatment of keratosis pilaris and its variants: a systematic review. *J Dermatolog Treat.* 2022;33(3):1231-1242.

Mannschreck D, Feig J, Selph J, Cohen B. Disseminated bullous impetigo and atopic dermatitis: case series and literature review. *Pediatr Dermatol.* 2020;37(1):103-108.

Melchionda V, Harman KE. Pemphigus vulgaris and pemphigus foliaceus: an overview of the clinical presentation, investigations and management. *Clin Exp Dermatol.* 2019;44(7):740-746.

Ohata C, Ishii N, Furumura M. Locations of acantholysis in pemphigus vulgaris and pemphigus foliaceus. *J Cutan Pathol.* 2014;41(11):880-889.

Porro AM, Seque CA, Ferreira MCC, Enokihara MMSES. Pemphigus vulgaris. *An Bras Dermatol.* 2019;94(3):264-278.

Quirk CJ, Heenan PJ. Grover's disease: 34 years on. *Australas J Dermatol.* 2004;45(2):83-86; quiz 87-8.

Rogner DF, Lammer J, Zink A, Hamm H. Darier and Hailey-Hailey disease: update 2021. *J Dtsch Dermatol Ges.* 2021;19(10):1478-1501.

Schmidt E, Kasperkiewicz M, Joly P. Pemphigus. *Lancet.* 2019;394(10201):882-894.

Zhao CY, Murrell DF. Pemphigus vulgaris: an evidence-based treatment update. *Drugs.* 2015;75(3):271-284.

4 Disorders of the Adnexae

- **4.1** Androgenetic Alopecia vs Alopecia Areata
- **4.2** Androgenetic Alopecia vs Telogen Effluvium
- **4.3** Telogen Effluvium vs Alopecia Areata
- **4.4** Alopecia Areata vs Trichotillomania
- **4.5** Discoid Lupus Erythematosus Alopecia vs Lichen Planopilaris
- **4.6** Central Centrifugal Cicatricial Alopecia vs Lichen Planopilaris
- **4.7** Acne Rosacea vs Acne Vulgaris
- **4.8** Favre-Racouchot Syndrome vs Acne Vulgaris
- **4.9** Hidradenitis Suppurativa vs Follicular Infundibular Cyst
- **4.10** Hidradenitis Suppurativa vs Acne Keloidalis Nuchae
- **4.11** Keratosis Pilaris vs Infectious Folliculitis

4.1 ANDROGENETIC ALOPECIA VS ALOPECIA AREATA

	Androgenetic Alopecia	**Alopecia Areata**
Age	Adults primarily. May first present in adolescence.	Any age, majority of patients under the age of 30 years.
Location	Scalp.	Scalp primarily involved. Alopecia totalis involves entire scalp. Ophiasis pattern has hair loss on posterior and lateral aspects of scalp. Alopecia universalis also involves nonscalp locations including eyelashes, eyebrows, beard, and pubic region.
Etiology	Androgen-mediated miniaturization of hair follicles in genetically predisposed individuals.	Autoimmune etiology postulated with genetic contribution and modification by environmental factors.
Presentation	Gradual patterned reduction in hair density typically involving the anterior, vertex, and temporal areas of the skin. Hair loss is a continual process that waxes and wanes and is not associated with appreciable inflammation.	Sudden onset of one or more, well-defined, round to oval, patches of hair loss. At the periphery of the patches, there are small, abnormal hair shafts that have thinned proximal ends that resemble an exclamation point. Nail pitting may accompany the hair loss.
Histology	1. Normal interfollicular epidermis *(Fig. 4.1.1)*. 2. Normal overall number of hair follicles with increased number of vellus follicles. Decreased terminal:vellus follicle ratio (less than 2:1) *(Figs. 4.1.1 and 4.1.3)*. 3. Anagen follicles of varying caliber with some rooted in dermis and superficial subcutis *(Figs. 4.1.1, 4.1.2, 4.1.4)*. Mildly increased number of telogen follicles. No significant increase in catagen follicles. 4. Fibrous streamers (stelae) present below miniaturized follicles *(Figs. 4.1.1 and 4.1.2)*. 5. No significant inflammation or scar formation.	1. Normal interfollicular epidermis *(Fig. 4.1.5)*. 2. Normal overall number of hair follicles with increased number of vellus follicles in late stages. Decreased terminal:vellus follicle ratio (less than 2:1) *(Figs. 4.1.5 and 4.1.7)*. 3. Fibrous streamers (stelae) present below miniaturized follicles *(Fig. 4.1.7)*. Streamers may contain lymphocytes and eosinophils. 4. Increased number of terminal catagen and telogen follicles *(Figs. 4.1.5 and 4.1.6)*. 5. Lymphocytic infiltrate in and around the bulb of anagen and catagen follicles ("swarm of bees") *(Figs. 4.1.7 and 4.1.8)*. 6. No scar formation.
Special studies	None.	None.
Treatment	Topical minoxidil and oral finasteride are efficacious for both male and female androgenetic alopecia. Hair transplantation is alternative treatment option.	Intralesional and potent topical corticosteroids are preferred for limited hair loss. Extensive hair loss may be treated with topical immunotherapy or systemic corticosteroids.
Prognosis	Response to treatment is highly variable. The disease typically progresses with cessation of therapy. Although complete baldness is common in males, it is not generally seen in females.	Unpredictable course. May show spontaneous regrowth of hair. Recurrences common. Some show progressive loss of hair without regrowth. Poor outcomes associated with extensive hair loss, ophiasis pattern, nail changes, early age of onset, family history, and concomitant autoimmune disease.

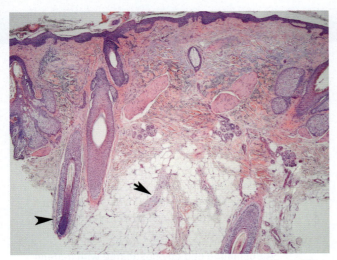

Figure 4.1.1 Androgenetic alopecia. Vertical section of scalp showing variation in caliber of anagen hair follicles with a diminutive anagen follicle rooted near dermal-subcutis interface (arrowhead). Presence of stela (arrow) is further evidence of miniaturization of follicles.

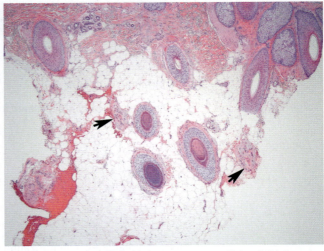

Figure 4.1.2 Androgenetic alopecia. Terminal anagen follicles of slightly varying caliber accompanied by stelae (arrows) indicative of miniaturization of follicles. Note that there is no appreciable inflammation.

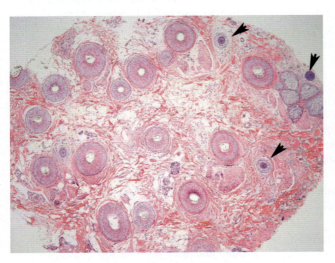

Figure 4.1.3 Androgenetic alopecia. Transverse section showing variation in caliber of anagen follicles with diminutive forms (arrows). There is no appreciable inflammation and no significant catagen/telogen shift.

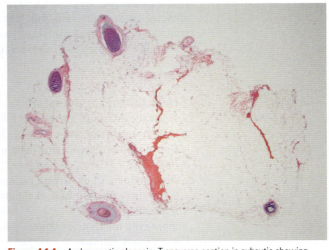

Figure 4.1.4 Androgenetic alopecia. Transverse section in subcutis showing reduced number of deeply rooted anagen follicles. Note that there is no inflammation associated with the residual bulbs.

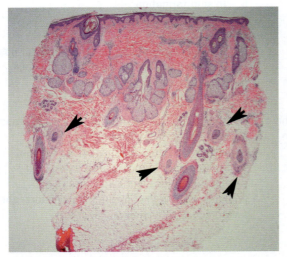

Figure 4.1.5 Alopecia areata. Vertical section of scalp with relatively normal overall number of follicular units. Dramatic increase in catagen follicles (arrows) with a few miniaturized follicles.

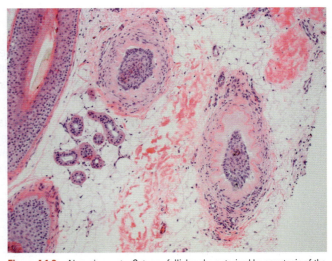

Figure 4.1.6 Alopecia areata. Catagen follicles characterized by apoptosis of the follicular epithelium and surrounding thickened fibrous root sheath.

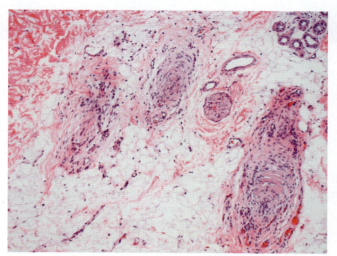 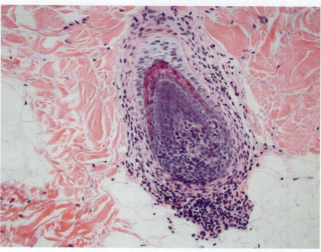

Figure 4.1.7 Alopecia areata. Like androgenetic alopecia, alopecia areata is characterized by miniaturization of follicles as evidenced by the presence of stelae. In alopecia areata, inflammatory cells are often seen in the stelae.

Figure 4.1.8 Alopecia areata. Active lymphocytic inflammation of an anagen bulb reminiscent of a "swarm of bees."

4.2 ANDROGENETIC ALOPECIA VS TELOGEN EFFLUVIUM

	Androgenetic Alopecia	**Telogen Effluvium**
Age	Adults primarily. May first present in adolescence.	Any age. In adults, females affected more than males.
Location	Scalp.	Scalp.
Etiology	Androgen-mediated miniaturization of hair follicles in genetically predisposed individuals.	Reactive disorder due to stress to the hair follicles resulting in altered regulation of follicular growth cycle. Triggering events include major illnesses, emotional stress, childbirth, metabolic disorders, drugs, and infections.
Presentation	Gradual patterned reduction in hair density typically involving the anterior, vertex, and temporal areas of the skin. Hair loss is a continual process that waxes and wanes and is not associated with appreciable inflammation.	Diffuse shedding of hair throughout entire scalp. Hair loss is not associated with erythema, scale, hair shaft abnormality, or scarring. May have insidious or abrupt onset.
Histology	1. Normal interfollicular epidermis *(Fig. 4.2.3)*. 2. Normal overall number of hair follicles with increased number of vellus follicles *(Figs. 4.2.2 and 4.2.3)*. Decreased terminal:vellus follicle ratio (less than 2:1) *(Fig. 4.2.4)*. 3. Anagen follicles of varying caliber with some rooted in dermis and superficial subcutis *(Figs. 4.2.1 and 4.2.2)*. Mildly increased number of telogen follicles. 4. Fibrous streamers present below miniaturized follicles *(Fig. 4.2.3)*. 5. No significant inflammation or scar formation.	1. Normal interfollicular epidermis *(Fig. 4.2.5)*. 2. Normal total number of hair follicles with no miniaturization of follicles or increase in number of vellus follicles (normal terminal:vellus ratio) *(Fig. 4.2.5)*. 3. Increased proportion of terminal catagen and telogen follicles (catagen/telogen shift) *(Figs. 4.2.5-4.2.8)*. 4. No significant inflammation.
Special studies	None.	None.
Treatment	Topical minoxidil and oral finasteride are efficacious for both male and female androgenetic alopecia. Hair transplantation is alternative treatment option.	Elimination or treatment of underlying trigger. Once cause is resolved, hair loss generally ceases and slow regrowth over months is expected.
Prognosis	Response to treatment is highly variable. The disease typically progresses with cessation of therapy. Although complete baldness is common in males, it is not generally seen in females.	Most cases show resolution with elimination of underlying cause. A minority of cases become chronic.

4.2 Androgenetic Alopecia vs Telogen Effluvium

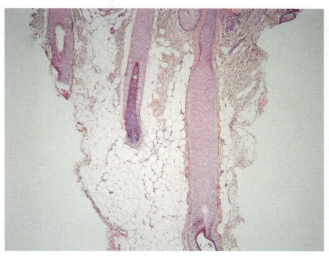

Figure 4.2.1 Androgenetic alopecia. Normal overall number of terminal anagen follicles with marked variation in the caliber of the follicles including diminutive follicle rooted in superficial subcutis.

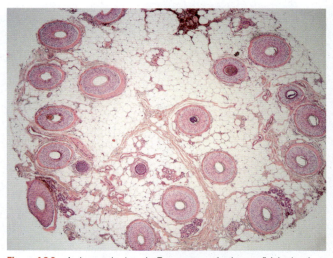

Figure 4.2.2 Androgenetic alopecia. Transverse section in superficial subcutis showing variation in caliber of terminal anagen follicles. Note that there is no appreciate catagen/telogen shift or inflammation.

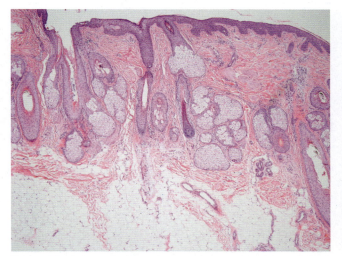

Figure 4.2.3 Androgenetic alopecia. Late stage characterized by miniaturization of follicular units; a feature not seen in telogen effluvium. Rare catagen/telogen follicles may be present, but the percentage is much less than that seen in telogen effluvium.

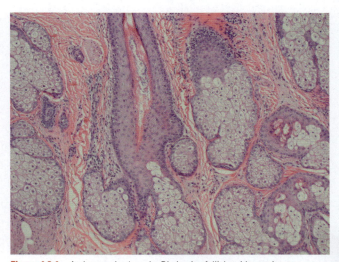

Figure 4.2.4 Androgenetic alopecia. Diminutive follicle with prominent sebaceous gland lobules.

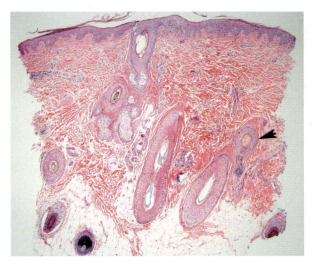

Figure 4.2.5 Telogen effluvium. Vertical section of scalp with normal overall number of hair follicles. The majority of follicles consist of terminal anagen follicles with an occasional telogen follicle (arrow).

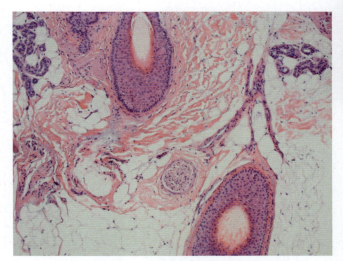

Figure 4.2.6 Telogen effluvium. Telogen follicles characterized by central cornified club hair shaft with serrated edge.

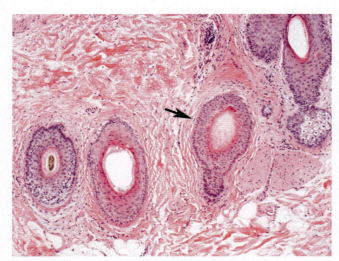

Figure 4.2.7 Telogen effluvium. Telogen follicle (arrow) adjacent to anagen follicles.

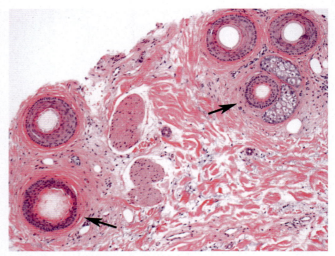

Figure 4.2.8 Telogen effluvium. Percentage of telogen and/or catagen follicles is best evaluated on transverse sections. In telogen effluvium, there is an increased percentage of telogen follicles, but typically less than 50%. In this section, there are two telogen follicles (arrows) and three anagen follicles.

4.3 TELOGEN EFFLUVIUM VS ALOPECIA AREATA

	Telogen Effluvium	**Alopecia Areata**
Age	Any age. In adults, females affected more than males.	Any age, majority of patients under the age of 30 years.
Location	Scalp.	Scalp primarily involved. Alopecia totalis involves entire scalp. Ophiasis pattern has hair loss on posterior and lateral aspects of scalp. Alopecia universalis also involves nonscalp locations including eyelashes, eyebrows, beard, and pubic region.
Etiology	Reactive disorder due to stress to the hair follicles resulting in altered regulation of follicular growth cycle. Triggering events include major illnesses, emotional stress, childbirth, metabolic disorders, drugs, and infections.	Autoimmune etiology postulated with genetic contribution and modification by environmental factors.
Presentation	Diffuse shedding of hair throughout entire scalp. Hair loss is not associated with erythema, scale, hair shaft abnormality, or scarring. May have insidious or abrupt onset.	Sudden onset of one or more, well-defined, round to oval, patches of hair loss. At the periphery of the patches, there are small, abnormal hair shafts that have thinned proximal ends that resemble an exclamation point. Nail pitting may accompany the hair loss.
Histology	1. Normal interfollicular epidermis *(Fig. 4.3.1)*. 2. Normal total number of hair follicles with no miniaturization of follicles or increase in number of vellus follicles (normal terminal:vellus ratio) *(Fig. 4.3.1)*. 3. Increased proportion of terminal catagen and telogen follicles *(Figs. 4.3.2-4.3.4)*. Percentage of telogen follicles typically less than 50%. 4. No significant inflammation.	1. Normal interfollicular epidermis *(Fig. 4.3.5)*. 2. Normal overall number of hair follicles with increased number of vellus follicles *(Fig. 4.3.5)*. Decreased terminal:vellus follicle ratio (less than 2:1). 3. Fibrous streamers (stelae) present below miniaturized follicles *(Figs. 4.3.5* and *4.3.8)*. Streamers may contain lymphocytes and eosinophils. 4. Increased number of terminal catagen and telogen follicles (catagen/telogen shift) *(Fig. 4.3.6)*. Percentage of catagen/telogen follicles typically greater than 50%. 5. Lymphocytic infiltrate in and around the bulb of anagen follicles ("swarm of bees") *(Figs. 4.3.5* and *4.3.7)*. 6. No scar formation.
Special studies	None.	None.
Treatment	Elimination or treatment of underlying trigger. Once cause is resolved, hair loss generally ceases and slow regrowth over months is expected.	Intralesional and potent topical corticosteroids are preferred for limited hair loss. Extensive hair loss may be treated with topical immunotherapy or systemic corticosteroids.

(continued)

	Telogen Effluvium	**Alopecia Areata**
Prognosis	Most cases show resolution with elimination of underlying cause. A minority of cases become chronic.	Unpredictable course. May show spontaneous regrowth of hair. Recurrences common. Some show progressive loss of hair without regrowth. Poor outcomes associated with extensive hair loss, ophiasis pattern, nail changes, early age of onset, family history, and concomitant autoimmune disease.

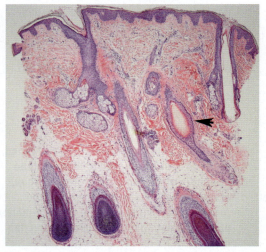

Figure 4.3.1 Telogen effluvium. Vertical section showing relatively normal number of hair follicles for scalp. The majority of follicles consist of terminal anagen follicles. There is a rare telogen follicle (arrow). Note that there is no appreciable inflammation around the anagen bulbs and no miniaturization of follicles.

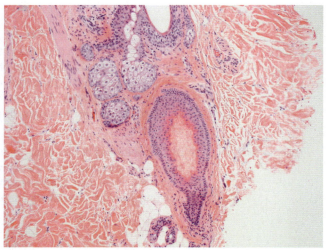

Figure 4.3.2 Telogen effluvium. Telogen effluvium is characterized by an increased number of telogen and/or catagen follicles. Telogen follicles are characterized by a club hair shaft that has a serrated contour that interdigitates with the follicular epithelium.

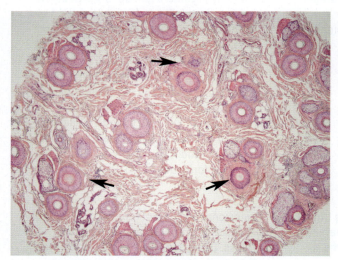

Figure 4.3.3 Telogen effluvium. Follicular counts are best performed on transverse sections. In telogen effluvium, there is an increase in telogen follicles (arrows) but typically representing less than 50%. The percentage of catagen/telogen follicles is greater in alopecia areata and accompanied by bulbar lymphocytic inflammation.

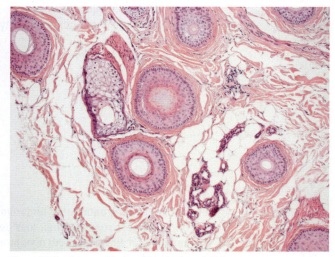

Figure 4.3.4 Telogen effluvium. Central telogen follicle on transverse section.

4.3 Telogen Effluvium vs Alopecia Areata

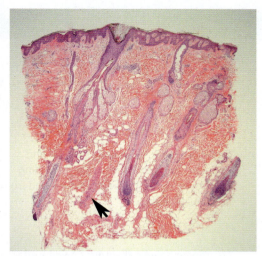

Figure 4.3.5 Alopecia areata. Vertical section of scalp with relatively normal overall number of follicular units. A peribulbar lymphocytic infiltrate is associated with anagen follicles. Rare stela (arrow) suggesting miniaturization of follicles.

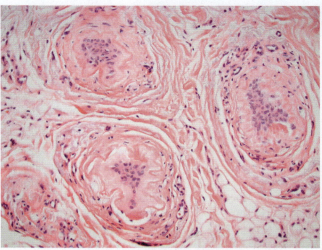

Figure 4.3.6 Alopecia areata. Like telogen effluvium, alopecia areata has an increased percentage of catagen/telogen follicles. The percentage of follicles in catagen, as seen here, is higher in alopecia areata, typically over 50%.

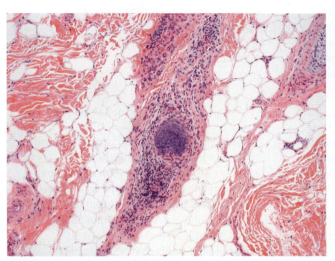

Figure 4.3.7 Alopecia areata. Lymphocytic infiltrate around bulb of anagen follicle with a "swarm of bees" appearance. Telogen effluvium does not have an appreciable inflammatory component.

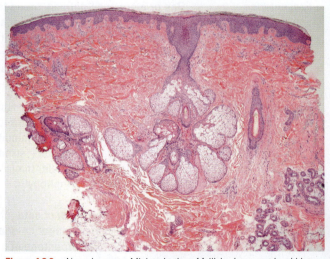

Figure 4.3.8 Alopecia areata. Miniaturization of follicles is present in mid-late stages of alopecia areata and is not a feature of telogen effluvium.

4.4 ALOPECIA AREATA VS TRICHOTILLOMANIA

	Alopecia Areata	**Trichotillomania**
Age	Any age, majority of patients under the age of 30 years.	Children, adolescents, and young adults. Females more commonly than males.
Location	Scalp primarily involved. Alopecia totalis involves entire scalp. Ophiasis pattern has hair loss on posterior and lateral aspects of scalp. Alopecia universalis also involves nonscalp locations including eyelashes, eyebrows, beard, and pubic region.	Scalp primarily, especially parietal and temporal regions. Other areas, including eyebrows, eyelashes, extremities, and trunk may be involved.
Etiology	Autoimmune etiology postulated with genetic contribution and modification by environmental factors.	Neuropsychologic disorder considered to be a component of obsessive-compulsive disorder characterized by repetitive, self-induced hair pulling.
Presentation	One or more, well-defined, round to oval, patches of hair loss. At the periphery of the patches, there are small, abnormal hair shafts that have thinned proximal ends that resemble an exclamation point. Nail pitting may accompany the hair loss.	Alopecic plaques of varying size, often geometric and sharply defined, that have hair of different lengths and various stages of regrowth.
Histology	1. Normal interfollicular epidermis *(Fig. 4.4.1)*. 2. Normal overall number of hair follicles with increased number of miniaturized follicles *(Fig. 4.4.1)*. Stelae ("streamers") are evidence of follicular miniaturization and may contain lymphocytic inflammation *(Figs. 4.4.4)*. 3. Increased proportion of catagen and telogen follicles (catagen/telogen shift) *(Figs. 4.4.1-4.4.3)*. Percentage of catagen/telogen follicles typically greater than 50%. 4. Lymphocytic infiltrate in and around the bulb of anagen and catagen follicles ("swarm of bees") *(Figs. 4.4.2 and 4.4.3)*. 5. No scar formation.	1. Normal overall number of hair follicles *(Fig. 4.4.5)*. 2. Mildly increased number of catagen and telogen follicles (less than 50%) *(Figs. 4.4.5 and 4.4.6)*. No miniaturization of follicles. 3. Distorted follicular anatomy with pigment casts, trichomalacia, fractured hair shafts, and melanin pigment in collapsed fibrous root sheaths *(Figs. 4.4.5, 4.4.7, 4.4.8)*. 4. Absence of peribulbar lymphocytic infiltrate.
Special studies	None.	None.
Treatment	Intralesional and potent topical corticosteroids are preferred for limited hair loss. Extensive hair loss may be treated with topical immunotherapy or systemic corticosteroids.	Cognitive behavior therapy is first line of therapy. Psychopharmacological treatment, primarily with selective serotonin reuptake inhibitors, may be indicated in cases with lack of response to cognitive behavior therapy.

4.4 Alopecia Areata vs Trichotillomania

	Alopecia Areata	**Trichotillomania**
Prognosis	Unpredictable course. May show spontaneous regrowth of hair. Recurrences common. Some show progressive loss of hair without regrowth. Poor outcomes associated with extensive hair loss, ophiasis pattern, nail changes, early age of onset, family history, and concomitant autoimmune disease.	Recurrent episodes with complete remission if adequately treated.

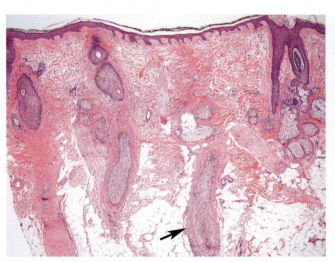

Figure 4.4.1 Alopecia areata. Scalp biopsy with relatively normal overall number of hair follicles. Note terminal catagen follicle (arrow) and miniaturized follicles.

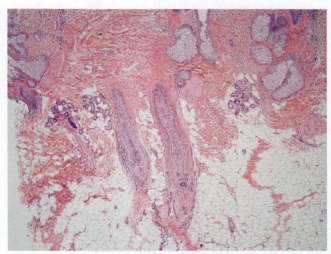

Figure 4.4.2 Alopecia areata. Terminal catagen hair follicles with peribulbar lymphomononuclear inflammatory infiltrate.

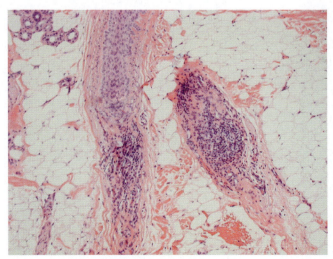

Figure 4.4.3 Alopecia areata. Peribulbar lymphocytic infiltrate surrounding catagen hair follicle ("swarm of bees") and within stela.

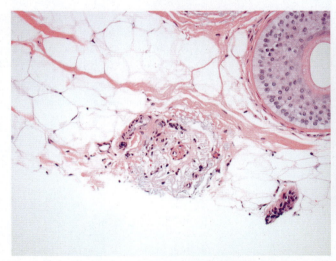

Figure 4.4.4 Alopecia areata. On transverse section, follicular stela ("streamer"), as evidence of follicular miniaturization, adjacent to a terminal anagen follicle.

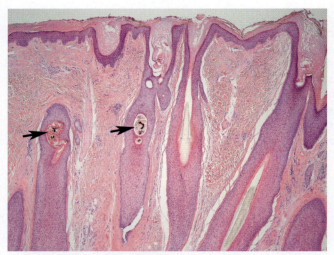

Figure 4.4.5 Trichotillomania. Normal total number of terminal anagen hair follicles. There is compact hyperkeratosis with infundibular dilatation suggestive of chronic rubbing. Two follicles have pigment casts (arrows). Note that there is minimal inflammation.

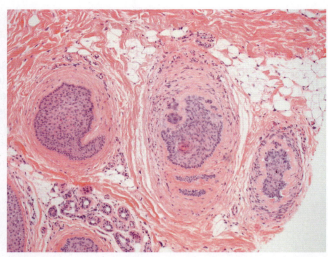

Figure 4.4.6 Trichotillomania. Mild increase in catagen follicles on transverse sections. No appreciable inflammation or miniaturization of hair follicles.

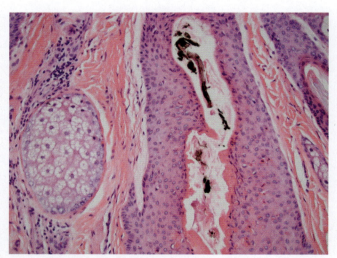

Figure 4.4.7 Trichotillomania. Pigment cast formation and trichomalacia in a mildly distorted follicular lumen.

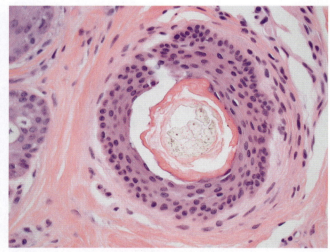

Figure 4.4.8 Trichotillomania. Trichomalacia with disruption of the inner root sheath from forcible pulling of hair shaft.

4.5 DISCOID LUPUS ERYTHEMATOSUS ALOPECIA VS LICHEN PLANOPILARIS

	Discoid Lupus Erythematosus Alopecia	**Lichen Planopilaris**
Age	Any age, predominately between 20 and 40 years of age.	Adults, between 40 and 60 years of age; predominately women.
Location	Scalp.	Scalp and, less commonly, hair on the face and body.
Etiology	Chronic autoimmune disease initiated by an environmental trigger in a genetic susceptible individual.	Unknown but theorized to be a follicle-specific autoimmune disorder due to activated T lymphocytes targeting follicular antigens and initiating a cell-mediated cytotoxic reaction. Exogenous or endogenous agents may function as triggers for the autoimmune response.
Presentation	Well-circumscribed, round-oval, erythematous indurated plaques. There may be associated follicular plugging, telangiectasia, atrophy, with central hypopigmentation and peripheral hyperpigmentation. Late-stage lesions show loss of follicular ostia and scar formation.	Multifocal areas of permanent hair loss (absent follicular ostia) that coalesce into larger patches. Perifollicular erythema and hyperkeratosis at the periphery of the patches. May have associated scalp pruritus, burning, or tenderness. Cutaneous and/or mucosa lesions of lichen planus may be present. Clinical variants include frontal fibrosing alopecia with band-like hair loss of frontotemporal scalp and Graham-Little syndrome characterized by scarring scalp alopecia, nonscarring alopecia of axillae and groin, and cutaneous lichenoid follicular papules.
Histology	1. Interface vacuolar change with necrotic basal keratinocytes, epidermal atrophy, and follicular plugging *(Figs. 4.5.2-4.5.4)*. 2. Superficial and deep, perivascular, perifollicular, and perieccrine lymphocytic infiltrate *(Fig. 4.5.1)*. 3. Reduced density of follicular units and sebaceous gland lobules with scar formation in late stage. 4. Mucin deposition in reticular dermis on colloidal iron stain *(Fig. 4.5.5)*. 5. Scar formation in late stage.	1. Normal interfollicular epidermis with generally no interface alteration *(Figs. 4.5.6 and 4.5.8)*. 2. Follicular hypergranulosis with lichenoid lymphomononuclear infiltrate affecting infundibulum and isthmus *(Figs. 4.5.7 and 4.5.8)*. No appreciate perivascular or perieccrine inflammation. 3. Asymmetric thinning of the follicular epithelium with diminished to absent sebaceous glands *(Figs. 4.5.8 and 4.5.9)*. 4. Concentric fibroplasia around affected follicles with artifactual clefting between follicular epithelium and stroma *(Figs. 4.5.8 and 4.5.9)*. 5. Scar formation where follicles have been destroyed. No appreciable mucin accumulation.
Special studies	Direct immunofluorescence shows granular IgG, IgM, and C3 deposition along the dermal-epidermal junction.	Direct immunofluorescence shows cytoid body staining with anti-IgM and anti-IgA.

(continued)

	Discoid Lupus Erythematosus Alopecia	Lichen Planopilaris
Treatment	Photoprotection. First-line therapies include topical and intralesional corticosteroids and hydroxychloroquine. Oral retinoids, methotrexate, thalidomide, and immunomodulatory agents may be used as second-line therapies.	Primary goals of treatment are to alleviate symptoms and to prevent additional hair loss. Topical and intralesional corticosteroids are first-line therapies. Systemic corticosteroids and hydroxychloroquine for recalcitrant or rapidly progressive cases.
Prognosis	Active disease generally responds well to therapy. Once scarring has occurred, the hair loss is permanent.	Chronic disorder with unpredictable course. Response to therapy is variable and generally only seen in active stages of disease. Treatment does not induce hair growth in areas of scarring.

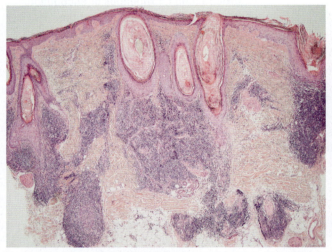

Figure 4.5.1 Discoid lupus erythematosus alopecia. Dense superficial and deep perivascular and periadnexal lymphocytic infiltrate. Note the prominent follicular plugging.

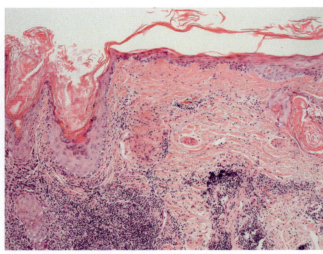

Figure 4.5.2 Discoid lupus erythematosus alopecia. Vacuolar interface alteration involving interfollicular epidermis and follicular units. There is epidermal atrophy.

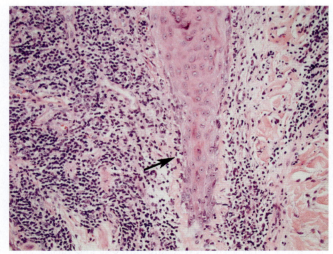

Figure 4.5.3 Discoid lupus erythematosus alopecia. Interface vacuolar change (arrow) involving follicular unit with surrounding dense lymphocytic infiltrate. Note that there is no appreciable perifollicular fibroplasia.

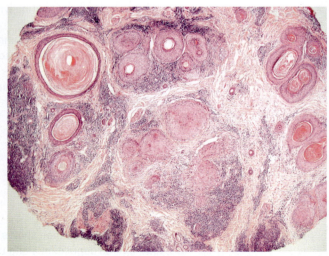

Figure 4.5.4 Discoid lupus erythematosus alopecia. Transverse section showing dense perifollicular inflammation and follicular plugging. Progressive destruction of follicles, as seen centrally, leads to scarring in later stages of the disease.

4.5 Discoid Lupus Erythematosus Alopecia vs Lichen Planopilaris

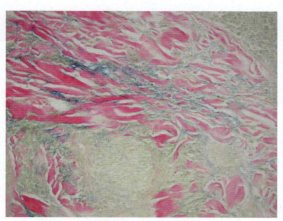

Figure 4.5.5 Discoid lupus erythematosus alopecia. Colloidal iron stain demonstrating mucin deposition in reticular dermis.

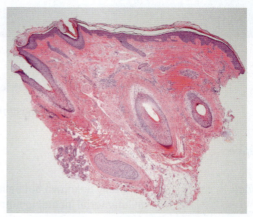

Figure 4.5.6 Lichen planopilaris. Scalp biopsy with lymphocytic inflammation associated with terminal hair follicles that have early concentric fibroplasia. Unlike lupus erythematosus, there is no appreciable deep perivascular or perieccrine inflammation. Note that there is no follicular plugging or mucin deposition.

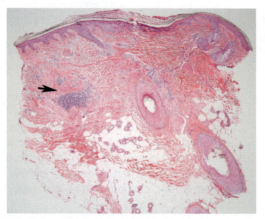

Figure 4.5.7 Lichen planopilaris. Scalp biopsy with reduced number of terminal hair follicles. Follicular unit replaced by scar (arrow) with residual lichenoid lymphocytic inflammation. The interfollicular epidermis is intact and without interface vacuolar alteration.

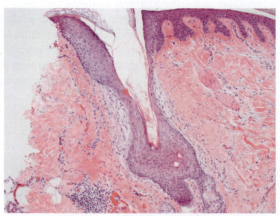

Figure 4.5.8 Lichen planopilaris. Interface vacuolar alteration of follicular infundibulum with thinning of the follicular epithelium. Note that there is no interfollicular epidermal vacuolar change and the epidermis is of normal thickness.

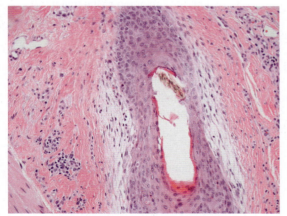

Figure 4.5.9 Lichen planopilaris. Interface vacuolar alteration with loss of the basal zone of the follicular epithelium. Thinning of the follicular epithelium with concentric loose fibroplasia.

4.6 CENTRAL CENTRIFUGAL CICATRICIAL ALOPECIA VS LICHEN PLANOPILARIS

	Central Centrifugal Cicatricial Alopecia	**Lichen Planopilaris**
Age	Middle-aged adults; most often African-American women.	Adults, between 40 and 60 years of age; predominately women.
Location	Scalp.	Scalp, less commonly, hair on the face and body.
Etiology	Generally unknown but believed to be multifactorial including autoimmune, genetic, environmental, and infectious causes. Use of chemical relaxers, hot combs, and other caustic chemicals has been implicated in the pathogenesis but has not been validated.	Unknown but theorized to be a follicle-specific autoimmune disorder due to activated T lymphocytes targeting follicular antigens and initiating a cell-mediated cytotoxic reaction. Exogenous or endogenous agents may function as triggers for the autoimmune response.
Presentation	Scarring alopecia that begins on the vertex or central crown of the scalp and progresses centrifugally in a symmetric fashion. Variable amount of associated erythema and crusting. Associated with tenderness and burning. May have islands of preserved follicles with polytrichia.	Multifocal areas of permanent hair loss (absent follicular ostia) that coalesce into larger patches. Perifollicular erythema and hyperkeratosis at the periphery of the patches. May have associated scalp pruritus, burning, or tenderness. Cutaneous and/or mucosa lesions of lichen planus may be present. Clinical variants include frontal fibrosing alopecia with band-like hair loss of frontotemporal scalp and Graham-Little syndrome characterized by scarring scalp alopecia, nonscarring alopecia of axillae and groin, and cutaneous lichenoid follicular papules.
Histology	1. Normal interfollicular epidermis *(Fig. 4.6.1)*. 2. Earliest feature is premature desquamation of the inner root sheath *(Figs. 4.6.1-4.6.3)*. 3. Eccentric follicular epithelial thinning and patchy lymphomononuclear infiltrate in the infundibular and isthmic regions *(Fig. 4.6.4)*. No significant interface vacuolar change, cytoid bodies, or hypergranulosis. 4. Concentric lamellar fibroplasia but no cleft formation between epithelium and stroma *(Fig. 4.6.4)*. 5. Destruction of hair follicles in late-stage lesions with scar formation, naked hair shafts, and polytrichia of residual follicles *(Fig. 4.6.5)*.	1. Normal interfollicular epidermis with no interface alteration *(Fig. 4.6.6)*. 2. Follicular hypergranulosis with lichenoid lymphomononuclear infiltrate affecting infundibulum and isthmus *(Figs. 4.6.6 and 4.6.7)*. 3. Asymmetric thinning of the follicular epithelium with diminished to absent sebaceous glands *(Figs. 4.6.8 and 4.6.9)*. 4. Concentric fibroplasia around affected follicles with artifactual clefting between follicular epithelium and stroma *(Fig. 4.6.8)*. 5. Scar formation where follicles have been destroyed *(Fig. 4.6.6)*.
Special studies	None.	Direct immunofluorescence shows cytoid body staining with anti-IgM and anti-IgA.

4.6 Central Centrifugal Cicatricial Alopecia vs Lichen Planopilaris

	Central Centrifugal Cicatricial Alopecia	**Lichen Planopilaris**
Treatment	Goals of treatment are to prevent further hair loss, minimize symptoms, and possibly stimulate regrowth of hair. First-line therapies include topical and intralesional corticosteroids combined with oral tetracycline antibiotics. Modification of hair care practices with avoidance of traction on hair follicles and discontinuation of the use of chemical relaxers.	Primary goals of treatment are to alleviate symptoms and to prevent additional hair loss. Topical and intralesional corticosteroids are first-line therapies. Systemic corticosteroids and hydroxychloroquine for recalcitrant or rapidly progressive cases.
Prognosis	Treatment is generally effective in active disease, before extensive scarring and destruction of hair follicles, with most experiencing decreased hair loss and improvement in symptoms.	Chronic disorder with unpredictable course. Response to therapy is variable and generally only seen in active stages of disease. Treatment does not induce hair growth in areas of scarring.

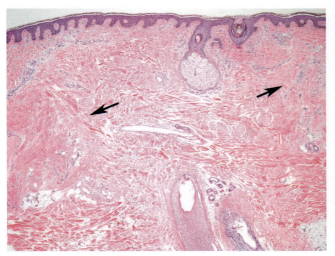

Figure 4.6.1 Central centrifugal cicatricial alopecia. Vertical section of scalp with reduced number of terminal anagen follicles. Follicular units replaced by scar (arrows).

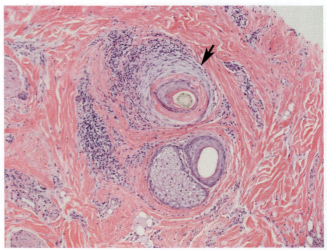

Figure 4.6.2 Central centrifugal cicatricial alopecia. Transverse section showing perifollicular lichenoid lymphocytic infiltrate and concentric lamellar fibroplasia (arrow). The follicular epithelium shows premature desquamation of the inner root sheath, the hallmark of the disorder.

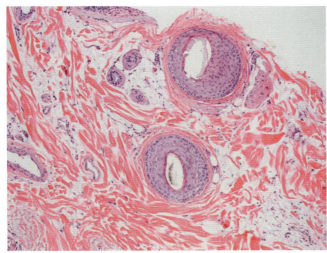

Figure 4.6.3 Central centrifugal cicatricial alopecia. Two follicles showing premature desquamation of the inner root sheath without significant inflammation, a feature not seen in lichen planopilaris.

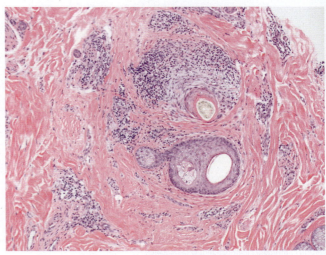

Figure 4.6.4 Central centrifugal cicatricial alopecia. Concentric fibroplasia and asymmetric thinning of the follicular epithelium. The hair shaft is in close approximation to the dermis.

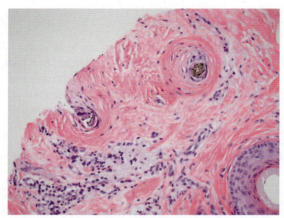

Figure 4.6.5 Central centrifugal cicatricial alopecia. Naked hair shafts in dermis due to destruction of follicular units.

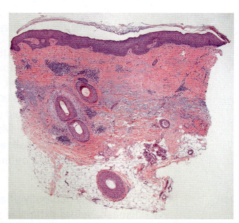

Figure 4.6.6 Lichen planopilaris. Vertical section of scalp showing decreased number of terminal follicular units and areas of scar. Residual units have associated lymphocytic inflammation.

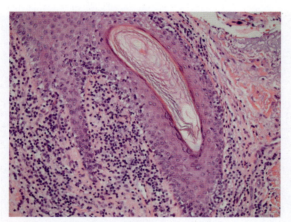

Figure 4.6.7 Lichen planopilaris. Active lymphocytic inflammation with interface vacuolization involving follicular infundibulum.

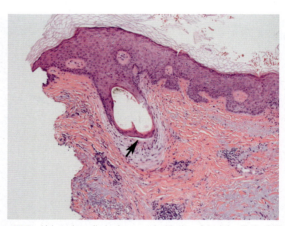

Figure 4.6.8 Lichen planopilaris. Asymmetric thinning of the infundibular follicular epithelium with surrounding fibroplasia and focal cleft formation between epithelium and fibroplasia (arrow). Similar features are seen in central centrifugal cicatricial alopecia but without clefting and accompanied by premature desquamation of the inner root sheath.

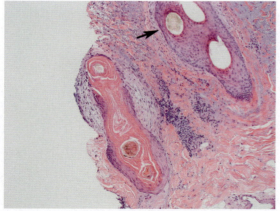

Figure 4.6.9 Lichen planopilaris. Pronounced thinning of the follicular epithelium with surrounding concentric fibroplasia and patchy lymphocytic inflammation. Fusion of follicular units (arrow) leads to polytrichia, a finding that may be seen in central centrifugal cicatricial alopecia as well.

4.7 ACNE ROSACEA VS ACNE VULGARIS

	Acne Rosacea	Acne Vulgaris
Age	Adults between 30 and 50 years of age.	Children and adolescents; particularly teenage years.
Location	Cheeks, nose, chin, and forehead.	Areas with high density of sebaceous glands including face, chest, and back.
Etiology	Multifactorial etiology that is incompletely understood. Involves genetic factors, dysregulation of innate immune system, vasoactive and neurocutaneous mechanisms, and altered colonization of *Demodex folliculorum* microorganisms. Precipitating factors include heat, stress, alcohol, hot beverages, spicy foods, and sun exposure.	Multifactorial etiology that involves keratinocyte hyperproliferation, androgen-induced increased sebum production, comedone formation, inflammation, and altered colonization of hair follicles with *Propionibacterium acnes*.
Presentation	Erythema with telangiectasia, papules, and pustules. Absence of comedones. Often with background of transient and nontransient facial flushing.	Primary lesion is the comedone, both open and closed, but may also have inflammatory papules, nodules, and pustules. Often associated with postinflammatory pigmentary changes and scarring. Telangiectasia generally not present.
Histology	1. Normal epidermis *(Fig. 4.7.1)*. 2. Perivascular and perifollicular inflammatory infiltrate of lymphocytes, plasma cells, and neutrophils *(Figs. 4.7.1-4.7.3)*. Neutrophils extend beyond the follicle in some cases. Loose perifollicular granulomas may be present *(Fig. 4.7.1)*. 3. Conspicuous number of *D. folliculorum* in lumen of hair follicles *(Fig. 4.7.3)*. 4. Telangiectasia and mild dermal edema *(Fig. 4.7.4)*.	1. Comedone formation consisting of dilated follicular lumen distended by keratin and bacteria *(Figs. 4.7.5* and *4.7.6)*. 2. Thinning of the follicular epithelium *(Fig. 4.7.7)*. 3. Perifollicular inflammation with neutrophils confined to follicle *(Figs. 4.7.6* and *4.7.7)*. 4. No apparent telangiectasia or significant perivascular inflammation.
Special studies	None.	May perform tissue Gram stain to demonstrate bacteria *(Fig. 4.7.8)* but generally not needed for assessment.
Treatment	Avoidance of triggering factors, gentle skin care, and photoprotection. Topical modalities including metronidazole and azelaic acid. Topical brimonidine and oxymetazoline for facial erythema. Laser and intense pulsed light therapies used for telangiectasias and erythema.	Topical therapies including benzoyl peroxide, retinoids, and antibiotics for mild disease. More severe cases may require oral antibiotics combined with topical benzoyl peroxide to reduce antibiotic resistance. Oral isotretinoin is highly effective for moderate to severe disease.
Prognosis	Chronic disease. Although benign, may be associated with low self-esteem, anxiety, and depression.	Severe cases may lead to scarring. Common, benign disease but may be associated with considerable psychological morbidity affecting quality of life.

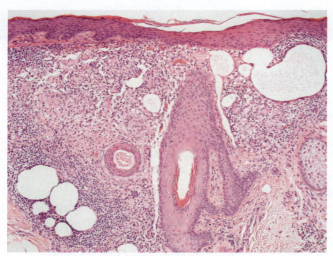

Figure 4.7.1 Acne rosacea. Dense perifollicular mixed inflammatory infiltrate. Infiltrate includes formation of loose noncaseating granulomas, neutrophils, lymphocytes, and plasma cells. Note the absence of comedone formation.

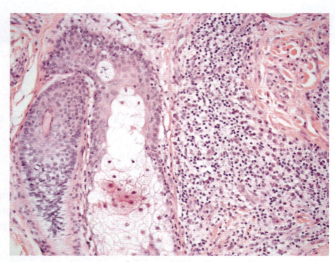

Figure 4.7.2 Acne rosacea. Sebaceous follicle with surrounding lymphoplasmacytic infiltrate.

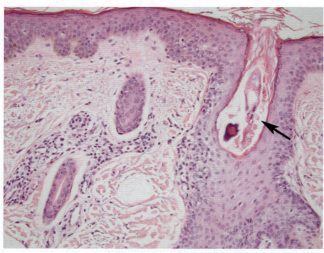

Figure 4.7.3 Acne rosacea. Follicular unit containing *Demodex folliculorum* within lumen (arrow). Inflammation extends beyond the follicle around the vascular plexus.

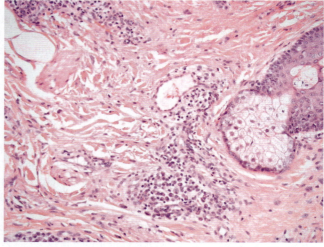

Figure 4.7.4 Acne rosacea. Perifollicular and perivascular infiltrate of lymphocytes and plasma cells. There is associated telangiectasia of vessels and mild edema.

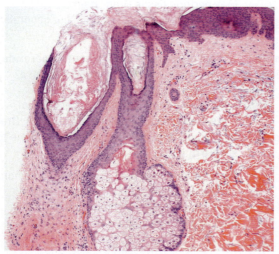

Figure 4.7.5 Acne vulgaris. Sebaceous hair follicles showing open comedone formation with dilated lumens filled with loose keratin.

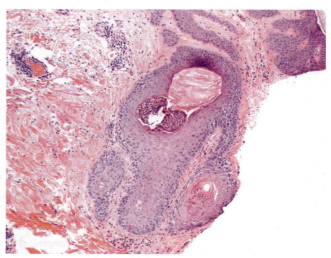

Figure 4.7.6 Acne vulgaris. Closed comedone formation with dilated follicular lumen distended by laminated keratin and neutrophils. Note that neutrophils are confined to follicle.

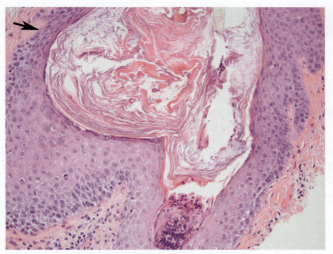

Figure 4.7.7 Acne vulgaris. Follicular lumen is distended by keratin, basophilic debris, and neutrophils. The follicular epithelium is thinned (arrow).

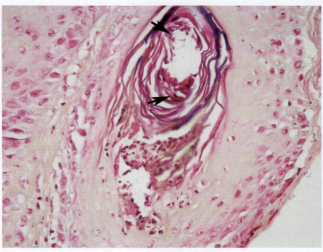

Figure 4.7.8 Acne vulgaris. Tissue Gram stain revealing gram-positive bacilli (arrows) within the lumen of the inflamed comedone.

4.8 FAVRE-RACOUCHOT SYNDROME VS ACNE VULGARIS

	Favre-Racouchot Syndrome	**Acne Vulgaris**
Age	Elderly. Males affected more than females.	Children and adolescents; particularly teenage years.
Location	Facial locations in areas of sun exposure, especially temples, periorbital regions, and lateral canthal areas. Less commonly seen on malar eminence, neck, earlobes, and postauricular regions.	Areas with high density of sebaceous glands including face, chest, and back.
Etiology	Excessive ultraviolet radiation, physical agents such as harsh weather, and ionizing radiation. Heavy smoking is also implicated in the pathogenesis.	Multifactorial etiology that involves keratinocyte hyperproliferation, androgen-induced increased sebum production, comedone formation, inflammation, and altered colonization of hair follicles with *Propionibacterium acnes*.
Presentation	Grouped, large open comedones and cystic nodules in actinically damaged skin that appears thickened and yellow with deep furrows.	Primary lesion is the comedone, both open and closed but may also have inflammatory papules, nodules, and pustules. Often associated with postinflammatory pigmentary changes and scarring. Telangiectasia typically not present.
Histology	1. Epidermal atrophy with prominent nodular elastosis and fragmented elastic fibers *(Figs. 4.8.1-4.8.3)*. 2. Dilation of follicular infundibulum with distention of the lumen by loose lamellar keratin (comedones) *(Figs. 4.8.1-4.8.3)*. Some follicles have cystic dilation. 3. Atrophy of the follicular epithelium with decreased/absent sebaceous glands *(Fig. 4.8.3)*. 4. Comedones may also contain bacteria and sebum.	1. Dilated follicular lumen distended by keratin and bacteria *(Figs. 4.8.4* and *4.8.5)*. 2. Thinning of the follicular epithelium *(Figs. 4.8.4, 4.8.5)*. 3. Variable inflammation that may be dense if comedone ruptures *(Figs. 4.8.4* and *4.8.5)*. 4. No significant dermal solar elastosis.
Special studies	None.	Tissue Gram stain may be performed to detect bacteria but generally not necessary.
Treatment	Topical tretinoin as well as manual treatments such as cryotherapy, CO_2 laser ablation, comedone extraction, salicylic acid peel, dermabrasion, curettage, and surgical excision. Sun protection and smoking cessation also recommended.	Topical therapies including benzoyl peroxide, retinoids, and antibiotics for mild disease. More severe cases may require oral antibiotics combined with topical benzoyl peroxide to reduce antibiotic resistance. Oral isotretinoin is highly effective for moderate to severe disease.
Prognosis	Benign condition that is not associated with increased risk of malignancy. Persists without treatment and may recur after therapy.	Severe cases may lead to scarring. Common, benign disease but may be associated with considerable psychological morbidity affecting quality of life.

4.8 Favre-Racouchot Syndrome vs Acne Vulgaris

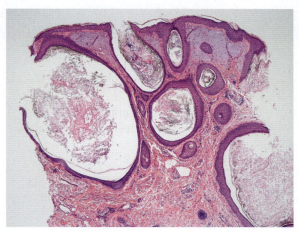

Figure 4.8.1 Favre-Racouchot syndrome. Open and closed comedones with small cysts in a background of chronic solar damage with nodular elastosis of the dermis.

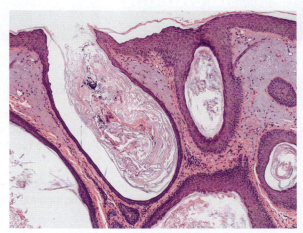

Figure 4.8.2 Favre-Racouchot syndrome. Comedones characterized by dilated follicular infundibula distended by keratin. The open comedone has thinned epithelium. Note the nodular elastosis in the surrounding dermis.

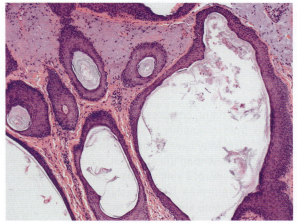

Figure 4.8.3 Favre-Racouchot syndrome. Formation of comedones and cysts containing keratinous debris. The surrounding dermis has nodular elastosis but generally no appreciable inflammation.

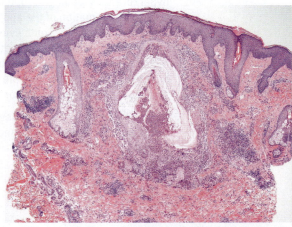

Figure 4.8.4 Acne vulgaris. Comedone formation with reactive epidermal changes. The central closed comedone is ruptured and there is a dense perifollicular mixed inflammatory infiltrate. Note that there is no appreciable elastosis in the dermis.

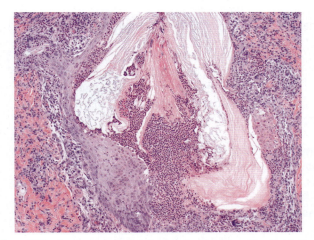

Figure 4.8.5 Acne vulgaris. Ruptured comedone with release of keratin into the dermis and dense mixed inflammation with neutrophils predominating within the follicular lumen.

4.9 HIDRADENITIS SUPPURATIVA VS FOLLICULAR INFUNDIBULAR CYST

	Hidradenitis Suppurativa	**Follicular Infundibular Cyst**
Age	Onset in postpuberty adolescence to early adulthood, with peak in second and third decades of life. Females affected more than males.	Typically young adults primarily between third and fourth decades of life. Rare before puberty.
Location	Intertriginous regions including axillae, inframammary folds, inguinal creases, and perineum.	May occur on any hair-bearing region but most common on face, neck, trunk, and scrotum.
Etiology	Multifactorial with contributions from genetic predisposition, obesity, metabolic syndrome, androgenic hormones, and smoking. Primary event is follicular dilatation and hyperkeratosis leading to rupture of the hair follicle, inflammation of the apocrine sweat glands, and scarring. Some evidence that interleukin-12-interleukin-23 pathway and tumor necrosis factor α are also involved, suggesting dysregulation of the immune system as a contributing factor.	Caused by plugging of a follicular ostium with resultant cystic dilatation of the follicular lumen and retention of keratin. Rupture of the cyst often occurs with liberation of keratin into the surrounding dermis. This triggers a foreign body giant cells reaction that is often misinterpreted clinically as infection.
Presentation	Deep-seated nodules, abscesses, and sinus tracts that become inflamed and lead to scarring.	Fluctuant, compressible mass ranging from millimeters to several centimeters in size. May have central open comedone representing the punctum and exude malodorous yellow friable material when compressed. If previously ruptured, may have erythema and tenderness.
Histology	1. Follicular dilation involving multiple follicles *(Fig. 4.9.1)*. Follicles have hyperkeratosis and plugging. 2. Sinus tract formation *(Fig. 4.9.2)*. 3. Mixed inflammation involving follicles and sweat glands *(Figs. 4.9.2 and 4.9.3)*. 4. Destruction of hair follicles and dermal scar formation.	1. Isolated dilated follicular infundibulum representing the punctum. 2. Cyst lined by stratified squamous epithelium that matures through a granular layer *(Figs. 4.9.4 and 4.9.5)*. No sinus tract formation. 3. Lumen filled with laminated orthokeratin *(Fig. 4.9.5)*. 4. Inflammation consisting of multinucleate, foreign body–type giant cells surrounding liberated keratin *(Figs. 4.9.6 and 4.9.7)*. 5. Fibrosis limited to vicinity of cystic follicle.
Special studies	None.	None.
Treatment	Initial management with topical clindamycin, oral tetracyclines, antiandrogenic therapy, and metformin. Oral antibiotics, retinoids, dapsone, and biologics may be initiated for moderate to severe and refractory disease. Surgical excision is reserved for severe disease.	Surgical excision is most effective treatment. Removal of the complete epithelial lining of the cyst is necessary to prevent recurrence.

4.9 Hidradenitis Suppurativa vs Follicular Infundibular Cyst

	Hidradenitis Suppurativa	**Follicular Infundibular Cyst**
Prognosis	Prognosis is best when disease is diagnosed early before extensive sinus tract and scar formation. Generally, it is a chronic disease that has acute symptomatic episodes. Usually has a dramatic effect on overall quality of life.	Benign lesion with rare reports of development of malignancy. Multiple lesions may be associated with familial adenomatous polyposis (Gardner) and basal cell nevus (Gorlin) syndromes.

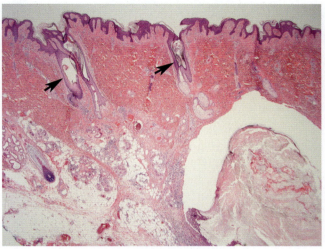

Figure 4.9.1 Hidradenitis suppurativa. Multiple hair follicles show dilatation and distension of the lumen by keratin (arrows). At the lower right of the image, there is a cystic follicle that is ruptured and inflamed. The inflammation extends into adjacent eccrine and apocrine sweat gland units.

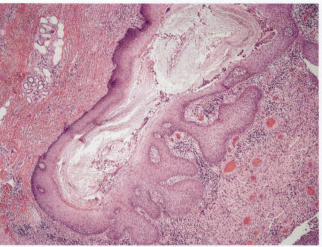

Figure 4.9.2 Hidradenitis suppurativa. Sinus tract formation with irregular hyperplasia of the squamous epithelium and associated edematous granulation tissue with mixed inflammation.

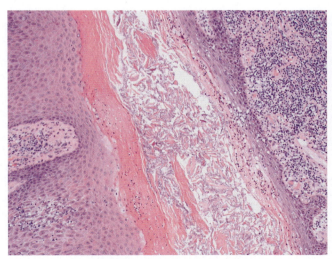

Figure 4.9.3 Hidradenitis suppurativa. Sinus tract containing keratin, granular debris, and inflammatory cells. The surrounding dermis has dense inflammation.

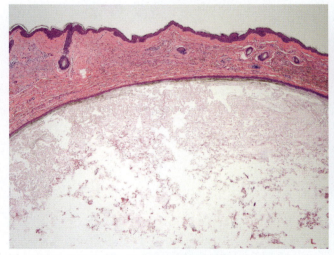

Figure 4.9.4 Follicular infundibular cyst. Although hidradenitis suppurativa is also characterized by cyst formation, the changes involve multiple follicular units rather than a single follicle as in a follicular infundibular cyst. In this image, there is a large dermal cyst lined by thinned squamous epithelium and filled with loose, laminated keratin.

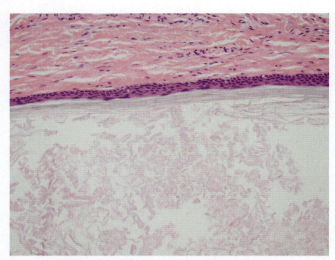

Figure 4.9.5 Follicular infundibular cyst. Uninterrupted cyst epithelium composed of this stratified squamous epithelium with an inner granular layer. The cyst contains loose keratin (not sebum as the colloquial clinical term "sebaceous cyst" would imply).

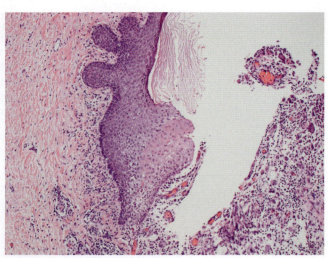

Figure 4.9.6 Follicular infundibular cyst. Example of a ruptured follicular infundibular cyst with mixed inflammation. Sinus tract formation is not a feature.

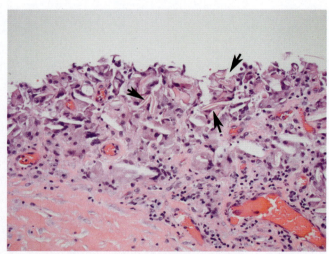

Figure 4.9.7 Follicular infundibular cyst. The inflammation associated with follicular cyst rupture is typically predominated by multinucleate foreign body–type giant cells surrounding keratin debris (arrows) liberated from the cyst lumen.

4.10 HIDRADENITIS SUPPURATIVA VS ACNE KELOIDALIS NUCHAE

	Hidradenitis Suppurativa	**Acne Keloidalis Nuchae**
Age	Onset in postpuberty adolescence to early adulthood, with peak in second and third decades of life. Females affected more than males.	Young adults. Males affected more than females. Predilection for dark skinned individuals.
Location	Intertriginous regions including axillae, inframammary folds, inguinal creases, and perineum.	Nape of the neck and occipital scalp.
Etiology	Multifactorial with contributions from genetic predisposition, obesity, metabolic syndrome, androgenic hormones, and smoking. Primary event is follicular dilatation and hyperkeratosis leading to rupture of the hair follicle, inflammation of the apocrine sweat glands, and scarring. Some evidence that interleukin-12-interleukin-23 pathway and tumor necrosis factor α are also involved, suggesting dysregulation of the immune system as a contributing factor.	Occlusion of hair follicles due to repeated irritation, mechanical trauma, and friction. Close haircuts and restrictive collars and headgear have been implicated.
Presentation	Deep-seated nodules, abscesses, and sinus tracts that become inflamed and lead to scarring.	Firm, dome-shaped, erythematous papules and pustules that coalescence into keloidal plaques.
Histology	1. Follicular dilation involving multiple follicles. Follicles have hyperkeratosis and plugging *(Fig. 4.10.1)*. 2. Sinus tract formation *(Figs. 4.10.1 and 4.10.2)*. 3. Mixed inflammation involving follicles and sweat glands *(Figs. 4.10.2 and 4.10.3)*. 4. Destruction of hair follicles and dermal scar formation.	1. Distorted hair follicles associated with acute and chronic inflammation and pustule formation *(Fig. 4.10.4)*. Destruction of sebaceous glands. 2. Naked portions of hair shaft within dermis associated with granulomatous inflammation *(Fig. 4.10.5)*. 3. Dense scar and lymphoplasmacytic infiltrate *(Figs. 4.10.6 and 4.10.7)*.
Special studies	None.	None.
Treatment	Initial management with topical clindamycin, oral tetracyclines, antiandrogenic therapy, and metformin. Oral antibiotics, retinoids, dapsone, and biologics may be initiated for moderate to severe and refractory disease. Surgical excision is reserved for severe disease.	Prevention by avoiding close and frequent haircuts and restrictive clothing. Mild disease treated with topical corticosteroids, antibiotics, and retinoids. Oral antibiotics and intralesional corticosteroids are used for moderate to severe inflammatory cases. Surgery, ablative laser resurfacing, and oral isotretinoin may be considered for recalcitrant disease.

(continued)

	Hidradenitis Suppurativa	**Acne Keloidalis Nuchae**
Prognosis	Prognosis is best when disease is diagnosed early before extensive sinus tract and scar formation. Generally, it is a chronic disease that has acute symptomatic episodes. Usually has a dramatic effect on overall quality of life.	Chronic disease with flares and remissions.

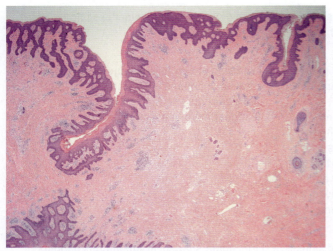

Figure 4.10.1 Hidradenitis suppurativa. Follicular dilatation and sinus tract formation with dense dermal scar. Sweat glands within the scar are inflamed and atrophic.

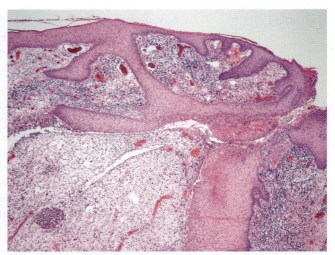

Figure 4.10.2 Hidradenitis suppurativa. Region of active inflammation involving the superficial portion of a sinus tract. The surrounding dermis is edematous and has a dense mixed inflammatory infiltrate and granulation tissue formation.

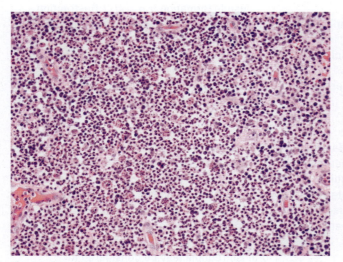

Figure 4.10.3 Hidradenitis suppurativa. Areas of suppurative inflammation with abscess formation are commonly present.

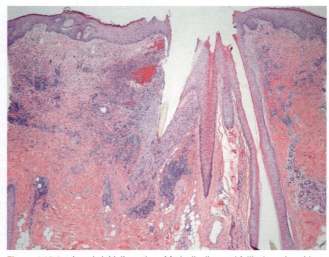

Figure 4.10.4 Acne keloidalis nuchae. Markedly distorted follicular units with destruction of follicular epithelium and sebaceous glands. There is a dense mixed inflammatory infiltrate.

4.10 Hidradenitis Suppurativa vs Acne Keloidalis Nuchae

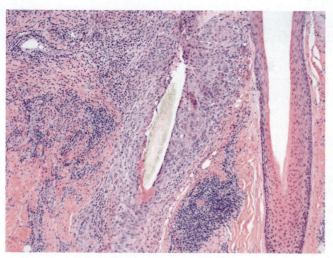

Figure 4.10.5 Acne keloidalis nuchae. Destruction of follicles leads to naked portions of hair shaft surrounded by inflammation including multinucleate giant cells.

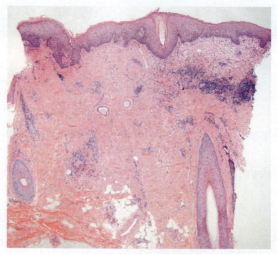

Figure 4.10.6 Acne keloidalis nuchae. Chronic phase with replacement of follicular units by dense scar and a plasma cell rich inflammatory infiltrate.

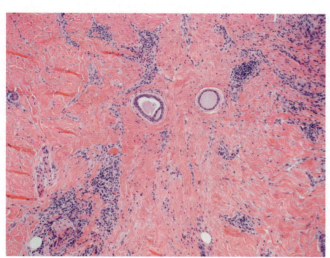

Figure 4.10.7 Acne keloidalis nuchae. Dense dermal scar with plasmacytic infiltrate and residual atrophic eccrine ducts. The histologic features overlap with those of hidradenitis suppurativa although the nape of the neck location, lack of prominent cyst/sinus formation, and plasma cell–rich infiltrate favor acne keloidalis nuchae.

4.11 KERATOSIS PILARIS VS INFECTIOUS FOLLICULITIS

	Keratosis Pilaris	**Infectious Folliculitis**
Age	Adolescents and adults.	Any age.
Location	Extensor surfaces of proximal extremities and buttocks.	Any hair-bearing region of the body.
Etiology	Unknown. Possibly due to altered loss of normal barrier function of the epidermis due to defects in filaggrin gene. This leads to mild follicular dilatation and plugging.	Infection of the hair follicle by a variety of bacterial, fungal, and viral organisms.
Presentation	Multiple, asymptomatic, skin-colored, keratotic, folliculocentric papules measuring 1-2 millimeters. Erythema and edema generally not present unless lesions have been manipulated.	Folliculocentric, erythematous papules and pustules.
Histology	1. Follicular dilatation and distention of the follicular lumen with orthokeratin *(Figs. 4.11.1-4.11.3)*. 2. Keratin plug extends above the surface of the follicle *(Figs. 4.11.1-4.11.3)*. 3. Mild perifollicular fibrosis and sparse chronic inflammation *(Fig. 4.11.3)*.	1. Follicular dilatation with exocytosis of neutrophils into the infundibular portion of the follicular epithelium *(Figs. 4.11.4 and 4.11.5)*. 2. May have superficial pustule formation *(Fig. 4.11.5)*. 3. Perifollicular mixed inflammation *(Fig. 4.11.4)*. Giant cells may be present if the follicular epithelium is disrupted.
Special studies	None.	Tissue Gram stain *(Figs. 4.11.6)* and PAS-diastase/GMS stain to detect bacterial and fungal organisms, respectively. Bacterial and fungal tissue culture. PCR or DFA testing for viral organisms.
Treatment	Treatment is generally not necessary. If treatment is desired, emollients and topical keratolytics may be used. Topical retinoids as second line therapy.	Topical or oral antibiotics depending upon offending organism and extent of infection.
Prognosis	Disease typically spontaneously improves with age. Symptoms may be ameliorated with treatment.	Resolution with identification of the causative organism and appropriate treatment regimen.

4.11 Keratosis Pilaris vs Infectious Folliculitis

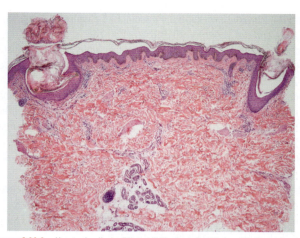

Figure 4.11.1 Keratosis pilaris. Dilated follicular infundibula with distension of the lumens by keratin. The keratin plug protrudes above the surface of the epidermis forming a spicule.

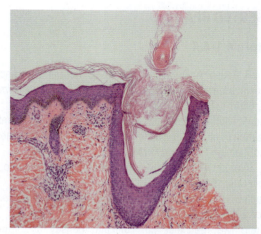

Figure 4.11.2 Keratosis pilaris. Dilated follicular infundibulum with spicule of keratin extending above the follicular ostium. Note that there is only sparse inflammation and no scarring.

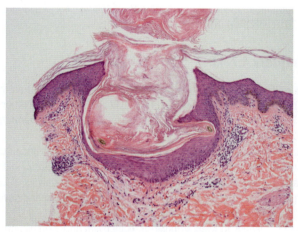

Figure 4.11.3 Keratosis pilaris. Dilated follicular infundibulum with plug of keratin that extends above the surface of the epidermis. There is a coiled hair shaft within the lumen.

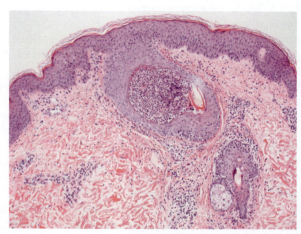

Figure 4.11.4 Infectious folliculitis. Follicular dilatation with exocytosis of neutrophils and formation of a superficial pustule. No comedone or keratin plug formation.

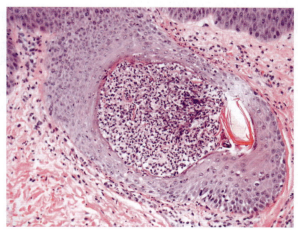

Figure 4.11.5 Infectious folliculitis. Exocytosis of neutrophils into the hair follicle with formation of a pustule.

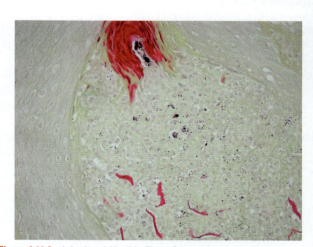

Figure 4.11.6 Infectious folliculitis. Tissue Gram stain reveals numerous gram-positive cocci within the lumen.

SUGGESTED READING

Chapters 4.1-4.4

Barton VR, Toussi A, Awasthi S, Kiuru M. Treatment of pediatric alopecia areata: A systematic review. *J Am Acad Dermatol.* 2022;86(6):1318-1334.

Bergfeld W, Mulinari-Brenner F, McCarron K, Embi C. The combined utilization of clinical and histological findings in the diagnosis of trichotillomania. *J Cutan Pathol.* 2002;29(4):207-214.

Eudy G, Solomon AR. The histopathology of noncicatricial alopecia. *Semin Cutan Med Surg.* 2006;25(1):35-40.

Hautmann G, Hercogova J, Lotti T. Trichotillomania. *J Am Acad Dermatol.* 2002;46(6):807-821; quiz 822-6.

Horenstein MG, Bacheler CJ. Follicular density and ratios in scarring and nonscarring alopecia. *Am J Dermatopathol.* 2013;35(8):818-826.

Piraccini BM, Alessandrini A. Androgenetic alopecia. *G Ital Dermatol Venereol.* 2014;149(1):15-24.

Pratt CH, King LEJr, Messenger AG, Christiano AM, Sundberg JP. Alopecia areata. *Nat Rev Dis Primers.* 2017;3:17011.

Rebora A. Telogen effluvium: a comprehensive review. *Clin Cosmet Investig Dermatol.* 2019;12:583-590.

Starace M, Orlando G, Alessandrini A, Piraccini BM. Female androgenetic alopecia: an update on diagnosis and management. *Am J Clin Dermatol.* 2020;21(1):69-84.

Stefanato CM. Histopathology of alopecia: a clinicopathological approach to diagnosis. *Histopathology.* 2010;56(1):24-38.

Sterkens A, Lambert J, Bervoets A. Alopecia areata: a review on diagnosis, immunological etiopathogenesis and treatment options. *Clin Exp Med.* 2021;21(2):215-230.

Strazzulla LC, Wang EHC, Avila L, et al. Alopecia areata: disease characteristics, clinical evaluation, and new perspectives on pathogenesis. *J Am Acad Dermatol.* 2018;78:1-12.

Zhou C, Li X, Wang C, Zhang J. Alopecia areata: an update on etiopathogenesis, diagnosis, and management. *Clin Rev Allergy Immunol.* 2021;61(3):403-423.

Chapters 4.5-4.6

Bernárdez C, Molina-Ruiz AM, Requena L. Histologic features of alopecias: part II – scarring alopecias. *Actas Dermosifiliogr.* 2015;106(4):260-270.

Bolduc C, Sperling LC, Shapiro J. Primary cicatricial alopecia: other lymphocytic primary cicatricial alopecias and neutrophilic and mixed primary cicatricial alopecias. *J Am Acad Dermatol.* 2016;75(6):1101-1117.

Fabbri P, Amato L, Chiarini C, Moretti S, Massi D. Scarring alopecia in discoid lupus erythematosus: a clinical, histopathologic and immunopathologic study. *Lupus.* 2004;13(6):455-462.

Fanti PA, Baraldi C, Misciali C, Piraccini BM. Cicatricial alopecia. *G Ital Dermatol Venereol.* 2018;153(2):230-242.

Filotico R, Mastrandrea V. Cutaneous lupus erythematosus: clinico-pathologic correlation. *G Ital Dermatol Venereol.* 2018;153(2):216-229.

Gong Y, Ye Y, Zhao Y, et al. Severe diffuse non-scarring hair loss in systemic lupus erythematosus: clinical and histopathological analysis of four cases. *J Eur Acad Dermatol Venereol.* 2013;27(5):651-654.

Kanti V, Röwert-Huber J, Vogt A, Blume-Peytavi U. Cicatricial alopecia. *J Dtsch Dermatol Ges.* 2018;16(4):435-461.

Otberg N, Wu WY, McElwee KJ, Shapiro J. Diagnosis and management of primary cicatricial alopecia: part I. *Skinmed.* 2008;7(1):19-26.

Sperling LC. Scarring alopecia and the dermatopathologist. *J Cutan Pathol.* 2001;28(7):333-342.

Sun CW, Motaparthi K, Hsu S. Central centrifugal cicatricial alopecia and lichen planopilaris can look identical on histopathology. *Skinmed.* 2020;18(6):365-366.

Whiting DA, Olsen EA. Central centrifugal cicatricial alopecia. *Dermatol Ther.* 2008;21(4):268-278.

Zampella JG, Kwatra SG, Alhariri J. Correlation of clinical and pathologic evaluation of scarring alopecia. *Int J Dermatol.* 2019;58(2):194-197.

Chapters 4.7-4.8

Gallo RL, Granstein RD, Kang S, et al. Standard classification and pathophysiology of rosacea: The 2017 update by the National Rosacea Society Expert Committee. *J Am Acad Dermatol.* 2018;78(1):148-155.

Hazarika N. Acne vulgaris: new evidence in pathogenesis and future modalities of treatment. *J Dermatolog Treat.* 2021;32(3):277-285.

Lee WJ, Jung JM, Lee YJ, et al. Histopathological analysis of 226 patients with rosacea according to rosacea subtype and severity. *Am J Dermatopathol.* 2016;38(5):347-352.

Moradi Tuchayi S, Makrantonaki E, Ganceviciene R, Dessinioti C, Feldman SR, Zouboulis CC. Acne vulgaris. *Nat Rev Dis Primers.* 2015;1:15029.

Patterson WM, Fox MD, Schwartz RA. Favre-Racouchot disease. *Int J Dermatol.* 2004;43(3):167-169.

Sánchez JL, Berlingeri-Ramos AC, Dueño DV. Granulomatous rosacea. *Am J Dermatopathol.* 2008;30(1):6-9.

Two AM, Wu W, Gallo RL, Hata TR. Rosacea: part I. Introduction, categorization, histology, pathogenesis, and risk factors. *J Am Acad Dermatol.* 2015;72(5):749-758. quiz 759-60.

Van Zuuren EJ. Rosacea. *N Engl J Med.* 2017;377(18):1754-1764.

Williams HC, Dellavalle RP, Garner S. Acne vulgaris. *Lancet.* 2012;379(9813):361-372.

Yeh C, Schwartz RA. Favre-Racouchot disease: protective effect of solar elastosis. *Arch Dermatol Res.* 2022;314(3):217-222.

Chapters 4.9-4.10

Brahe C, Peters K, Meunier N. Acne keloidalis nuchae in the armed forces. *Cutis*. 2020;105(5):223-226.

Goldburg SR, Strober BE, Payette MJ. Hidradenitis suppurativa: epidemiology, clinical presentation, and pathogenesis. *J Am Acad Dermatol*. 2020;82(5):1045-1058.

Maranda EL, Simmons BJ, Nguyen AH, Lim VM, Keri JE. Treatment of acne keloidalis nuchae: a systematic review of the literature. *Dermatol Ther (Heidelb)*. 2016;6(3):363-378.

Sabat R, Jemec GBE, Matusiak Ł, Kimball AB, Prens E, Wolk K. Hidradenitis suppurativa. *Nat Rev Dis Primers*. 2020;6(1):18.

Saunte DML, Jemec GBE. Hidradenitis suppurativa: advances in diagnosis and treatment. *JAMA*. 2017;318(20):2019-2032.

Smith SDB, Okoye GA, Sokumbi O. Histopathology of hidradenitis suppurativa: a systematic review. *Dermatopathology (Basel)*. 2022;9(3):251-257.

Chapter 4.11

Hwang S, Schwartz RA. Keratosis pilaris: a common follicular hyperkeratosis. *Cutis*. 2008;82(3):177-180.

Lateef A, Schwartz RA. Keratosis pilaris. *Cutis*. 1999;63(4):205-207.

Laureano AC, Schwartz RA, Cohen PJ. Facial bacterial infections: folliculitis. *Clin Dermatol*. 2014;32(6):711-714.

Levy AL, Simpson G, Skinner RB. Medical pearl: circle of desquamation — a clue to the diagnosis of folliculitis and furunculosis caused by Staphylococcus aureus. *J Am Acad Dermatol*. 2006;55(6):1079-1080.

Neubert U, Jansen T, Plewig G. Bacteriologic and immunologic aspects of gram-negative folliculitis: a study of 46 patients. *Int J Dermatol*. 1999;38:270-274.

Wang JF, Orlow SJ. Keratosis pilaris and its subtypes: associations, new molecular and pharmacologic etiologies, and therapeutic options. *Am J Clin Dermatol*. 2018;19(5):733-757.

5 Disorders of the Subcutis

- **5.1** Erythema Nodosum vs Nodular Vasculitis
- **5.2** Erythema Nodosum vs Behcet Disease
- **5.3** Erythema Nodosum vs Traumatic Panniculitis
- **5.4** Lipodermatosclerosis vs Traumatic Panniculitis
- **5.5** Lipodermatosclerosis vs Morphea
- **5.6** Eosinophilic Fasciitis vs Scleroderma
- **5.7** Lupus Panniculitis vs Subcutaneous Panniculitis-Like T-Cell Lymphoma
- **5.8** Cold Panniculitis vs Lupus Panniculitis
- **5.9** Pancreatic Panniculitis vs Infectious Panniculitis
- **5.10** Pancreatic Panniculitis vs Alpha-1 Antitrypsin Deficiency Panniculitis
- **5.11** Calciphylaxis vs Monckeberg Medial Calcific Sclerosis
- **5.12** Nodular Vasculitis vs Polyarteritis Nodosa

5.1 ERYTHEMA NODOSUM VS NODULAR VASCULITIS

	Erythema Nodosum	**Nodular Vasculitis**
Age	Any age; most commonly between 25 and 40 years of age; women more often than men.	Adults; more common in women than in men.
Location	Extensor surfaces of legs and knees; less commonly on thighs, arms, calves, and face.	Posterior lower legs/calves.
Etiology	Delayed-type hypersensitivity due to exposure to a variety of antigens. Underlying causes include infection, medications, malignancy, inflammatory bowel disease, and other inflammatory processes. Between 30% and 50% of cases are idiopathic.	Immune-mediated hypersensitivity reaction most frequently associated with tuberculosis. Other infections, inflammatory processes, and medications less commonly associated. Minority of idiopathic cases.
Presentation	Abrupt onset of tender, erythematous, nonulcerated, fixed nodules on bilateral shins. May have prodrome of fever, fatigue, and arthralgias.	Unilateral or bilateral, tender, erythematous nodules that typically ulcerate.
Histology	1. Septal panniculitis with edema and mixed inflammatory infiltrate *(Fig. 5.1.1)*. 2. Inflammation includes lymphocytes, histiocytes, neutrophils, and eosinophils, especially in early lesions *(Figs. 5.1.2 and 5.1.4)*. 3. Noncaseating granulomas including Miescher radial granulomas characterized by macrophages surrounding cleft-like spaces with or without clusters of neutrophils *(Figs. 5.1.3 and 5.1.5)*. 4. Septal fibrosis with mild extension of inflammation into fat lobules *(Figs. 5.1.2 and 5.1.3)*. 5. No vasculitis.	1. Lobular or mixed lobular and septal panniculitis with mixed inflammatory infiltrate consisting of lymphocytes, plasma cells, histiocytes, neutrophils, and eosinophils *(Figs. 5.1.6-5.1.8)*. 2. Granuloma formation may be present but less frequent than erythema nodosum. 3. Vasculitis involving variably sized arterial and venous vessels with fibrinoid necrosis and leukocytoclasis *(Fig. 5.1.9)*.
Special studies	PAS or GMS and AFB stains to exclude fungal and mycobacterial infection.	Histochemical stains to exclude bacterial, fungal, and mycobacterial infection.
Treatment	Treatment is not generally necessary but nonsteroidal anti-inflammatory agents and potassium iodide may be used for symptomatic relief. Intralesional or systemic glucocorticoids are alternative therapies for nonresponsive cases.	Identification and treatment of underlying cause, including therapy for active or latent tuberculosis if present. Nonsteroidal anti-inflammatory medications and rest for symptomatic relief. Oral potassium iodide provides rapid response in most cases.
Prognosis	Nodules spontaneously resolve within 2 months but may have postinflammatory hyperpigmentation.	Variable course. Resolution of disease with treatment of underlying cause, but cases associated with tuberculosis may recur. Idiopathic cases may persist for months to years.

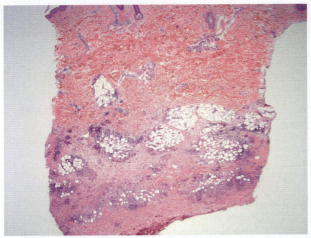

Figure 5.1.1 Erythema nodosum. Marked thickening of the subcutaneous septae by fibrosis and inflammation.

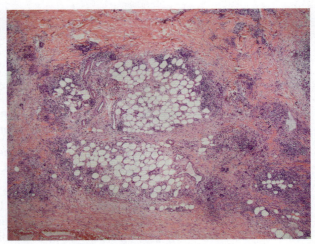

Figure 5.1.2 Erythema nodosum. Septal fibrosis and edema with mixed inflammatory infiltrate. The inflammation and fibrosis encroaches upon the lobules. Note that the vessels are dilated but there is no vasculitis.

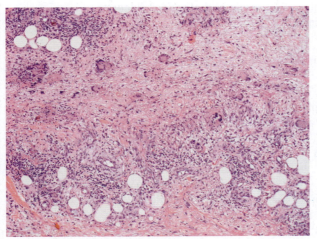

Figure 5.1.3 Erythema nodosum. Granuloma formation characterized by loose aggregates of multinucleate giant cells without necrosis. Septae are markedly thickened by fibrosis with reactive vessels.

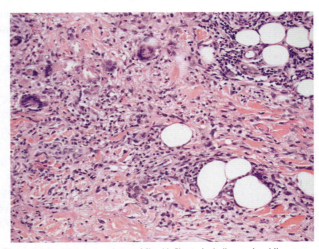

Figure 5.1.4 Erythema nodosum. Mixed infiltrate including eosinophils, lymphocytes, and plasma cells in addition to multinucleate histiocytes.

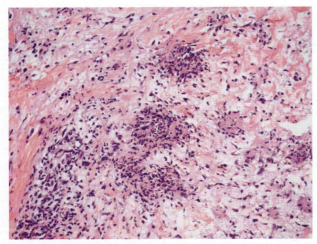

Figure 5.1.5 Erythema nodosum. Miescher radial granulomas characterized by macrophages surrounding small cleft-like spaces with clusters of neutrophils.

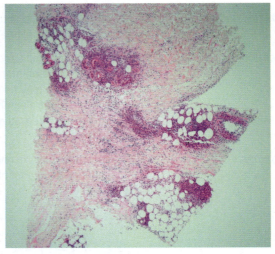

Figure 5.1.6 Nodular vasculitis. Predominantly lobular infiltrate with septal edema but no significant septal fibrosis.

5.1 Erythema Nodosum vs Nodular Vasculitis

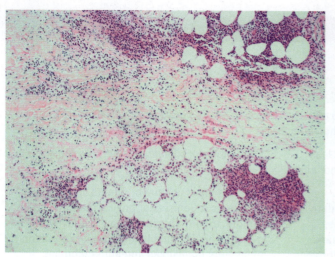

Figure 5.1.7 Nodular vasculitis. Mixed inflammatory infiltrate with a predominance of neutrophils within fat lobules and extending into septae.

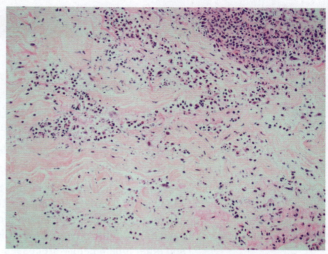

Figure 5.1.8 Nodular vasculitis. Neutrophils and leukocytoclasis with smaller numbers of eosinophils, lymphocytes, and histiocytes. No granuloma formation.

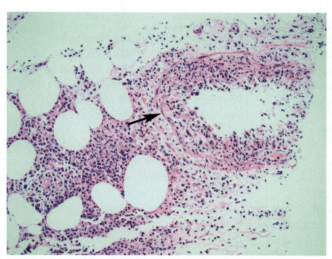

Figure 5.1.9 Nodular vasculitis. Hallmark of nodular vasculitis is infiltration of the walls of variably sized arterial and venous vessels with destruction of the vessel wall. At the arrow, a small vein is infiltrated by neutrophils with mild fibrinoid necrosis of the wall.

5.2 ERYTHEMA NODOSUM VS BEHCET DISEASE

	Erythema Nodosum	**Behcet Disease**
Age	Any age; most commonly between 25 and 40 years of age; women more often than men.	Young adults between 20 and 40 years of age.
Location	Extensor surfaces of legs and knees; less commonly on thighs, arms, calves, and face.	Extremities, predominantly anterior legs.
Etiology	Delayed-type hypersensitivity due to exposure to a variety of antigens. Underlying causes include infection, medications, malignancy, inflammatory bowel disease, and other inflammatory processes. Between 30% and 50% of cases are idiopathic.	Exact cause is unknown. Agents, including infectious organisms or environmental factors, trigger aberrant immune activity in genetically susceptible individuals. Formation of immune complexes and autoantibodies, in the presence of vascular endothelial and neutrophil activation, leads to vasculitis.
Presentation	Abrupt onset of tender, erythematous, nonulcerated, fixed nodules on bilateral shins. May have prodrome of fever, fatigue, and arthralgias.	The erythema nodosum–like lesions present as discrete, erythematous nodules with edema. Other associated clinical features include aphthous ulcers and uveitis.
Histology	1. Septal panniculitis with edema and mixed inflammatory infiltrate *(Figs. 5.2.1* and *5.2.2)*. 2. Inflammation includes lymphocytes, histiocytes, neutrophils, and eosinophils, especially in early lesions *(Figs. 5.2.2* and *5.2.3)*. 3. Noncaseating granulomas including Miescher radial granulomas characterized by macrophages surrounding cleft-like spaces with or without clusters of neutrophils *(Fig. 5.2.4)*. 4. Septal fibrosis with slight extension of inflammation into fat lobules *(Figs. 5.2.1* and *5.2.2)*. 5. No vasculitis.	1. Primarily lobular or mixed septal and lobular panniculitis with neutrophil-predominant infiltrate *(Figs. 5.2.5* and *5.2.6)*. 2. Lymphocytic and neutrophilic inflammation of medium-sized vessels with thrombus formation and erythrocyte extravasation *(Fig. 5.2.8)*. 3. Lymphocytes and histiocytes extend into lobules and are associated with fat necrosis *(Fig. 5.2.7)*.
Special studies	PAS or GMS and AFB stains to exclude fungal and mycobacterial infection.	No specific laboratory tests. May have elevated erythrocyte sedimentation rate and C-reactive protein with active disease.
Treatment	Treatment is not generally necessary but nonsteroidal anti-inflammatory agents and potassium iodide may be used for symptomatic relief. Intralesional or systemic glucocorticoids are alternative therapies for nonresponsive cases.	Topical corticosteroids for mild cases. Prednisone, azathioprine, colchicine, dapsone, thalidomide, or methotrexate for severe or refractory disease.
Prognosis	Nodules spontaneously resolve within 2 months but may have postinflammatory hyperpigmentation.	Chronic disease with waxing and waning course. Involvement of other organ systems may be associated with significant morbidity and mortality.

5.2 Erythema Nodosum vs Behcet Disease

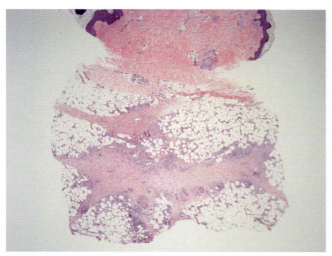

Figure 5.2.1 Erythema nodosum. Thickening of subcutaneous septae with inflammation that extends minimally into the periphery of fat lobules. The lobules are generally preserved.

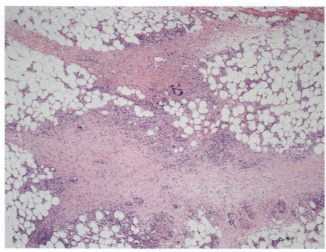

Figure 5.2.2 Erythema nodosum. Septal fibrosis with reactive vascular proliferation and mixed inflammatory infiltrate. Multinucleate histiocytes are conspicuous. Vessels show reactive change but there is no vasculitis.

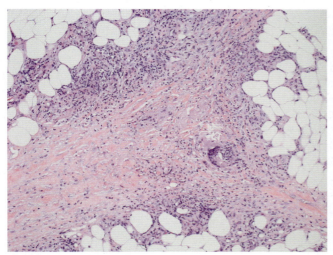

Figure 5.2.3 Erythema nodosum. Fibrosis of septa with mixed infiltrate including eosinophils, lymphocytes, histiocytes, and multinucleate giant cells. Neutrophils present but do not predominate.

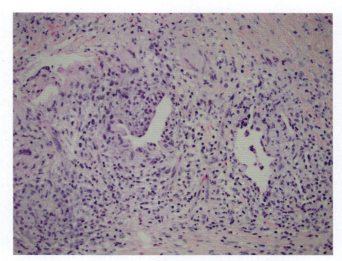

Figure 5.2.4 Erythema nodosum. Miescher radial granulomas characterized by macrophages surrounding cleft-like spaces with few neutrophils.

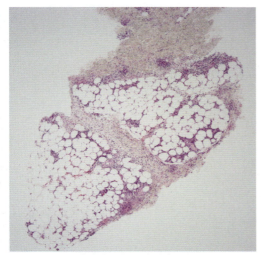

Figure 5.2.5 Behcet disease. Predominately lobular inflammatory infiltrate with mild edema of septae.

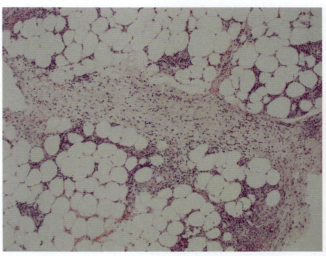

Figure 5.2.6 Behcet disease. Mixed lobular infiltrate with septal edema and mild inflammation.

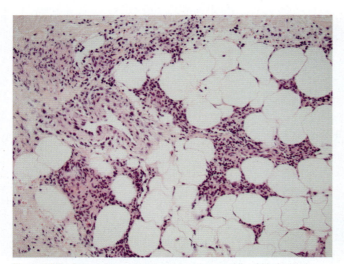

Figure 5.2.7 Behcet disease. Lymphocytes and neutrophils within fat lobule. There is mild erythrocyte extravasation.

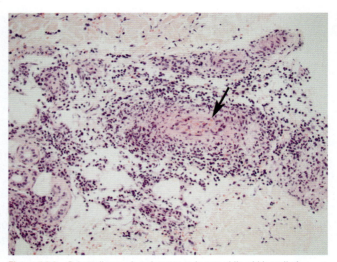

Figure 5.2.8 Behcet disease. Lymphocytes and neutrophils within wall of medium-sized vessel with occlusion of the lumen (arrow) and erythrocyte extravasation.

5.3 ERYTHEMA NODOSUM VS TRAUMATIC PANNICULITIS

	Erythema Nodosum	**Traumatic Panniculitis**
Age	Any age; most commonly between 25 and 40 years of age; women more often than men.	Any age.
Location	Extensor surfaces of legs and knees; less commonly on thighs, arms, calves, and face.	Any site but most commonly involves shins, forearms, and breasts.
Etiology	Delayed-type hypersensitivity due to exposure to a variety of antigens. Underlying causes include infection, medications, malignancy, inflammatory bowel disease, and other inflammatory processes. Between 30% and 50% of cases are idiopathic.	Blunt trauma in fatty zones.
Presentation	Abrupt onset of tender, erythematous, nonulcerated, fixed nodules on bilateral shins. May have prodrome of fever, fatigue, and arthralgias.	Indurated, erythematous subcutaneous plaques or nodules. Hypertrichosis has been reported in some cases.
Histology	1. Septal panniculitis with edema and mixed inflammatory infiltrate *(Figs. 5.3.1* and *5.3.2)*. 2. Inflammation includes lymphocytes, histiocytes, neutrophils, and eosinophils *(Fig. 5.3.2)*. 3. Noncaseating granulomas including Miescher radial granulomas characterized by macrophages surrounding cleft-like spaces with or without clusters of neutrophils *(Fig. 5.3.3)*. 4. Septal fibrosis with slight extension of inflammation into fat lobules *(Figs. 5.3.1* and *5.3.2)*. 5. No significant fat necrosis or calcification.	1. Normal epidermis and dermis. 2. Lobular infiltrate of histiocytes, including foamy histiocytes and giant cells, surrounding fat microcysts (lipophagic fat necrosis) *(Figs. 5.3.5* and *5.3.6)*. 3. Microcysts vary in size and shape *(Fig. 5.3.5)*. 4. Lipomembranous change with variable fibrosis and dystrophic calcification *(Fig. 5.3.6)*. Lipomembranous change consists of feathery eosinophilic material at the periphery of cystic spaces. 5. Fibrosis may form a capsule around the fat necrosis *(Fig. 5.3.4)*.
Special studies	PAS or GMS and AFB stains to exclude fungal and mycobacterial infection.	None.
Treatment	Treatment is not generally necessary but nonsteroidal anti-inflammatory agents and potassium iodide may be used for symptomatic relief. Intralesional or systemic glucocorticoids are alternative therapies for nonresponsive cases.	Symptomatic treatment only.
Prognosis	Nodules spontaneously resolve within 2 months but may have postinflammatory hyperpigmentation.	Self-limited disorder. May recur in individuals susceptible to repeat trauma.

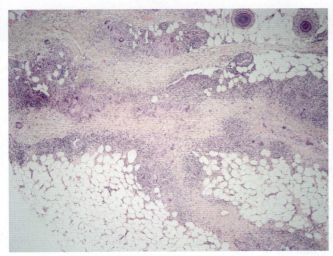

Figure 5.3.1 Erythema nodosum. Fibrosis and thickening of subcutaneous septae with dense mixed infiltrate that extends minimally into the periphery of the fat lobules.

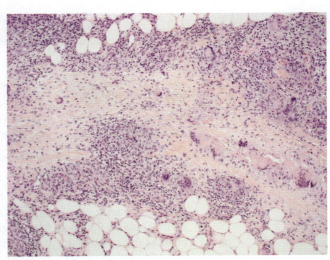

Figure 5.3.2 Erythema nodosum. Thickened septae with mixed infiltrate predominated by lymphocytes and histiocytes with few eosinophils. Multinucleate giant cells are conspicuous.

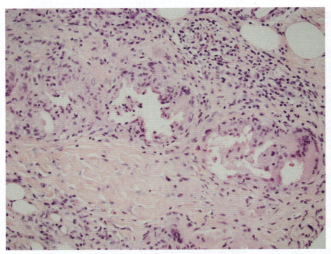

Figure 5.3.3 Erythema nodosum. Miescher radial granulomas formed by multinucleate giant cells surrounding irregular cleft-like spaces.

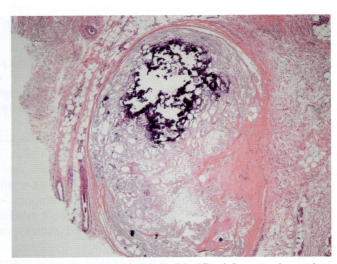

Figure 5.3.4 Traumatic panniculitis. Hyalinized fibrosis forms capsule around area of fat necrosis with calcification.

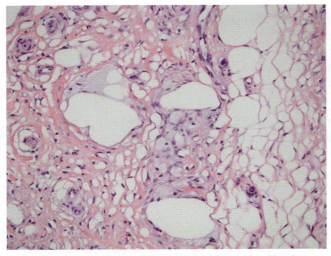

Figure 5.3.5 Traumatic panniculitis. Fat necrosis with formation of fat microcysts of varying size. Foamy histiocytes surround the fat cells and microcysts (lipophagic fat necrosis). No discrete granuloma formation.

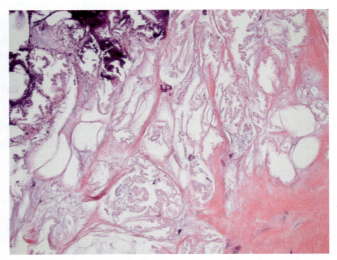

Figure 5.3.6 Traumatic panniculitis. Lipomembranous change characterized by feathery eosinophilic material at the periphery of cystic spaces. There is a peripheral hyalinized fibrotic capsule (lower right) and prominent calcification (upper left).

5.4 LIPODERMATOSCLEROSIS VS TRAUMATIC PANNICULITIS

	Lipodermatosclerosis	**Traumatic Panniculitis**
Age	Middle-aged adults; women affected more than men.	Any age.
Location	Lower legs.	Any site but most commonly involves shins, forearms, and breasts.
Etiology	Chronic venous insufficiency.	Blunt trauma in fatty zones.
Presentation	Early phase of red to violaceous, mildly tender plaques that evolve into indurated, thick, hyperpigmented skin involving the lower third of the leg. Constriction in the ankle region imparts an "inverted champagne bottle" appearance to the leg. May be associated with other features of chronic venous stasis including edema, varicosities, and ulceration.	Indurated, erythematous subcutaneous plaques or nodules. Hypertrichosis has been reported in some cases.
Histology	1. Grouped, thick-walled vessels within the superficial dermis *(Fig. 5.4.5)*. 2. Erythrocyte extravasation and hemosiderin deposition may be evident in superficial dermis. 3. Subcutaneous septal fibrosis *(Fig. 5.4.1)*. 4. Membranocystic (lipomembranous) fat necrosis with lipogranuloma formation and xanthomatous macrophages *(Figs. 5.4.2 and 5.4.3)*. 5. Siderophages (hemosiderin-laden macrophages) in septae *(Fig. 5.4.4)*.	1. Normal epidermis and dermis. 2. Lobular infiltrate of histiocytes, including foamy histiocytes and giant cells, surrounding fat microcysts *(Figs. 5.4.6 and 5.4.9)*. 3. Microcysts vary in size and shape *(Figs. 5.4.6 and 5.4.7)*. 4. Lipomembranous change with variable fibrosis and dystrophic calcification *(Fig. 5.4.7)*. Lipomembranous change consists of feathery eosinophilic material at the periphery of cystic spaces. 5. Fibrosis may form a capsule around the fat necrosis *(Fig. 5.4.8)*.
Special studies	Iron stain may be performed to detect siderophages.	None.
Treatment	Compression therapy is the conventional treatment for chronic venous insufficiency and lipodermatosclerosis. Anabolic steroids are also utilized for their fibrinolytic properties in some cases.	Symptomatic treatment only.
Prognosis	Progressive disease that is chronic and recurring. May be associated with other complications of chronic venous insufficiency including chronic ulceration and secondary infection.	Self-limited disorder. May recur in individuals susceptible to repeat trauma.

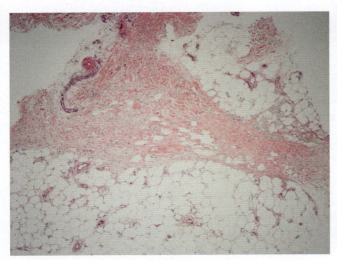

Figure 5.4.1 Lipodermatosclerosis. Fibrosis and thickening of subcutaneous septae with minimal inflammation.

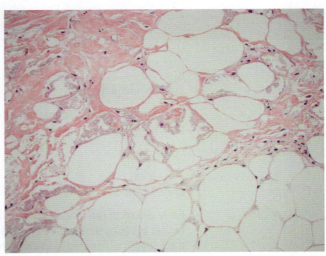

Figure 5.4.2 Lipodermatosclerosis. Lipomembranous fat necrosis characterized by feathery eosinophilic material at the periphery of fat cells and fat microcysts.

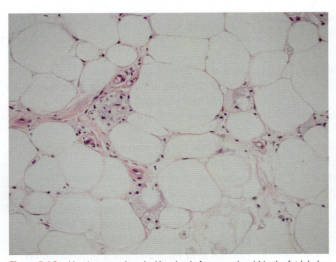

Figure 5.4.3 Lipodermatosclerosis. Lipophagic fat necrosis within the fat lobules with foamy, xanthomatous histiocytes surrounding fat cells of varying size.

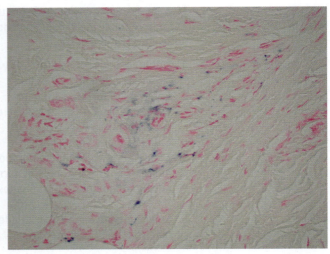

Figure 5.4.4 Lipodermatosclerosis. Siderophages (hemosiderin-laden macrophages) within the septae as highlighted with iron stain.

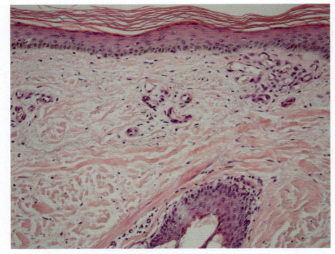

Figure 5.4.5 Lipodermatosclerosis. Features of chronic venous stasis within the superficial dermis with grouped, thick-walled vessels.

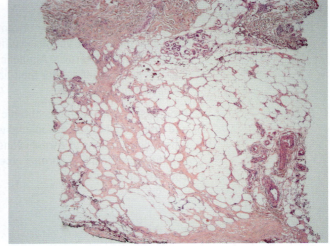

Figure 5.4.6 Traumatic panniculitis. Fat necrosis with formation of fat microcysts of varying size. Septae and lobules are distorted by hyalinized sclerosis. No significant inflammation.

5.4 Lipodermatosclerosis vs Traumatic Panniculitis

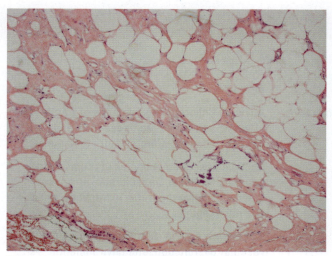

Figure 5.4.7 Traumatic panniculitis. Fat microcysts with intervening sclerosis and dystrophic calcification.

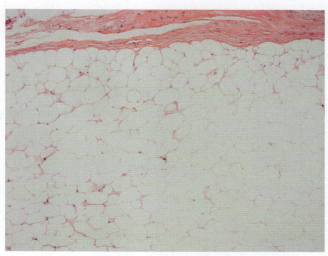

Figure 5.4.8 Traumatic panniculitis. Areas of fat necrosis characterized by anucleate adipocytes and few foamy histiocytes surrounded by dense collagen.

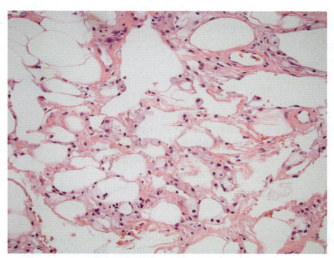

Figure 5.4.9 Traumatic panniculitis. Lipophagic fat necrosis with fat microcysts associated with foamy histiocytes.

5.5 LIPODERMATOSCLEROSIS VS MORPHEA

	Lipodermatosclerosis	**Morphea**
Age	Middle-aged adults; women affected more than men.	Any age. Children between ages of 7 and 11 years; adults between ages of 44 and 47 years. Females affected more than males.
Location	Lower legs.	Multiple described subtypes (circumscribed, generalized, linear, pansclerotic, and mixed) that may involve the trunk, extremities, head and neck regions.
Etiology	Chronic venous insufficiency.	Not entirely known. Autoimmune, genetic, vascular dysfunction, and environmental factors play a role.
Presentation	Early phase of red to violaceous, mildly tender plaques that evolve into indurated, thick, hyperpigmented skin involving the lower third of the leg. Constriction in the ankle region imparts an "inverted champagne bottle" appearance to the leg. May be associated with other features of chronic venous stasis including edema, varicosities, and ulceration.	Yellow-white indurated plaque with erythematous, violaceous border and hyper- or hypopigmentation. Lesions may be solitary or multiple.
Histology	1. Grouped, thick-walled vessels within the superficial dermis *(Fig. 5.5.6)*. 2. Erythrocyte extravasation and hemosiderin deposition *(Fig. 5.5.6)*. 3. Subcutaneous septal fibrosis *(Figs. 5.5.1 and 5.5.5)*. 4. Membranocystic (lipomembranous) fat necrosis with lipogranuloma formation and xanthomatous macrophages *(Figs. 5.5.2-5.5.4)*.	1. Biopsy appears "squared off" due to expansion of dermis *(Fig. 5.5.7)*. 2. Epidermis and stratum corneum generally unremarkable. 3. Perivascular and interstitial infiltrate of lymphocytes and plasma cells; eosinophils and histiocytes in early lesions *(Fig. 5.5.9)*. 4. Sclerosis of collagen bundles in reticular dermis and subcutaneous septae with loss of normal fenestrations between collagen bundles *(Figs. 5.5.7 and 5.5.8)*. 5. Loss of fat around adnexal structures and entrapment of adnexa by sclerosis *(Fig. 5.5.10)*. Progressive replacement of subcutaneous fat by sclerosis.
Special studies	None.	None.
Treatment	Compression therapy is the conventional treatment for chronic venous insufficiency and lipodermatosclerosis. Anabolic steroids are also utilized for their fibrinolytic properties in some cases.	Therapy is based upon subtype, level of disease activity, depth of skin involvement, and quality of life impairment. For limited, superficial disease, topical corticosteroids are first-line therapy. Phototherapy or methotrexate is indicated for widespread superficial disease. Methotrexate is used in cases with deep extension of the sclerosis. Systemic corticosteroids are indicated in cases with rapid progression or development of contractures.

	Lipodermatosclerosis	**Morphea**
Prognosis	Progressive disease that is chronic and recurring. May be associated with other complications of chronic venous insufficiency including chronic ulceration and secondary infection.	Superficial, circumscribed disease has a good prognosis and often resolves in 3-6 years but may have recurrent disease. Variants that involve deep soft tissue may lead to functional problems and cosmetic issues. Linear morphea, particularly in childhood, can lead to development of contractures and limb length discrepancies.

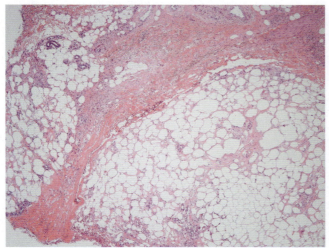

Figure 5.5.1 Lipodermatosclerosis. Septal thickening by fibrosis with lobular fat necrosis.

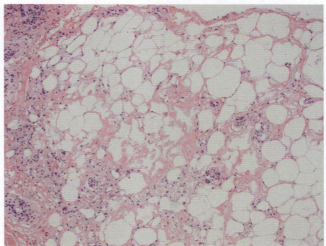

Figure 5.5.2 Lipodermatosclerosis. Lipomembranous fat necrosis characterized by eosinophilic feathery material at the periphery of fat cysts.

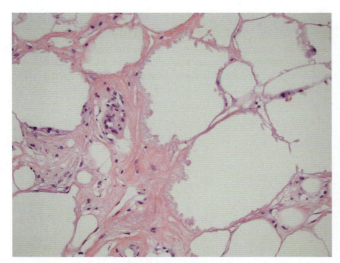

Figure 5.5.3 Lipodermatosclerosis. Lipomembranous fat necrosis with minimal inflammation.

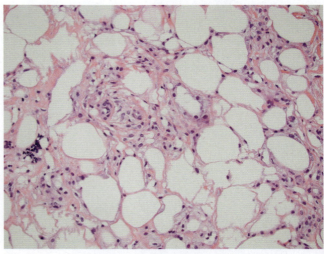

Figure 5.5.4 Lipodermatosclerosis. Lipophagic fat necrosis with foamy (xanthomatized) histiocytes surrounding adipocytes and fat cysts.

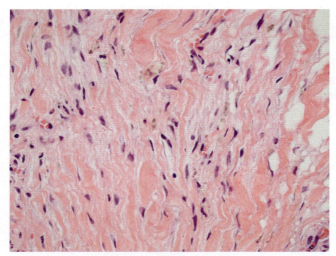

Figure 5.5.5 Lipodermatosclerosis. Septal fibrosis with hemosiderin deposition (siderophages).

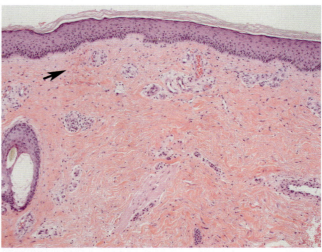

Figure 5.5.6 Lipodermatosclerosis. Features of chronic venous stasis with thick-walled, grouped vessels in the superficial dermis that are associated with erythrocyte extravasation (arrow).

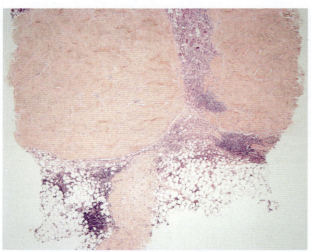

Figure 5.5.7 Morphea. "Squared-off" biopsy due to expansion of the dermis by sclerotic collagen bundles. The sclerosis extends into the subcutis with thickening of the septae. Perieccrine and deep perivascular inflammation that extends into the fat lobules.

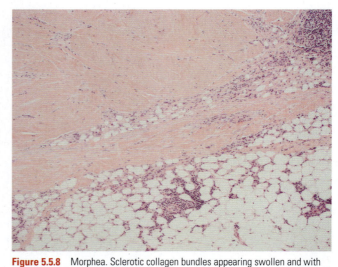

Figure 5.5.8 Morphea. Sclerotic collagen bundles appearing swollen and with loss of usual fenestrations. The sclerosis encroaches upon the subcutaneous adipose tissue with obliteration of the fat. No appreciable lipomembranous or lipophagic fat necrosis.

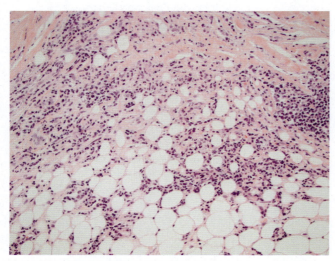

Figure 5.5.9 Morphea. Infiltrate of small lymphocytes and plasma cells within the deep dermis at the interface with the subcutis.

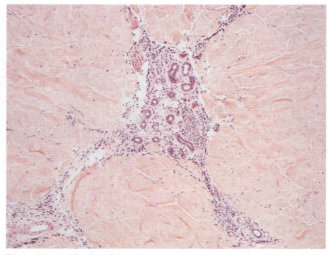

Figure 5.5.10 Morphea. Sclerosis replaces normal fat around eccrine unit and is accompanied by a lymphoplasmacytic infiltrate.

5.6 EOSINOPHILIC FASCIITIS VS SCLERODERMA

	Eosinophilic Fasciitis	**Scleroderma**
Age	Adults, typically in fourth and fifth decades of life.	All ages, but most commonly between 30 and 50 years of age. There is a female predominance.
Location	Extremities are symmetrically involved with exclusion of hands and feet. Trunk and neck involvement may be seen in widespread disease.	Fingers, hands, and face followed by distal extremities. Trunk and proximal extremities are typically spared.
Etiology	Unknown. Trauma and strenuous exercise have been postulated as etiologic factors.	Disease of unknown cause involving immune dysregulation, microangiopathy, and excess synthesis of extracellular matrix with deposition of increased amounts of collagen in the skin.
Presentation	Acute or subacute onset of erythema and pitting edema. Deep sclerosis creates diffuse induration and "peau d'orange" appearance as well as "groove sign" (collapse of superficial veins with elevation of extremity). Cutaneous symptoms may be accompanied by myalgias, weakness, and weight loss. No Raynaud phenomenon.	Slowly progressive thickening and hardening of the skin. Skin edema and erythema is followed by induration and mottled pigmentation. Often associated with abnormal nailfold capillaries and Raynaud phenomenon. Late-stage lesions may have calcinosis and ulceration.
Histology	1. Full-thickness biopsy, including fascia, is necessary for diagnosis. Superficial findings in deep dermis and superficial subcutis of sclerosis and lymphoplasmacytic infiltrate may mimic morphea/scleroderma *(Figs. 5.6.1* and *5.6.2)*. 2. Fibrosis and thickening of the subcutis and fascia with an infiltrate of eosinophils, plasma cells, and histiocytes *(Figs. 5.6.3* and *5.6.4)*. Sclerosis extends into dermis only in extensive, severe cases. 3. Eosinophils may be transient and even absent in late stages of the disease or if systemic corticosteroids have been administered.	1. Biopsy appears "squared off" at low magnification *(Fig. 5.6.5)*. 2. Dermis is expanded by sclerotic collagen bundles that appear swollen and smudgy with loss of intervening fenestrations *(Fig. 5.6.6)*. Sclerosis extends into subcutis but not into fascia. 3. Sclerotic collagen bundles obliterate fat surrounding adnexal structures *(Fig. 5.6.7)*. Adnexae are atrophic or absent in late-stage lesions. 4. Patchy perivascular and interstitial infiltrate of lymphocytes and plasma cells *(Fig. 5.6.8)*. Eosinophils generally not prominent.
Special studies	Testing for increased absolute eosinophil count and elevated inflammatory markers (erythrocyte sedimentation rate and C-reactive protein) may be useful in initial diagnosis and for detection of disease reactivation.	Serology for systemic sclerosis-related autoantibodies including antinuclear antibody, anti-centromere, anti-topoisomerase I (anti-Scl-70), and anti-RNA polymerase III. No peripheral eosinophilia.

(continued)

	Eosinophilic Fasciitis	**Scleroderma**
Treatment	High-dose systemic corticosteroids are first-line therapy. Other immunosuppressant agents, such as methotrexate, are used as steroid-sparing agents and in nonresponsive cases.	Methotrexate or mycophenolate mofetil are treatments of choice for extensive skin disease without visceral involvement. Cyclophosphamide may be used for refractory cases and rapidly progressive disease, and in patients with associated pulmonary fibrosis.
Prognosis	A majority of patients show response to corticosteroid therapy, especially if treatment is initiated in early phases of the disease. Patients unresponsive to corticosteroids or other immunosuppressive therapy may have chronic skin thickening and develop contractures.	Dependent upon extent of cutaneous disease and presence of other organ involvement. Increased mortality is linked to extensive skin disease; cardiac, pulmonary, and/or renal disease; and presence of anti-topoisomerase I antibodies.

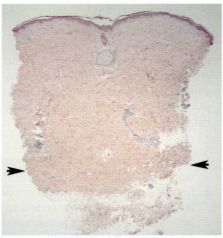

Figure 5.6.1 Eosinophilic fasciitis. Superficial portion of biopsy showing expansion of the dermis into the subcutis by sclerotic collagen (arrows). There is a patchy perivascular and perieccrine infiltrate of lymphocytes and plasma cells. These features are similar to those seen in morphea/scleroderma.

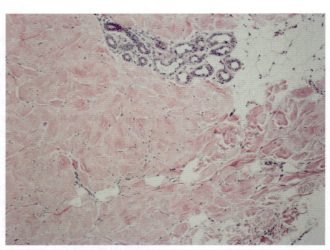

Figure 5.6.2 Eosinophilic fasciitis. Sclerotic collagen bundles, with loss of normal fenestrated pattern, encroaching upon the eccrine unit.

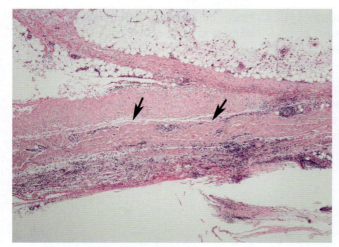

Figure 5.6.3 Eosinophilic fasciitis. Deeper component of biopsy showing portion of fascia (arrows) with moderately dense inflammatory infiltrate.

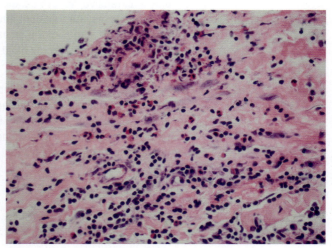

Figure 5.6.4 Eosinophilic fasciitis. Infiltrate within fascia consists of lymphocytes, plasma cells, and many eosinophils. Eosinophils may be only focally present, or transient, so ample sampling of fascia may be necessary to demonstrate them.

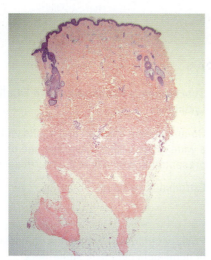

Figure 5.6.5 Scleroderma. Sclerotic collagen expanding the reticular dermis and extending into the subcutis along septae.

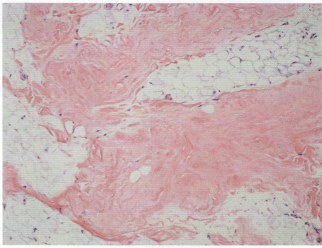

Figure 5.6.6 Scleroderma. Sclerotic collagen bundles appearing swollen and smudgy with loss of intervening fenestrations. Sclerosis obliterates the subcutaneous adipose tissue but does not extend into the fascia.

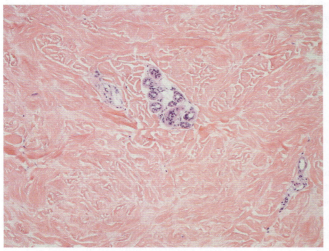

Figure 5.6.7 Scleroderma. Sclerotic collagen of reticular dermis encroaching upon the eccrine unit and replacing the normal cuff of fat surrounding the eccrine unit.

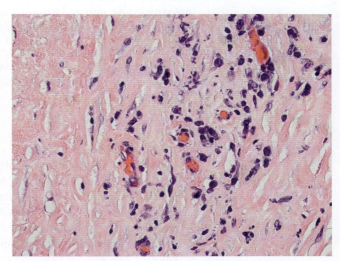

Figure 5.6.8 Scleroderma. Lymphoplasmacytic infiltrate in the sclerotic collagen of the deep dermis. Note that eosinophils are not present.

5.7 LUPUS PANNICULITIS VS SUBCUTANEOUS PANNICULITIS-LIKE T-CELL LYMPHOMA

	Lupus Panniculitis	**Subcutaneous Panniculitis-Like T-Cell Lymphoma**
Age	Variable age of presentation but typically between 30 and 60 years of age. More frequent in women.	Occurs in both children and adults with a wide range of ages. Average age of presentation typically in the fourth decade.
Location	Most commonly involves upper arms and shoulders but can involve trunk, buttocks, chest, face, and scalp.	Extremities and trunk primarily.
Etiology	Autoimmune disorder caused by failure of the mechanisms that maintain self-tolerance. Genetic and environmental factors, including ultraviolet radiation, sex hormones, and medications, contribute to the pathogenesis. Autoantibodies, directed toward a variety of nuclear proteins, mediate tissue injury.	Primary cutaneous lymphoma composed of neoplastic cytotoxic alpha-beta T-cell lymphocytes that migrate to the subcutaneous adipose tissue.
Presentation	Tender, deep-seated, indurated, erythematous nodules or plaques. Lesions may be solitary or arise in crops involving multiple regions.	Multiple, painless nodules or indurated plaques with dull erythematous surface. Individuals, especially those with concomitant hemophagocytic syndrome, may have associated fever, chills, myalgias, weight loss, and cytopenias.
Histology	1. Variable superficial changes of hyperkeratosis, interface vacuolar degeneration, perivascular lymphocytic infiltrate, and dermal mucin deposition *(Fig. 5.7.6)*. In many cases, the epidermis and dermis are unremarkable. 2. Predominantly lobular infiltrate of small lymphocytes without cytologic atypia *(Figs. 5.7.1-5.7.3)*. May have associated germinal center formation and plasma cells. Lymphocytes do not show rimming of adipocytes. 3. Lymphocytic vasculopathy with infiltration of subcutaneous vessel walls by lymphocytes, endothelial swelling, and erythrocyte extravasation *(Fig. 5.7.4)*. 4. Hyaline sclerosis and myxoid change of collagen of deep dermis and subcutaneous septa *(Figs. 5.7.1* and *5.7.5)*. 5. Lipomembranous fat necrosis occasionally involving subcutaneous fat lobules.	1. May have epidermal vacuolar interface change and mucin deposition, but less commonly than lupus panniculitis. Generally, the overlying epidermis and dermis are unremarkable. 2. Subcutaneous lobular lymphocytic infiltrate that spares the septa *(Fig. 5.7.7)*. 3. Neoplastic lymphocytes are enlarged and have hyperchromatic nuclei with irregular nuclear contours *(Figs. 5.7.9* and *5.7.10)*. Plasma cells are rare, and germinal center formation is not present. 4. Atypical lymphocytes rim individual fat cells, and there are associated histiocytes with karyorrhectic debris ("bean bag cells") *(Figs. 5.7.8-5.7.10)*.

	Lupus Panniculitis	**Subcutaneous Panniculitis-Like T-Cell Lymphoma**
Special studies	Immunohistochemistry shows admixed CD4+ and CD8+ T cells with aggregates of CD20+ B cells. T-cell receptor (TCR) gene rearrangement generally polyclonal.	Neoplastic T-cell lymphocytes show CD3+, CD4−, CD8+, CD56− immunoprofile with expression for cytotoxic markers including granzyme B, TIA1, and perforin. Ki-67 hotspots may also help to distinguish from lupus panniculitis. The lymphocytes are TCR beta F1 positive and TCR gamma-1 negative.
Treatment	Administration of antimalarial drugs, such as hydroxychloroquine, is first-line therapy. Short-term systemic corticosteroids may be added. Steroid-sparing immunosuppressive agents, such as methotrexate, azathioprine, or cyclophosphamide, may be added for severe disease or those cases associated with systemic symptoms.	High-dose systemic corticosteroids generally result in long-term remission. Chemotherapy and stem cell transplantation may be necessary for aggressive, refractory, or recurrent cases.
Prognosis	Chronic, relapsing course. Patients may have concomitant discoid or systemic lupus erythematosus. May lead to lipoatrophy and calcinosis, which may be severe and cause disfigurement.	Generally indolent course. Occasionally shows spontaneous resolution. Extension to lymph nodes and visceral organs is rare. Cases with hemophagocytic lymphohistiocytosis have worse prognosis.

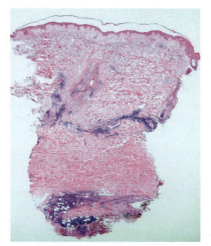

Figure 5.7.1 Lupus panniculitis. Lobular inflammatory infiltrate with extension along the deep vascular plexus in the reticular dermis and around adnexae. Note hyalinization of subcutis.

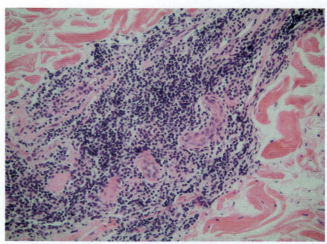

Figure 5.7.2 Lupus panniculitis. Infiltrate of lymphocytes and plasma cells around the eccrine unit.

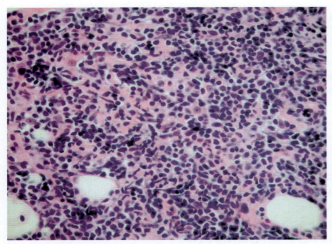

Figure 5.7.3 Lupus panniculitis. Lymphocytic infiltrate within fat lobules consists of small lymphocytes with round to slightly irregular nuclei and no significant atypia. Lymphocytes do not show rimming of fat cells.

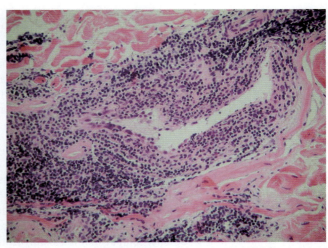

Figure 5.7.4 Lupus panniculitis. Lymphocytic vasculopathy with infiltration of vessel wall by lymphocytes.

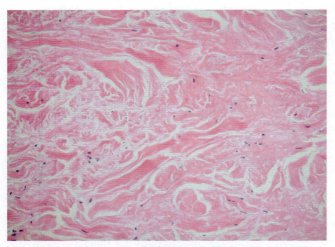

Figure 5.7.5 Lupus panniculitis. Hyalinized collagen within deep dermis and subcutaneous fat lobules.

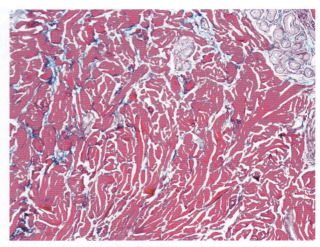

Figure 5.7.6 Lupus panniculitis. Colloidal iron stain demonstrating mucin deposition in the hyalinized stroma of the deep dermis and superficial subcutis.

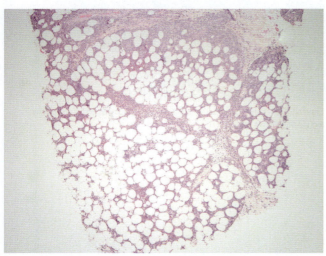

Figure 5.7.7 Subcutaneous panniculitis-like T-cell lymphoma. Dense lobular infiltrate with preservation of the adipocytes. Note that the infiltrate is primarily within the lobules.

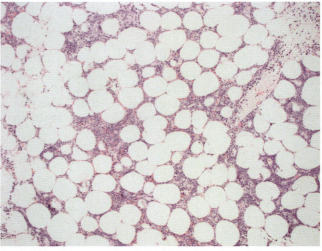

Figure 5.7.8 Subcutaneous panniculitis-like T-cell lymphoma. Infiltrate of lymphocytes that show "rimming" of the adipocytes but no significant fat necrosis.

5.7 Lupus Panniculitis vs Subcutaneous Panniculitis-Like T-Cell Lymphoma

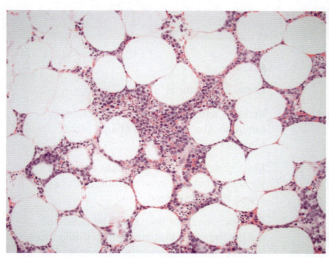

Figure 5.7.9 Subcutaneous panniculitis-like T-cell lymphoma. Rimming of adipocytes by large, hyperchromatic lymphocytes accompanied by histiocytes containing cellular debris ("bean bag cells").

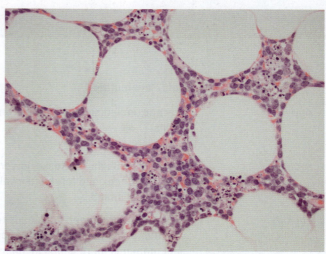

Figure 5.7.10 Subcutaneous panniculitis-like T-cell lymphoma. Lymphocytes are enlarged and show atypia with discernible nucleoli and mitotic activity. Note histiocytes with karyorrhectic debris ("bean bag cells").

5.8 COLD PANNICULITIS VS LUPUS PANNICULITIS

	Cold Panniculitis	**Lupus Panniculitis**
Age	Any age, including infants, children, and adults.	Variable age of presentation but typically between 30 and 60 years of age. More frequent in women.
Location	Typically on thighs, buttocks, lower abdomen in adults. Cheek and forehead involved primarily in infants.	Most commonly involves upper arms and shoulders but can involve trunk, buttocks, chest, face, and scalp.
Etiology	Exposure to prolonged cold leads to vascular damage and crystallization of the subcutaneous fat resulting in inflammation in the area.	Autoimmune disorder caused by failure of the mechanisms that maintain self-tolerance. Genetic and environmental factors, including ultraviolet radiation, sex hormones, and medications, contribute to the pathogenesis. Autoantibodies, directed toward a variety of nuclear proteins, mediate tissue injury.
Presentation	Erythematous or violaceous, indurated, ill-defined nodules. May have ulceration. Pruritus and burning variably present. Lesions typically evolve 24-48 hours after cold exposure. Associated with horse riding in women, ice pack use, and eating cold items in young children.	Tender, deep-seated, indurated, erythematous nodules or plaques. Lesions may be solitary or arise in crops involving multiple regions.
Histology	1. Superficial and deep perivascular lymphocytic infiltrate in the dermis *(Figs. 5.8.1* and *5.8.3)*. 2. Lymphocytic lobular infiltrate within the subcutis with lipophagic features *(Fig. 5.8.4)*. 3. Perieccrine and perineural lymphocytic inflammation *(Fig. 5.8.2)*. 4. Lymphocytic vasculopathy may be evident. 5. Mucin deposition *(Fig. 5.8.5)* may be present as in lupus erythematosus; therefore, clinical correlation is necessary.	1. Variable superficial changes of hyperkeratosis, interface vacuolar degeneration, perivascular lymphocytic infiltrate, and dermal mucin deposition. In many cases, the epidermis and dermis are unremarkable. 2. Predominantly lobular infiltrate of small lymphocytes without cytologic atypia *(Figs. 5.8.6* and *5.8.7)*. May have associated germinal center formation and plasma cells. 3. Lymphocytic vasculopathy with infiltration of subcutaneous vessel walls by lymphocytes, endothelial swelling, and erythrocyte extravasation *(Fig. 5.8.8)*. 4. Hyaline sclerosis and myxoid change of collagen of deep dermis and subcutaneous septa *(Figs. 5.8.9* and *5.8.10)*. 5. Lipomembranous fat necrosis involving subcutaneous fat lobules occasionally seen.

	Cold Panniculitis	**Lupus Panniculitis**
Special studies	Colloidal iron stain to demonstrate mucin deposition in dermis. Immunohistochemistry for CD123 to demonstrate plasmacytoid dendritic cells. Neither of these stains, however, are helpful in distinguishing from lupus panniculitis.	Colloidal iron stain to demonstrate mucin deposition in dermis. Immunohistochemistry for CD123 to demonstrate plasmacytoid dendritic cells. Neither of these stains, however, are helpful in distinguishing from cold panniculitis.
Treatment	Therapy is generally supportive and based upon symptomatology with use of nonsteroidal anti-inflammatory medications for pain. Gradual warming of the exposed areas generally aids in resolution of lesions.	Administration of antimalarial drugs, such as hydroxychloroquine, is first-line therapy. Short-term systemic corticosteroids may be added. Steroid-sparing immunosuppressive agents, such as methotrexate, azathioprine, or cyclophosphamide, may be added for severe disease or those cases associated with systemic symptoms.
Prognosis	Generally a self-limiting condition without sequelae.	Chronic, relapsing course. Patients may have concomitant discoid or systemic lupus erythematosus. May lead to lipoatrophy and calcinosis, which may be severe and cause disfigurement.

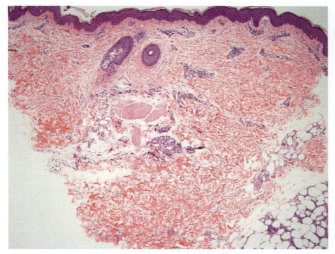

Figure 5.8.1 Cold panniculitis. Lobular subcutaneous infiltrate (lower right) with superficial and deep perivascular and periadnexal infiltrate within the dermis. Note that there is no hyalinization of the reticular dermis or subcutis.

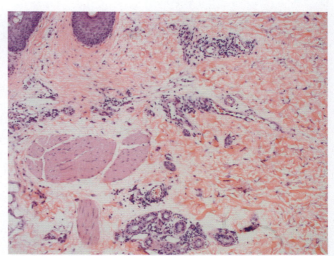

Figure 5.8.2 Cold panniculitis. Lymphocytic infiltrate around vascular plexus and eccrine units in dermis. The infiltrate is generally less dense than in lupus panniculitis.

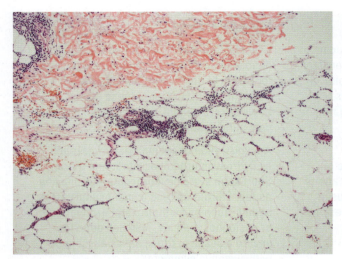

Figure 5.8.3 Cold panniculitis. Lobular lymphocytic infiltrate in subcutis consisting primarily of small lymphocytes. Blood vessels are unremarkable.

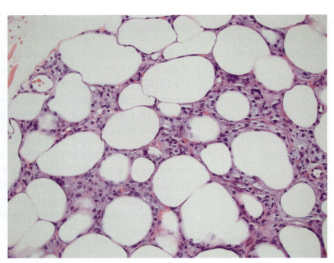

Figure 5.8.4 Cold panniculitis. Area of lipophagic fat necrosis with foamy histiocytes surrounding adipocytes and fat cysts.

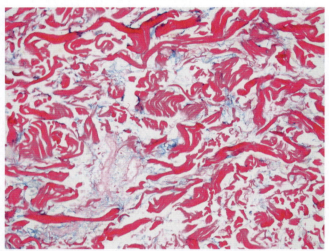

Figure 5.8.5 Cold panniculitis. Mucin deposition in reticular dermis on colloidal iron stain. This and other features overlap with lupus panniculitis; therefore, clinic correlation is essential.

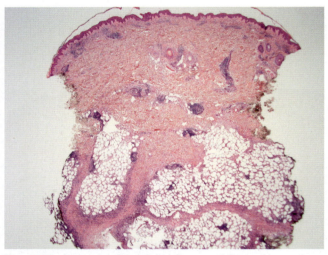

Figure 5.8.6 Lupus panniculitis. Lobular inflammatory infiltrate with extension into septae and, more superficially, around the vascular plexus and adnexae.

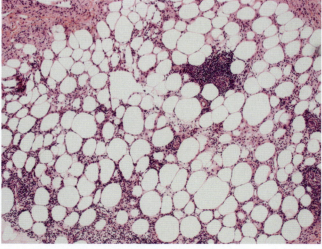

Figure 5.8.7 Lupus panniculitis. Moderately dense lobular lymphocytic infiltrate.

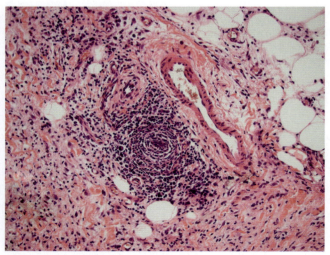

Figure 5.8.8 Lupus panniculitis. Lymphocytic vasculopathy characterized by lymphocytes permeating the vessel wall without appreciable fibrinoid necrosis.

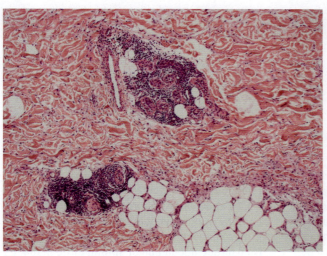

Figure 5.8.9 Lupus panniculitis. Hyalinization of deep dermis and fat lobules along with a moderately dense lymphocytic infiltrate around the deep plexus and eccrine unit.

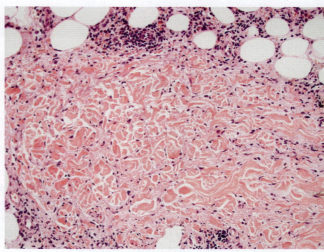

Figure 5.8.10 Lupus panniculitis. Hyalinization of subcutaneous lobule with infiltrate of small lymphocytes.

5.9 PANCREATIC PANNICULITIS VS INFECTIOUS PANNICULITIS

	Pancreatic Panniculitis	**Infectious Panniculitis**
Age	Middle-aged and elderly adults.	Any age.
Location	Lower extremities typically involved. May also extend to buttocks, trunk, upper extremities, and scalp.	Lower extremities often involved but also buttocks, abdomen, intertriginous regions, and upper extremities.
Etiology	Systemically released pancreatic enzymes, such as amylase and lipase, cause necrosis of subcutaneous adipocytes and recruitment of neutrophilic inflammation. Most commonly associated with acute and chronic pancreatitis and pancreatic carcinoma.	Infection of the subcutaneous tissues from a wide variety of organisms including bacteria, fungi, mycobacteria, as well as protozoa and viruses. Infection can result from direct inoculation or spread through the bloodstream.
Presentation	Tender, ill-defined, edematous, erythematous nodules that ulcerate and exude viscous, oily brown material. Often associated with arthralgias. Skin lesions may develop prior to diagnosis of pancreatic disease.	Swelling and erythema often precede development of one or more fluctuant nodules that ulcerate. More commonly seen in individuals with diabetes mellitus or immunosuppression.
Histology	1. Lobular infiltrate with mixed inflammatory cells predominated by neutrophils *(Fig. 5.9.2)*. 2. Coagulative necrosis of adipocytes with saponification and "ghost" cells representing fat cell remnants *(Figs. 5.9.1, 5.9.3, 5.9.4)*. 3. Basophilic granular calcification *(Figs. 5.9.1 and 5.9.3)*. 4. Viable fat lobules with acute and chronic inflammation and lipophages.	1. Epidermal acanthosis and parakeratosis. 2. Dermal edema with diffuse neutrophilic infiltrate. 3. Mixed septal and lobular inflammation with neutrophils predominating *(Figs. 5.9.5 and 5.9.6)*. Granulomas may be seen especially with fungal and mycobacterial causes *(Fig. 5.9.7)*. 4. Vascular proliferation with hemorrhage *(Fig. 5.9.5)*. 5. Fat necrosis may be present but generally no coagulative necrosis or saponification.
Special studies	Elevated levels of amylase, lipase, and trypsin are usually present and aid in confirming the diagnosis. Eosinophilia is seen in a majority of cases.	Tissue Gram, PAS or GMS, and AFB or Fite stains to identify bacteria, fungi, and mycobacteria, respectively *(Fig. 5.9.8)*. Microbiologic culture to increase sensitivity of detection of organisms.
Treatment	Primarily supportive and directed toward treatment of underlying pancreatic disease.	Systemic antibiotics are generally necessary to clear infection. Surgical excision and/or debridement may be an option for isolated lesions.
Prognosis	Dependent upon associated pancreatic disease. Panniculitis usually resolves with clearing of pancreatic inflammation in cases associated with pancreatitis. Individuals with pancreatic carcinoma have a more prolonged course and high mortality rate. The triad of pancreatitis, arthralgias, and peripheral eosinophilia is associated with a poor prognosis.	Dependent upon organism, extent of infection, and comorbidities. Some fungal and mycobacterial infections may be difficult to clear and require long duration of antimicrobial therapy.

5.9 Pancreatic Panniculitis vs Infectious Panniculitis

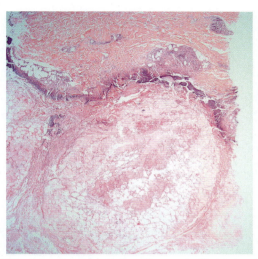

Figure 5.9.1 Pancreatic panniculitis. Extensive necrosis of fat lobules with ghost-like outlines of adipocyte nuclei.

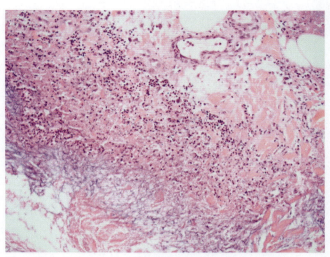

Figure 5.9.2 Pancreatic panniculitis. Inflammatory infiltrate predominated by neutrophils surrounding areas of lobular fat necrosis.

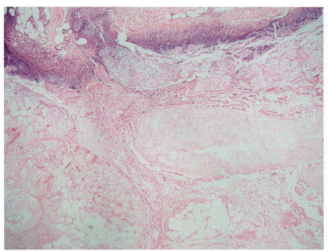

Figure 5.9.3 Pancreatic panniculitis. Extensive necrosis and saponification of fat lobules.

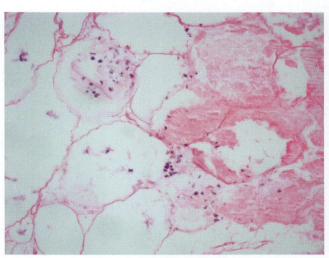

Figure 5.9.4 Pancreatic panniculitis. Necrosis and saponification of fat lobules with degenerated neutrophils.

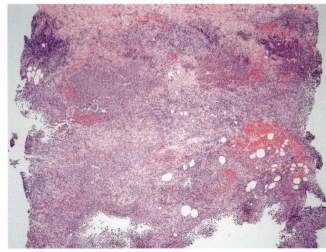

Figure 5.9.5 Infectious panniculitis. Dense mixed inflammatory infiltrate within lobules that is associated with vascular proliferation and hemorrhage.

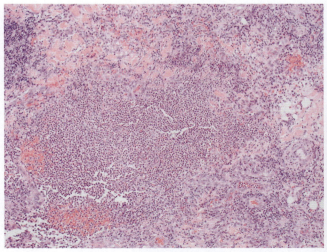

Figure 5.9.6 Infectious panniculitis. Neutrophils predominate in the lobular infiltrate and form sheets surrounded by reactive blood vessels.

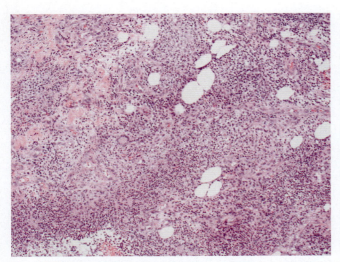

Figure 5.9.7 Infectious panniculitis. Histiocytes and a few multinucleate giant cells form loose and ill-defined granulomas.

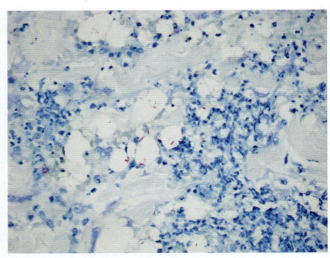

Figure 5.9.8 Infectious panniculitis. Acid-fast bacilli identified with AFB stain within the fat lobules.

5.10 PANCREATIC PANNICULITIS VS ALPHA-1 ANTITRYPSIN DEFICIENCY PANNICULITIS

	Pancreatic Panniculitis	**Alpha-1 Antitrypsin Deficiency Panniculitis**
Age	Middle-aged and elderly adults.	Generally presents in adults, between third and fifth decades of life, but may present in childhood in individuals with genotypes associated with greater deficiency.
Location	Lower extremities typically involved. May also extend to buttocks, trunk, upper extremities, and scalp.	Extremities most commonly involved but trunk, buttocks, abdomen, and face may also be affected.
Etiology	Systemically released pancreatic enzymes, such as amylase and lipase, cause necrosis of subcutaneous adipocytes and recruitment of neutrophilic inflammation. Most commonly associated with acute and chronic pancreatitis and pancreatic carcinoma.	Due to deficiency of serine protease inhibitor alpha-1 antitrypsin. Reduced circulating alpha-1 antitrypsin leads to impaired neutrophil elastase and exaggerated neutrophilic and proteolytic response.
Presentation	Tender, ill-defined, edematous, erythematous nodules that ulcerate and exude viscous, oily brown material. Often associated with arthralgias. Skin lesions may develop prior to diagnosis of pancreatic disease.	Tender, erythematous subcutaneous nodules that may ulcerate and have oily, yellow discharge. Lesions may arise spontaneously, or after minor trauma, and heal with atrophy and scarring. May be associated with chronic obstructive pulmonary disease, hepatitis, and glomerulonephritis.
Histology	1. Lobular infiltrate with mixed inflammatory cells predominated by neutrophils *(Figs. 5.10.1 and 5.10.2)*. 2. Coagulative necrosis of adipocytes with saponification and "ghost" cells representing fat cell remnants *(Fig. 5.10.3)*. 3. Basophilic granular calcification *(Fig. 5.10.3)*. 4. Viable fat lobules with acute and chronic inflammation and lipophages.	1. Septal and lobular neutrophilic infiltrate *(Figs. 5.10.4 and 5.10.5)*. 2. Neutrophils splay collagen bundles in the deep reticular dermis *(Fig. 5.10.6)*. 3. Fat necrosis with aggregates of histiocytes and lipophages *(Fig. 5.10.7)*. 4. Areas of normal subcutis adjacent to inflamed and necrotic subcutis *(Fig. 5.10.4)*.
Special studies	Elevated levels of amylase, lipase, and trypsin are usually present and aid in confirming the diagnosis. Eosinophilia is seen in a majority of cases.	Serum alpha-1 antitrypsin level. Alpha-1 antitrypsin phenotyping or genotyping.
Treatment	Primarily supportive and directed toward treatment of underlying pancreatic disease.	Dapsone is the preferred oral therapy, but glucocorticoids, tetracyclines, and other immunosuppressants show efficacy. Intravenous alpha-1 antitrypsin may be used in severe or refractory cases.

(continued)

	Pancreatic Panniculitis	Alpha-1 Antitrypsin Deficiency Panniculitis
Prognosis	Dependent upon associated pancreatic disease. Panniculitis usually resolves with clearing of pancreatic inflammation in cases associated with pancreatitis. Individuals with pancreatic carcinoma have a more prolonged course and high mortality rate. The triad of pancreatitis, arthralgias, and peripheral eosinophilia is associated with a poor prognosis.	Untreated, severe cases can lead to death. Resolution of disease is typically seen with adequate treatment, although relapses may occur.

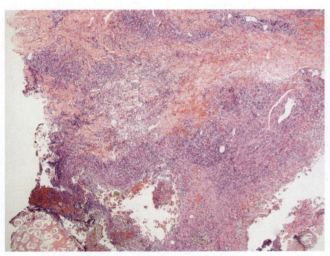

Figure 5.10.1 Pancreatic panniculitis. Dense deep dermal and lobular subcutaneous inflammatory infiltrate with reactive vascular proliferation and hemorrhage. Note area of fat necrosis at lower left corner of image.

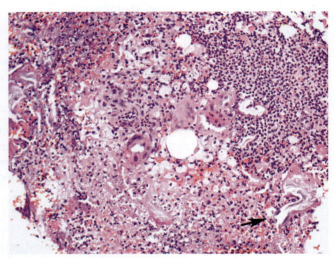

Figure 5.10.2 Pancreatic panniculitis. Lobular infiltrate predominated by neutrophils. Necrosis with focal calcification (arrow).

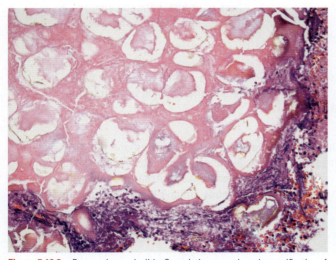

Figure 5.10.3 Pancreatic panniculitis. Coagulative necrosis and saponification of fat lobules with peripheral rim of neutrophilic inflammation.

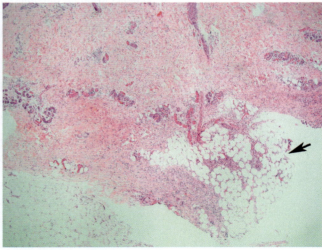

Figure 5.10.4 Alpha-1 antitrypsin deficiency panniculitis. Inflammation of subcutaneous septae and fat lobule (arrow). Note relatively uninvolved fat lobule at lower left.

5.10 Pancreatic Panniculitis vs Alpha-1 Antitrypsin Deficiency Panniculitis

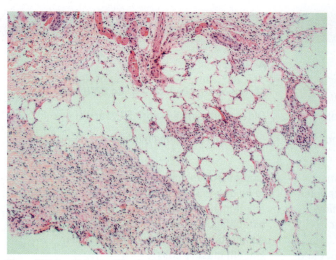

Figure 5.10.5 Alpha-1 antitrypsin deficiency panniculitis. Mixed lobular infiltrate of neutrophils with histiocytes and few lipophages.

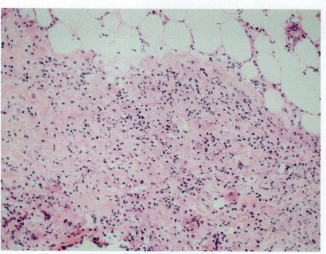

Figure 5.10.6 Alpha-1 antitrypsin deficiency panniculitis. Neutrophilic inflammation splays collagen of subcutaneous fibrous septae.

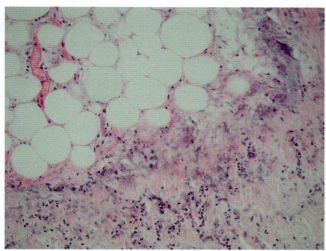

Figure 5.10.7 Alpha-1 antitrypsin deficiency panniculitis. Lipophagic fat necrosis with neutrophilic inflammation and basophilic degeneration of collagen.

5.11 CALCIPHYLAXIS VS MONCKEBERG MEDIAL CALCIFIC SCLEROSIS

	Calciphylaxis	**Monckeberg Medial Calcific Sclerosis**
Age	Adults between ages of 50 and 70 years.	Older adults, rare before 50 years of age.
Location	Typically involves buttocks, thighs, and abdomen.	Extremities primarily involved.
Etiology	Multifactorial mechanisms resulting in calcification of the media of small arterioles and capillaries. Obstruction of blood flow leads to thrombus formation, vascular occlusion, ischemia, and ulceration. Elevation in calcium/phosphate product and increased parathyroid hormone levels are seen in many patients.	Exact mechanism is unknown but postulated to be due to stimulation of migratory adventitial myofibroblasts that acquire an osteoblastic phenotype secondary to the elaboration of osteopontin by vascular smooth muscle cells.
Presentation	Painful, indurated, dusky plaques, livedo, or purpura. Lesions rapidly progress to ulcers with eschar. Highly associated with chronic renal disease and dialysis, but nonuremic cases do occur.	Generally an incidental and asymptomatic condition. It is highly associated with aging, diabetes mellitus, and chronic kidney disease. Radiographic images of involved distal extremities produce a characteristic "railroad track" pattern.
Histology	1. Epidermal ischemic necrosis with or without ulceration *(Fig. 5.11.1)*. 2. Mural calcification of small arterioles and capillaries in subcutaneous adipose tissue *(Figs. 5.11.3 and 5.11.4)*. 3. Intravascular thrombi and fibrointimal hyperplasia with erythrocyte extravasation *(Figs. 5.11.2 and 5.11.3)*.	1. Epidermis and dermis are generally normal and without ischemic changes. 2. Calcification in the tunica media of small and medium-sized arteries of the deep dermis and subcutaneous tissues *(Fig. 5.11.5)*. 3. Lumina of vessels are patent and the calcification is not associated with thrombus formation or erythrocyte extravasation *(Fig. 5.11.6)*.
Special studies	Von Kossa stain to confirm presence of vascular calcification in cases with subtle findings.	None needed. Calcifications are typically large and, therefore, von Kossa stain is not necessary.
Treatment	Wound care, pain management, and antibiotics for secondary infection. Sodium thiosulfate, hyperbaric oxygen, bisphosphonates, and parathyroidectomy have also been used for management.	No treatment is indicated.
Prognosis	Poor prognosis with considerable morbidity due to pain and chronic ulcerations. High mortality rate secondary to infection and sepsis.	Although Monckeberg medial calcific sclerosis does not cause vascular occlusion, as in atherosclerosis, it has been shown to be a risk factor for cardiovascular and peripheral vascular disease.

5.11 Calciphylaxis vs Monckeberg Medial Calcific Sclerosis

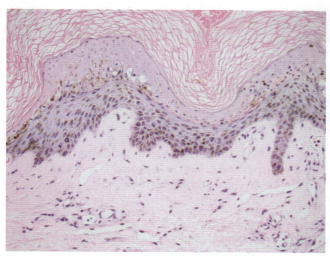

Figure 5.11.1 Calciphylaxis. Ischemic necrosis of superficial epidermis with ghost-like outlines of nuclei and pyknosis.

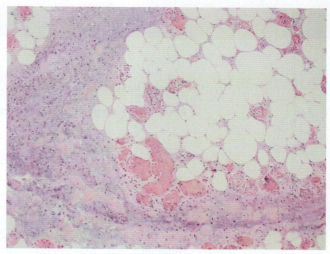

Figure 5.11.2 Calciphylaxis. Vascular congestion and thrombosis with necrosis of fat lobules and septae.

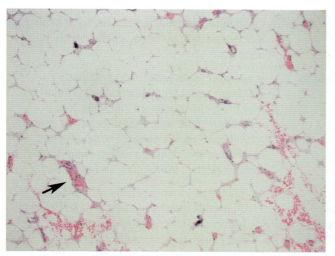

Figure 5.11.3 Calciphylaxis. Mural calcification of small capillaries within subcutaneous adipose tissue. There is vascular congestion and thrombus formation (arrow) with erythrocyte extravasation.

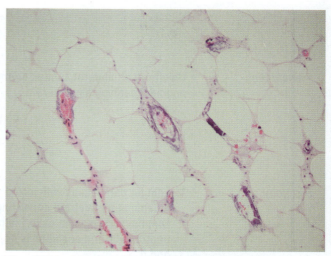

Figure 5.11.4 Calciphylaxis. Plate-like calcifications within the walls of small capillaries in subcutaneous fat lobules. There is surrounding fat necrosis.

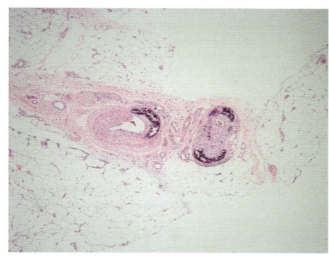

Figure 5.11.5 Monckeberg medial calcific sclerosis. Calcification in the tunica media of medium-sized arteries within the subcutis. Note that there is no associated fat necrosis.

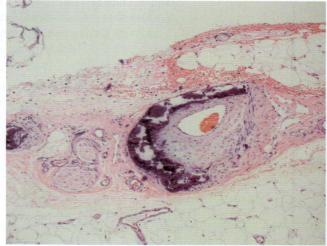

Figure 5.11.6 Monckeberg medial calcific sclerosis. Calcification in the tunica media of a medium-sized vessel with intimal thickening but no occlusion of the lumen. The erythrocyte extravasation is procedural.

5.12 NODULAR VASCULITIS VS POLYARTERITIS NODOSA

	Nodular Vasculitis	**Polyarteritis Nodosa**
Age	Adults; more common in women than men.	All ages, but most common in middle-aged to older adults.
Location	Posterior lower legs/calves.	Most commonly involves the lower extremities with less frequent involvement of the upper extremities, trunk, and head and neck regions.
Etiology	Immune-mediated hypersensitivity reaction most frequently associated with tuberculosis. Other infections, inflammatory processes, and medications less commonly associated. Minority of idiopathic cases.	Immune complex–mediated vasculitis hypothesized to be due to development of anti-phosphatidylserine-prothrombin complex antibodies and activation of classical complement pathway. Underlying inflammatory bowel disease, infection, malignancy, and medication use have been associated with cutaneous polyarteritis nodosa.
Presentation	Unilateral or bilateral, tender, erythematous nodules that typically ulcerate.	Initially presents with livedo reticularis and tender subcutaneous nodules. These may progress to purpura, necrosis, and ulceration of the skin. May experience digital infarction in severe cases. Extracutaneous manifestations include malaise, weight loss, fever, myalgias, arthralgias, and neuropathy.
Histology	1. Lobular panniculitis with mixed inflammatory infiltrate consisting of lymphocytes, plasma cells, histiocytes, neutrophils, and eosinophils *(Figs. 5.12.1 and 5.12.2)*. 2. Granuloma formation may be present. 3. Vasculitis involving variably sized arterial and venous vessels with fibrinoid necrosis and leukocytoclasis *(Fig. 5.12.3)*. Vasculitis not limited to medium-sized vessels. 4. Lipophagic fat necrosis with formation of microcysts *(Fig. 5.12.4)*.	1. Intact epidermis is relatively normal. Ulceration may be present in older lesions. 2. Transmural infiltration of the walls of medium-sized vessels of the deep reticular dermis and subcutis by infiltrate predominated by neutrophils *(Fig. 5.12.5)*. No granuloma formation. 3. Fibrinoid degeneration of the vessel walls with inflammation surrounding affected vessel *(Fig. 5.12.6)*. Intraluminal thrombus may be present. 4. No significant involvement of the fat lobules.
Special studies	Histochemical stains to exclude bacterial, fungal, and mycobacterial infection.	Direct immunofluorescence is relatively nonspecific but may show deposition of C3 and IgM around medium-sized vessels. May have mild anemia, leukocytosis, and elevated erythrocyte sedimentation rate. Serologies to exclude other forms of vasculitis involving medium-sized vessels may be indicated; not associated with anti-neutrophil cytoplasmic antibodies.

5.12 Nodular Vasculitis vs Polyarteritis Nodosa

	Nodular Vasculitis	**Polyarteritis Nodosa**
Treatment	Identification and treatment of underlying cause, including therapy for active or latent tuberculosis if present. Nonsteroidal anti-inflammatory medications and rest for symptomatic relief. Oral potassium iodide provides rapid response in most cases.	Mild cases may be treated with nonsteroidal anti-inflammatory drugs, topical corticosteroids, or colchicine. More severe disease may require systemic corticosteroids with or followed by colchicine, dapsone, hydroxychloroquine, azathioprine, methotrexate, or cyclophosphamide.
Prognosis	Variable course. Resolution of disease with treatment of underlying cause, but cases associated with tuberculosis may recur. Idiopathic cases may persist for months to years.	Typically has a chronic, relapsing, and remitting course. Course of disease may last months to years with flares lasting for weeks. Rarely, there is progression to systemic involvement of liver, kidneys, adrenals, joints, and heart.

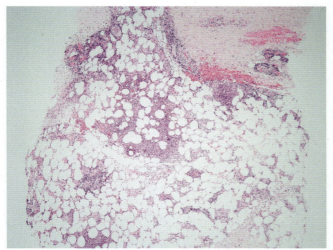

Figure 5.12.1 Nodular vasculitis. Dense mixed lobular inflammatory infiltrate with areas of hemorrhage.

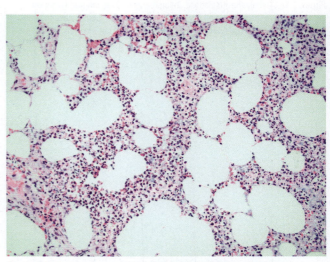

Figure 5.12.2 Nodular vasculitis. Mixed lobular infiltrate predominated by neutrophils but including eosinophils, lymphocytes, and plasma cells.

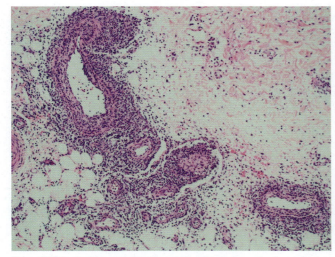

Figure 5.12.3 Nodular vasculitis. Neutrophils infiltrate the walls of vessels of varying size with mural fibrinoid change and leukocytoclastic debris. Note that the vasculitic change involves both arterial and venous vessels, not exclusively medium-sized arterioles.

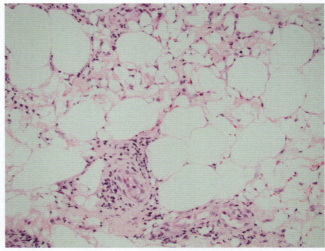

Figure 5.12.4 Nodular vasculitis. Lobules show lipophagic fat necrosis with formation of fat cysts associated with foamy macrophages.

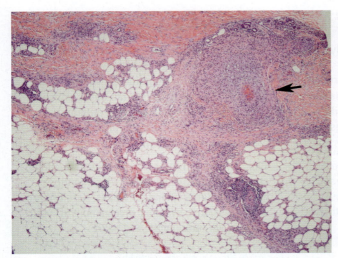

Figure 5.12.5 Polyarteritis nodosa. Inflammation of medium-sized arteriole with necrosis of the vessel wall (arrow). Note that the fat lobules have minimal inflammation and necrosis. Small vessels and veins are not involved.

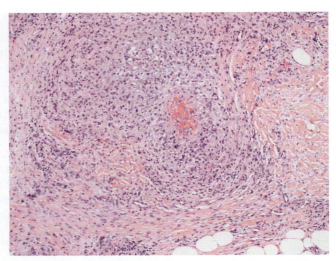

Figure 5.12.6 Polyarteritis nodosa. Infiltration of the wall of medium-sized arteriole by neutrophils and lymphomononuclear cells with destruction of the wall and erythrocyte extravasation.

SUGGESTED READING

Chapters 5.1-5.5

Bielsa Marsol I. Update on the classification and treatment of localized scleroderma. *Actas Dermosifiliogr.* 2013;104(8):654-666.

Choonhakarn C, Chaowattanapanit S, Julanon N. Lipodermatosclerosis: a clinicopathologic correlation. *Int J Dermatol.* 2016;55(3):303-308.

Davatchi F, Chams-Davatchi C, Shams H, et al. Behcet's disease: epidemiology, clinical manifestations, and diagnosis. *Expert Rev Clin Immunol.* 2017;13(1):57-65.

De Simone C, Caldarola G, Scaldaferri F, et al. Clinical, histopathological, and immunological evaluation of a series of patients with erythema nodosum. *Int J Dermatol.* 2016;55(5):e289-e294.

Ferrara G, Stefanato CM, Gianotti R, Kubba A, Annessi G. Panniculitis with vasculitis. *G Ital Dermatol Venereol.* 2013;148(4):387-394.

Grassi S, Rosso R, Tomasini C, Pezzini C, Merlino M, Borroni G. Post-surgical lipophagic panniculitis: a specific model of traumatic panniculitis and new histopathological findings. *G Ital Dermatol Venereol.* 2013;148(4):435-441.

Huang TM, Lee JYY. Lipodermatosclerosis: a clinicopathologic study of 17 cases and differential diagnosis from erythema nodosum. *J Cutan Pathol.* 2009;36(4):453-460.

Miteva M, Romanelli P, Kirsner RS. Lipodermatosclerosis. *Dermatol Ther.* 2010;23(4):375-388.

Moreno A, Marcoval J, Peyri J. Traumatic panniculitis. *Dermatol Clin.* 2008;26(4):481-483, vii.

Penmetsa GK, Sapra A. *Morphea.* In: *StatPearls.* StatPearls Publishing; 2022.

Pérez-Garza DM, Chavez-Alvarez S, Ocampo-Candiani J, Gomez-Flores M. Erythema nodosum: a practical approach and diagnostic algorithm. *Am J Clin Dermatol.* 2021;22(3):367-378.

Requena L, Sánchez Yus E. Panniculitis. Part II. Mostly lobular panniculitis. *J Am Acad Dermatol.* 2001;45(3):325-361; quiz 362-4.

Requena L, Sánchez Yus E. Erythema nodosum. *Semin Cutan Med Surg.* 2007;26(2):114-125.

Santos-Juanes J, Coto P, Galache C, Sánchez del Río J, Soto de Delás J. Encapsulated fat necrosis: a form of traumatic panniculitis. *J Eur Acad Dermatol Venereol.* 2007;21(3):405-406.

Wick MR. Panniculitis: a summary. *Semin Diagn Pathol.* 2017;34(3):261-272.

Winkelmann RK, Barker SM. Factitial traumatic panniculitis. *J Am Acad Dermatol.* 1985;13(6):988-994.

Chapter 5.6

Bielsa Marsol I. Update on the classification and treatment of localized scleroderma. *Actas Dermosifiliogr.* 2013;104(8):654-666.

Careta MF, Romiti R. Localized scleroderma: clinical spectrum and therapeutic update. *An Bras Dermatol.* 2015;90(1):62-73.

Lamback EB, Resende FSS, Lenzi TCR. Eosinophilic fasciitis. *An Bras Dermatol.* 2016;91(5 suppl 1):57-59.

Mazori DR, Femia AN, Vleugels RA. Eosinophilic fasciitis: an updated review on diagnosis and treatment. *Curr Rheumatol Rep.* 2017;19(12):74.

Mertens JS, Seyger MMB, Thurlings RM, Radstake TRDJ, de Jong EMGJ. Morphea and Eosinophilic fasciitis: an update. *Am J Clin Dermatol.* 2017;18(4):491-512.

Yano H, Kinjo M. Eosinophilic fasciitis. *JAMA Dermatol.* 2020;156(5):582.

Chapters 5.7-5.8

Ferrara G, Cerroni L. Cold-associated perniosis of the thighs ("Equestrian-Type" Chilblain): a reappraisal based on a clinicopathologic and immunohistochemical study of 6 cases. *Am J Dermatopathol.* 2016;38(10):726-731.

Fraga J, García-Díez A. Lupus erythematosus panniculitis. *Dermatol Clin.* 2008;26(4):453-463, vi.

Gallardo F, Pujol RM. Subcutaneous panniculitic-like T-cell lymphoma and other primary cutaneous lymphomas with prominent subcutaneous tissue involvement. *Dermatol Clin.* 2008;26(4):529-540, viii.

LeBlanc RE, Tavallaee M, Kim YH, Kim J. Useful parameters for distinguishing subcutaneous panniculitis-like T-cell lymphoma from lupus erythematosus panniculitis. *Am J Surg Pathol.* 2016;40(6):745-754.

Pincus LB, LeBoit PE, McCalmont TH, et al. Subcutaneous panniculitis-like T-cell lymphoma with overlapping clinicopathologic features of lupus erythematosus: coexistence of 2 entities? *Am J Dermatopathol.* 2009;31:520-526.

Quesada-Cortés A, Campos-Muñoz L, Díaz-Díaz RM, Casado-Jiménez M. Cold panniculitis. *Dermatol Clin.* 2008;26(4):485-489, vii.

West SE, McCalmont TH, North JP. Ice-pack dermatosis: a cold-induced dermatitis with similarities to cold panniculitis and perniosis that histopathologically resembles lupus. *JAMA Dermatol.* 2013;149(11):1314-1318.

Willemze R. Cutaneous lymphomas with a panniculitic presentation. *Semin Diagn Pathol.* 2017;34(1):36-43.

Chapters 5.9-5.10

Blanco I, Lipsker D, Lara B, Janciauskiene S. Neutrophilic panniculitis associated with alpha-1-antitrypsin deficiency: an update. *Br J Dermatol.* 2016;174(4):753-62.

Cutlan RT, Wesche WA, Jenkins JJ III, Chesney TM. A fatal case of pancreatic panniculitis presenting in a young patient with systemic lupus. *J Cutan Pathol.* 2000;27(9):466-471.

Franciosi AN, Ralph J, O'Farrell NJ, et al. Alpha-1 antitrypsin deficiency-associated panniculitis. *J Am Acad Dermatol.* 2022;87(4):825-832.

Johnson EF, Tolkachjov SN, Gibson LE. Alpha-1 antitrypsin deficiency panniculitis: clinical and pathologic characteristics of 10 cases. *Int J Dermatol.* 2018;57(8):952-958.

Llamas-Velasco M, Fraga J, Sánchez-Schmidt JM, et al. Neutrophilic infiltrates in panniculitis: comprehensive review and diagnostic algorithm proposal. *Am J Dermatopathol.* 2020;42(10):717-730.

Marcos P, Kieselova K, Cunha M. Pancreatic panniculitis. *Am J Gastroenterol.* 2017;112(8):1218.

Nosewicz J, Hyde J, McGrath M, Kaffenberger BH, Trinidad JC, Chung CG. Infectious panniculitis: an inpatient cohort. *Int J Dermatol*. 2022;61(12):e483-e485.

Patterson JW, Brown PC, Broecker AH. Infection-induced panniculitis. *J Cutan Pathol*. 1989;16(4):183-193.

Rongioletti F, Caputo V. Pancreatic panniculitis. *G Ital Dermatol Venereol*. 2013;148(4):419-425.

Chapter 5.11

Bahrani E, Perkins IU, North JP. Diagnosing calciphylaxis: a review with emphasis on histopathology. *Am J Dermatopathol*. 2020;42(7):471-480.

Nigwekar SU, Thadhani R, Brandenburg VM. Calciphylaxis. *N Engl J Med*. 2018;378(18):1704-1714.

Rick J, Strowd L, Pasieka HB, et al. Calciphylaxis: part I. Diagnosis and pathology. *J Am Acad Dermatol*. 2022;86(5):973-982.

Stack A, Sheffield S, Seegobin K, Maharaj S. Mönckeberg medial sclerosis. *Cleve Clin J Med*. 2020;87(7):396-397.

Yamamoto Y, Ishikawa Y, Shimpo M, Matsumura M. Mönckeberg's sclerosis. *J Gen Fam Med*. 2021;22(1):55-56.

Chapter 5.12

Morgan AJ, Schwartz RA. Cutaneous polyarteritis nodosa: a comprehensive review. *Int J Dermatol*. 2010;49(7):750-756.

Morimoto A, Chen KR. Reappraisal of histopathology of cutaneous polyarteritis nodosa. *J Cutan Pathol*. 2016;43(12):1131-1138.

Wee E, Kelly RI. The histopathology of cutaneous polyarteritis nodosa and its relationship with lymphocytic thrombophilic arteritis. *J Cutan Pathol*. 2017;44(4):411.

6
Alterations of the Epidermis and Dermis

- **6.1** Vitiligo vs Postinflammatory Hypomelanosis
- **6.2** Chondrodermatitis Nodularis Helicis vs Prurigo Nodularis
- **6.3** Acanthosis Nigricans vs Granular Parakeratosis
- **6.4** Acanthosis Nigricans vs Confluent and Reticulated Papillomatosis
- **6.5** Porokeratosis vs Lichen Planus–like Keratosis
- **6.6** Ichthyosis Vulgaris vs X-Linked Ichthyosis
- **6.7** Scleredema vs Pretibial Myxedema
- **6.8** Scleroderma vs Scleredema
- **6.9** Scleroderma vs Nephrogenic Systemic Fibrosis
- **6.10** Scleromyxedema vs Pretibial Myxedema
- **6.11** Focal Cutaneous Mucinosis vs Cutaneous Myxoma
- **6.12** Focal Cutaneous Mucinosis vs Digital Mucous Cyst
- **6.13** Calcinosis Cutis vs Gouty Tophus
- **6.14** Gouty Tophus vs Nodular Amyloidosis
- **6.15** Nodular Amyloidosis vs Adult Colloid Milium
- **6.16** Pseudoxanthoma Elasticum vs Solar Elastosis
- **6.17** Pseudoxanthoma Elasticum vs Mid-Dermal Elastolysis
- **6.18** Hypertrophic Scar vs Keloid
- **6.19** Tattoo vs Tumoral Melanosis
- **6.20** Exogenous Ochronosis vs Minocycline-Induced Hyperpigmentation

6.1 VITILIGO VS POSTINFLAMMATORY HYPOMELANOSIS

	Vitiligo	**Postinflammatory Hypomelanosis**
Age	Any age, especially children and young adults.	Any age.
Location	Any region of the skin and mucosa. Typically classified as segmental, nonsegmental, and mixed forms. Generalized, acrofacial, and acral nonsegmental forms most common. Nonsegmental forms have predilection for face, hands, and genital skin.	Any area of the body may be involved. Distribution dependent upon preceding inflammatory process.
Etiology	Multifactorial etiology with contributions from genetics, autoimmunity, oxidative stress, and infection. Considered to be autoimmune process with destruction of melanocytes by antimelanocytic cytotoxic T cells.	Inflammatory diseases of the skin (such as eczema, psoriasis, sarcoidosis, lichen sclerosus, and lupus erythematosus) alter steps involved in melanogenesis including melanosome formation, melanin production, melanosome transport, and transfer of melanin from melanocytes to keratinocytes.
Presentation	Asymptomatic, well-delineated, depigmented, white macules and patches without erythema or scale. Nonsegmental forms are generally bilateral and symmetric. Segmental forms are unilateral and may be dermatomal. Highlighted by Wood's light examination. Shows Koebner phenomenon with extension of lesions in areas of trauma.	Localized or widespread macules or patches with decrease, but not total loss, of pigmentation.
Histology	1. Skin appears relatively unremarkable at low magnification *(Fig. 6.1.1)*. 2. No melanocytes discernible along basal zone *(Fig. 6.1.2)*. 3. Absence of melanocytes with SOX10 stain *(Fig. 6.1.3)*. 4. No melanin pigment present with Fontana-Masson stain *(Fig. 6.1.4)*. 5. Patchy lymphocytic inflammation in early lesions; no appreciable inflammation in late-stage lesions.	1. Normal stratum corneum and epidermis *(Fig. 6.1.5)*. 2. Melanocytes present in relatively normal density as opposed to absent *(Fig. 6.1.6)*. 3. Mild perivascular lymphocytic infiltrate *(Figs. 6.1.5 and 6.1.6)*. 4. Melanin pigment preserved, but focally reduced in quantity, within epidermis with Fontana-Masson stain. Melanin is also present within melanophages residing in the superficial dermis *(Fig. 6.1.7)*. 5. Reparative dermal changes of mild fibrosis and reactive vessels may or may not be present depending upon preceding inflammatory process.
Special studies	Melanocyte marker (Melan A/MART1, SOX10, or HMB45) to demonstrate absence of melanocytes. Fontana-Masson stain to demonstrate lack of melanin pigment.	Fontana-Masson stain to demonstrate melanin within epidermis and dermal melanophages. Melanocyte marker may be performed to quantitate melanocytes, and distinguish from vitiligo, if not definitively evident on H&E-stained sections.

6.1 Vitiligo vs Postinflammatory Hypomelanosis

	Vitiligo	**Postinflammatory Hypomelanosis**
Treatment	Combination therapies more efficacious including topical or oral corticosteroids, calcineurin inhibitors, and phototherapy. Camouflage may be used for limited disease in cosmetically sensitive areas. Depigmentation of residual, normal pigmented skin alternative for individuals with extensive and recalcitrant disease.	Treatment of underlying inflammatory disorder. UV radiation exposure and phototherapy may hasten repigmentation.
Prognosis	Chronic disease with unpredictable clinical course. Progression more commonly seen in nonsegmental forms and correlated with early onset. Response to treatment is slow and highly variable. Often affects quality of life. Associated with an increased risk of development of other autoimmune diseases.	Benign condition that may have significant cosmetic and psychosocial effects. Generally, resolves in weeks to months with treatment of the causative inflammatory disorder.

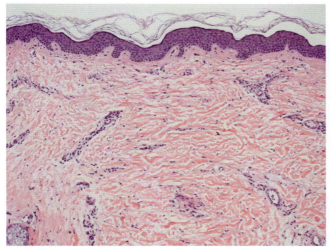

Figure 6.1.1 Vitiligo. Sections of late-stage lesion stained with H&E show minimal pathology with epidermis of normal thickness and rete ridge architecture. The vessels in the superficial dermis have mild reactive changes, and there is no appreciable inflammation.

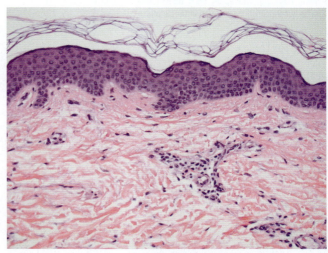

Figure 6.1.2 Vitiligo. At higher magnification, there is a notable lack of melanocytes along the dermal-epidermal junction.

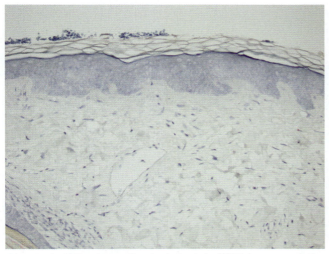

Figure 6.1.3 Vitiligo. Immunohistochemical stain for SOX10 demonstrates lack of melanocytes within the epidermis.

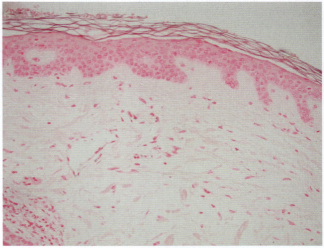

Figure 6.1.4 Vitiligo. Fontana-Masson stain showing absence of melanin within the epidermis. There are a few melanin pigment granules within macrophages within the dermis.

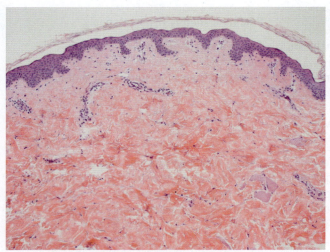

Figure 6.1.5 Postinflammatory hypomelanosis. Sections stained with H&E show minimal pathology with epidermis of normal thickness and rete ridge architecture. Sparse lymphocytic inflammation in the dermis.

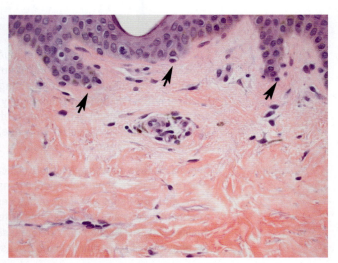

Figure 6.1.6 Postinflammatory hypomelanosis. At higher magnification, melanocytes are present and appear relatively normal in number and morphology (arrows). Melanophages are present within the dermis around superficial vessel.

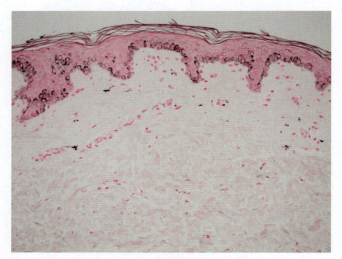

Figure 6.1.7 Postinflammatory hypomelanosis. Fontana-Masson stain demonstrates present, but focally reduced, melanin pigment along the basal zone of the epidermis. Melanin is also present within melanophages residing in the superficial dermis.

6.2 CHONDRODERMATITIS NODULARIS HELICIS VS PRURIGO NODULARIS

	Chondrodermatitis Nodularis Helicis	**Prurigo Nodularis**
Age	Adults.	Any age, but most commonly in middle-aged adults in the sixth and seventh decades.
Location	Helix and antihelix of the ear.	Any area of the body that is easily accessible to rubbing and scratching. Predilection for extensor surfaces of extremities and occipital scalp. Ear is unusual site.
Etiology	Chronic pressure on the ear leading to ischemia, degeneration of the collagen and cartilage, and transepidermal elimination of the degenerative material. Other contributing factors include trauma, chronic sun exposure, and hypothermia.	Chronic rubbing and scratching, due to unobstructed itch-scratch cycle and long-standing pruritus. Contribution from various underlying dermatologic, systemic, neuropsychologic, and infectious diseases.
Presentation	Rapid development of firm, painful nodule with central crust and rolled edges on the helix or antihelix. Often unilateral and involving the ear of same side sleeping or headgear.	Firm, dome-shaped, skin-colored to erythematous nodules ranging from millimeters to centimeters in diameter. May have areas of crust if scratching more than rubbing. Patients may endorse burning, itching, and stinging sensations.
Histology	1. Epidermal hyperplasia and central ulcer/channel with overlying hyperkeratosis and parakeratosis *(Fig. 6.2.1)*. 2. Epidermis lining the channel has dyskeratotic cells with pyknotic nuclei *(Fig. 6.2.2)*. 3. Subepidermal fibrin and fibrinoid degenerated collagen overlying cartilage *(Figs. 6.2.2* and *6.2.3)*. 4. Reactive vascular proliferation resembling granulation tissue adjacent to degenerative material *(Fig. 6.2.4)*.	1. Marked compact hyperkeratosis with parakeratosis and crust *(Figs. 6.2.5-6.2.7)*. 2. Irregular epidermal hyperplasia that may appear pseudoepitheliomatous *(Figs. 6.2.5* and *6.2.6)*. The epidermal hyperplasia has a "crescendo-decrescendo" appearance at scanning magnification. 3. Keratinocytes have reactive changes with hypergranulosis. May have focal areas of superficial necrosis and erosion, but no discrete channel *(Fig. 6.2.7)*. 4. Vertically oriented collagen bundles within widened papillae *(Fig. 6.2.8)*. No fibrinoid degeneration of collagen. 5. Nonspecific sparse mixed dermal inflammation.
Special studies	None. Sometimes need multiple sections to visualize channel.	None.
Treatment	Strategies to reduce pressure on the affected ear. Intralesional corticosteroids for pain relief. Surgical excision or ablative measures may be necessary for complete resolution.	Topical corticosteroids under occlusion, intralesional corticosteroids, and topical calcineurin inhibitors are first-line therapies. Phototherapy and systemic immunosuppressants for severe or recalcitrant disease. Antihistamines, mild cleansers, and emollients to reduce itch.
Prognosis	Benign condition that generally resolves with adequate treatment.	Chronic and recurrent disease that may severely impact quality of life.

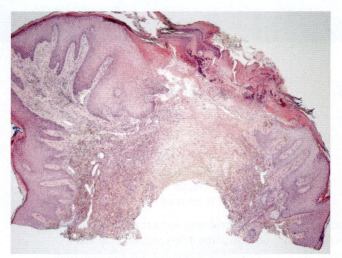

Figure 6.2.1 Chondrodermatitis nodularis helicis. Central crateriform ulcer/channel with overlying hemorrhagic crust. The adjacent epidermis shows reactive hyperplasia and parakeratosis.

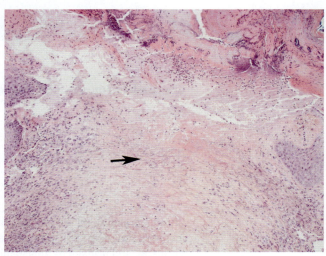

Figure 6.2.2 Chondrodermatitis nodularis helicis. Fibrinoid degenerative change of the collagen beneath the ulcer (arrow). Epidermis forming lining of channel has dyskeratotic/pyknotic cells.

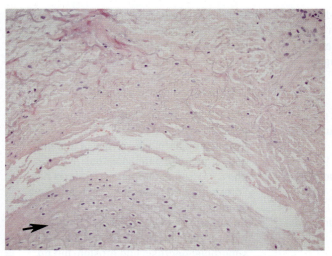

Figure 6.2.3 Chondrodermatitis nodularis helicis. Higher magnification of fibrinoid degenerative change of the collagen with underlying uninvolved cartilage (arrow).

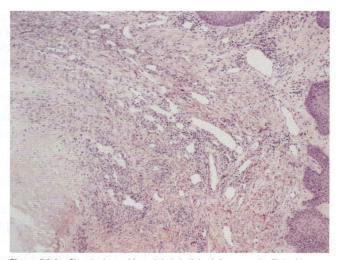

Figure 6.2.4 Chondrodermatitis nodularis helicis. Adjacent to the fibrinoid degeneration, there is granulation tissue and mild chronic inflammation.

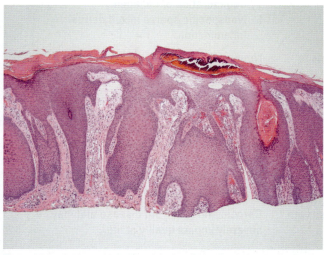

Figure 6.2.5 Prurigo nodularis. Marked irregular epidermal hyperplasia with elongated and thickened rete ridges. Overlying stratum corneum has compact hyperkeratosis, parakeratosis, and hemorrhagic crust.

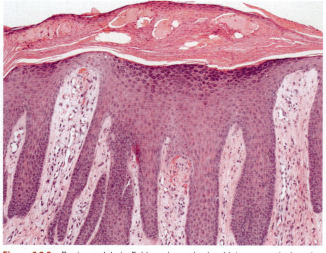

Figure 6.2.6 Prurigo nodularis. Epidermal acanthosis with hypergranulosis and hemorrhagic crust.

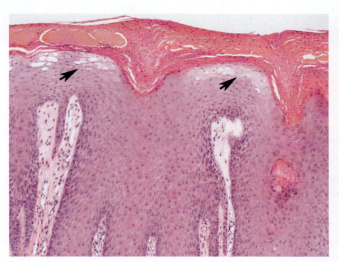 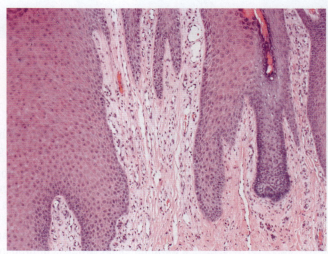

Figure 6.2.7 Prurigo nodularis. Areas of degenerative/ischemic change (arrows) in the superficial epidermis beneath the crust due to chronic rubbing.

Figure 6.2.8 Prurigo nodularis. Dermal papillae are widened by thick bundles of collagen oriented in a vertical array.

6.3 ACANTHOSIS NIGRICANS VS GRANULAR PARAKERATOSIS

	Acanthosis Nigricans	**Granular Parakeratosis**
Age	Any age.	All ages, but most common in adults.
Location	Axillae, neck, popliteal and antecubital fossae, inframammary region, and groin.	Axillae and intertriginous areas.
Etiology	Inherited or acquired with the majority of acquired cases associated with obesity and endocrine/metabolic disorders associated with insulin resistance. Less frequently associated with malignancy as a paraneoplastic process or drug induced. Insulin and insulin-like growth factor, fibroblast growth factor, and epidermal growth factor receptor promote stimulation of epidermal keratinocytes and dermal fibroblasts.	Unknown. Most likely a reactive process due to skin irritation from various factors including occlusion, maceration, sweat, and external agents.
Presentation	Symmetric, thickened, velvety gray-brown plaques.	Hyperkeratotic, red-brown papules that coalesce into plaques. May be malodorous and pruritic.
Histology	1. Basket weave and laminated hyperkeratosis with no parakeratosis *(Figs. 6.3.1 and 6.3.2)*. 2. Undulating papillomatous epidermis with squared rete ridges *(Figs. 6.3.1 and 6.3.2)*. 3. Mild basal hyperpigmentation *(Fig. 6.3.2)*. 4. No appreciable inflammation *(Figs. 6.3.1 and 6.3.2)*.	1. Hyperkeratosis and compact parakeratosis *(Figs. 6.3.3 and 6.3.4)*. 2. Retention of keratohyalin granules in parakeratotic cells *(Figs. 6.3.3 and 6.3.4)*. 3. Mild epidermal hyperplasia *(Fig. 6.3.3)*. 4. Sparse lymphohistiocytic infiltrate in superficial dermis *(Fig. 6.3.3)*.
Special studies	None.	None.
Treatment	Treatment of underlying cause with weight loss, medications for insulin resistance, discontinuation of offending medication, or treatment of malignancy is the first step in treatment. Topical therapies, including retinoids, calcipotriol, and keratolytics, may also be utilized.	Elimination of contributing factors. Topical treatments including corticosteroids, vitamin D analogues, and retinoids.
Prognosis	Chronic disease that persists if underlying cause is not addressed. Malignancy-associated form has poor prognosis as it is generally indicative of advanced stage.	Most often self-limiting, resolving within a year. Not associated with malignancy.

6.3 Acanthosis Nigricans vs Granular Parakeratosis

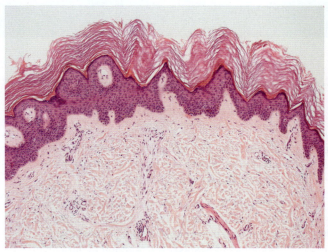

Figure 6.3.1 Acanthosis nigricans. Hyperkeratosis with basket-weave orthokeratosis and no parakeratosis. Epidermis is mildly acanthotic with low papillomatosis. No appreciable inflammation.

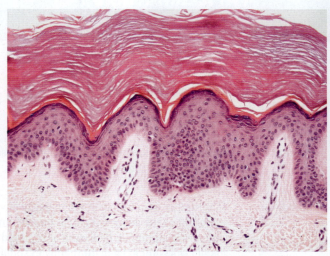

Figure 6.3.2 Acanthosis nigricans. Mild epidermal hyperplasia with low papillomatosis and thickened basket-weave stratum corneum.

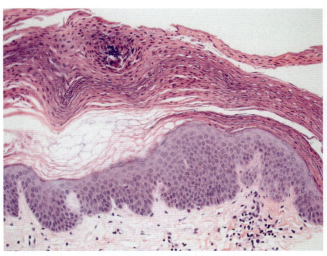

Figure 6.3.3 Granular parakeratosis. Confluent parakeratosis with mild epidermal hyperplasia and preserved, thin granular layer. Stratum corneum has a bluish tincture in addition to the parakeratotic nuclei.

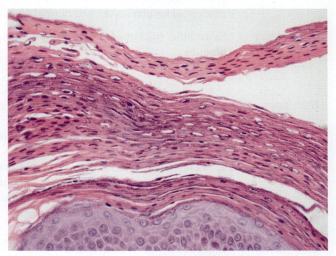

Figure 6.3.4 Granular parakeratosis. Higher magnification of the parakeratotic stratum corneum shows retained keratohyalin granules within the parakeratosis that is the hallmark of this condition.

6.4 ACANTHOSIS NIGRICANS VS CONFLUENT AND RETICULATED PAPILLOMATOSIS

	Acanthosis Nigricans	**Confluent and Reticulated Papillomatosis**
Age	Any age.	Individuals in the second and third decades of life predominately affected.
Location	Axillae, neck, popliteal and antecubital fossae, inframammary region, and groin.	Upper trunk and axillae most commonly. May involve shoulders and upper arms, as well as antecubital and popliteal fossae.
Etiology	Inherited or acquired with the majority of acquired cases associated with obesity and endocrine/metabolic disorders associated with insulin resistance. Less frequently associated with malignancy as a paraneoplastic process or drug induced. Insulin and insulin-like growth factor, fibroblast growth factor, and epidermal growth factor receptor promote stimulation of epidermal keratinocytes and dermal fibroblasts.	Not definitively known. Postulated to be disorder of keratinization. Various theories have suggested that abnormal keratinization is in response to *Malassezia*, reaction to ultraviolet radiation, associated with endocrinopathy including diabetes mellitus, or immune dysregulation.
Presentation	Symmetric, thickened, velvety gray-brown plaques.	Tan-brown macules or thin, scaly papules that coalesce into confluent patches and plaques with peripheral reticulated pigmentation. Generally asymptomatic.
Histology	1. Basket-weave to laminated hyperkeratosis with no parakeratosis *(Figs. 6.4.1-6.4.3)*. 2. Undulating papillomatous epidermis with squared rete ridges *(Figs. 6.4.1-6.4.3)*. 3. Basal hyperpigmentation is typically present, a feature less frequently seen in confluent and reticulated papillomatosis *(Figs. 6.4.2* and *6.4.3)*. 4. No appreciable inflammation *(Fig. 6.4.1)*.	1. Basket-weave to laminated hyperkeratosis with no appreciable parakeratosis *(Figs. 6.4.4-6.4.6)*. 2. Mild epidermal hyperplasia with papillomatosis. No appreciable basal hyperpigmentation *(Figs. 6.4.4-6.4.6)*. 3. Follicular plugging may be present. 4. Sparse superficial perivascular lymphomononuclear infiltrate *(Fig. 6.4.5)*.
Special studies	None.	PAS stain to exclude superficial fungal infection, including tinea versicolor and dermatophytosis, given overlap of clinical presentation.
Treatment	Treatment of underlying cause with weight loss, medications for insulin resistance, discontinuation of offending medication, or treatment of malignancy is the first step in treatment. Topical treatments, including retinoids, calcipotriol, and keratolytics, may also be utilized.	Treatment is not necessary unless desired due to cosmetic or symptomatic concerns. Minocycline is first-line therapy. Alternative antibiotics may be used including macrolides, doxycycline, and amoxicillin. Topical therapies, such as tretinoin, tazarotene, calcipotriol, and tacrolimus, may be utilized for refractory cases.
Prognosis	Chronic disease that persists if underlying cause not addressed. Malignancy-associated form has poor prognosis as it is generally indicative of advanced stage.	Benign disease with no significant morbidity. Slow resolution with treatment, typically taking between 1 and 3 y to resolve.

6.4 Acanthosis Nigricans vs Confluent and Reticulated Papillomatosis

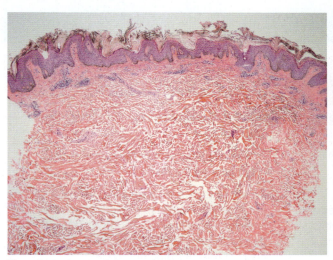

Figure 6.4.1 Acanthosis nigricans. Epidermal acanthosis with papillomatosis and basket-weave hyperkeratosis.

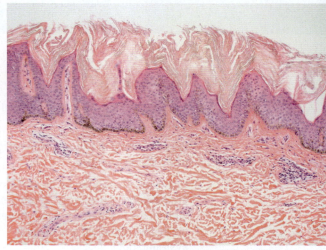

Figure 6.4.2 Acanthosis nigricans. Mild epidermal acanthosis with papillomatosis. Basal layer has increased melanin pigment, a feature less frequently seen in confluent and reticulated papillomatosis. The stratum corneum has hyperkeratosis.

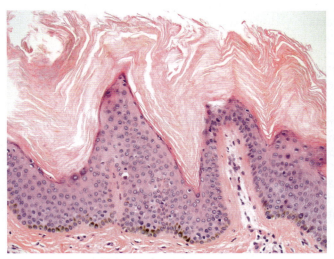

Figure 6.4.3 Acanthosis nigricans. Loose basket-weave hyperkeratosis, epidermal papillomatosis, and basal hyperpigmentation.

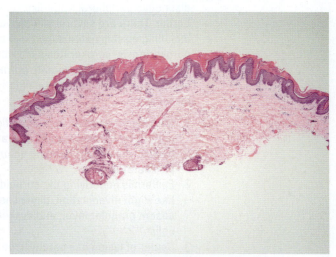

Figure 6.4.4 Confluent and reticulated papillomatosis. Hyperkeratosis overlying epidermal acanthosis with low papillomatosis. The features may be indistinguishable from acanthosis nigricans.

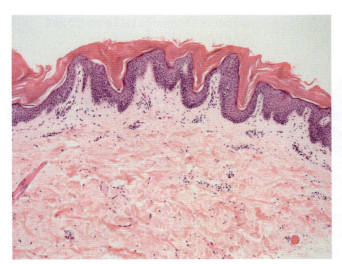

Figure 6.4.5 Confluent and reticulated papillomatosis. Orthohyperkeratosis with mild epidermal acanthosis and low papillomatosis. Very sparse mononuclear infiltrate in superficial dermis.

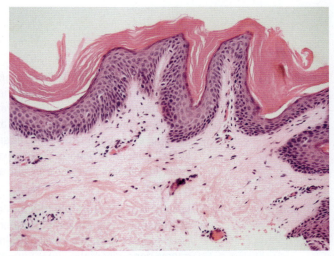

Figure 6.4.6 Confluent and reticulated papillomatosis. Features may be subtle but consist of basket-weave hyperkeratosis overlying low epidermal papillomatosis.

6.5 POROKERATOSIS VS LICHEN PLANUS–LIKE KERATOSIS

	Porokeratosis	**Lichen Planus–like Keratosis**
Age	Any age, but most frequently in middle-aged adults.	Adults, generally between the ages of 30 and 80 y.
Location	Predominately in sun-exposed regions of trunk and extremities.	Trunk and upper extremities, primarily, but may occur on the face.
Etiology	Unknown. Thought to be an abnormal proliferation of epidermal keratinocytes with possible contributions from genetics, ultraviolet radiation, and immune dysregulation.	Proposed to represent an immunological or regressive response to preexisting solar lentigines or seborrheic keratoses. May be triggered by sun exposure, trauma, medications, or irritation.
Presentation	Keratotic papule that expands to an annular plaque with central atrophy and distinctive peripheral ridge-like keratotic border. There are several clinical variants including disseminated superficial actinic porokeratosis, porokeratosis of Mibelli, linear porokeratosis, punctate porokeratosis, and porokeratosis plantaris palmaris et disseminata.	Solitary, erythematous, red-brown, scaly papule or plaque. Dermoscopy may show an annular granular pattern with coarse, regular gray dots around follicular ostia.
Histology	1. Mild hyperkeratosis with formation of peripheral cornoid lamella characterized by discrete inward bending column of parakeratosis *(Figs. 6.5.1-6.5.3)*. 2. Epidermis underlying the cornoid lamella has slight invagination, diminished to absent granular layer, and dyskeratotic cells *(Fig. 6.5.3)*. 3. Center of lesion has patchy lichenoid inflammation, atrophy, and interface vacuolar change *(Fig. 6.5.4)*.	1. Orthohyperkeratosis and focal or confluent parakeratosis. No discrete cornoid lamella formation *(Figs. 6.5.5-6.5.7)*. 2. Variable epidermal acanthosis with blunted rete ridge architecture *(Figs. 6.5.5 and 6.5.7)*. Remnants of solar lentigo or seborrheic keratosis at the periphery. 3. Patchy lichenoid inflammatory infiltrate composed of lymphocytes, histiocytes, and eosinophils *(Figs. 6.5.5 and 6.5.7)*. Melanophages may be present in late-stage lesions. 4. Interface vacuolar change with a variable number of necrotic basal keratinocytes *(Fig. 6.5.8)*.
Special studies	None.	None.
Treatment	Topical therapies include fluorouracil, imiquimod, retinoids, and calcipotriol. Destructive modalities such as cryotherapy, curettage and electrodesiccation, and surgical excision may be used for single or limited number of lesions. Severe cases may require systemic therapy with isotretinoin or acitretin.	Benign and slow-growing lesions; therefore, treatment is generally not necessary. Often biopsied due to clinical appearance similar to basal cell carcinoma. If removal is desired, cryotherapy, shave excision, and curettage with electrodesiccation may be utilized.
Prognosis	Lesions typically persist without treatment. Malignant transformation to squamous cell carcinoma is seen in a small percentage of cases, generally of the linear variant.	Excellent. Lesions often resolve spontaneously. There are no reports of malignant transformation.

6.5 Porokeratosis vs Lichen Planus–like Keratosis

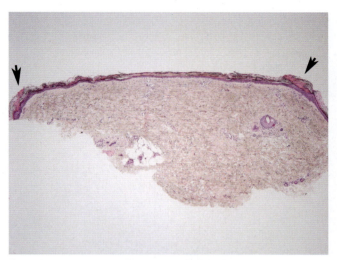

Figure 6.5.1 Porokeratosis. Epidermal atrophy flanked by angulate columns of parakeratosis (arrows) at periphery of lesion.

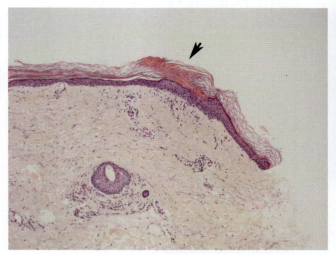

Figure 6.5.2 Porokeratosis. Cornoid lamella (arrow) angulated toward center of lesion and consisting of a discrete column of parakeratosis.

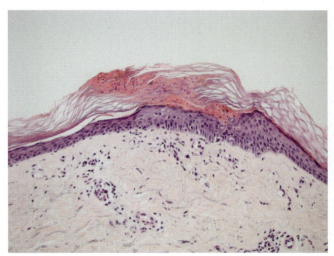

Figure 6.5.3 Porokeratosis. Cornoid lamella situated over slightly invaginated epidermis with diminished granular layer and dyskeratotic cells.

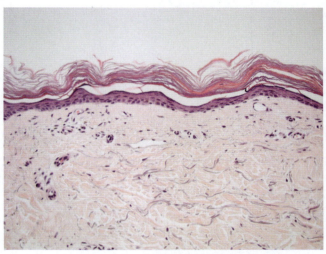

Figure 6.5.4 Porokeratosis. Center of lesion of disseminated superficial actinic porokeratosis has epidermal atrophy, sparse inflammation, and solar elastosis.

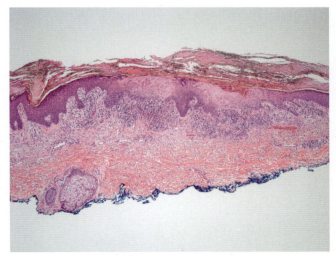

Figure 6.5.5 Lichen planus–like keratosis. Hyperkeratosis and parakeratosis overlying acanthotic epidermis with tapered rete ridges. Dermal-epidermal junction is partially obscured by lichenoid inflammation.

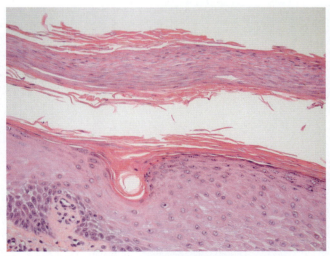

Figure 6.5.6 Lichen planus–like keratosis. Parakeratosis is frequently irregular with confluent areas. No discrete columns of parakeratosis. The epidermis has hypergranulosis.

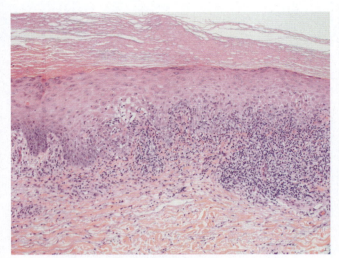

Figure 6.5.7 Lichen planus–like keratosis. Dense band of inflammation obscuring the dermal-epidermal junction and associated with vacuolar interface change.

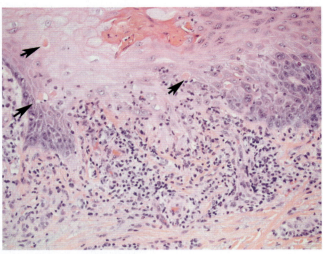

Figure 6.5.8 Lichen planus–like keratosis. Vacuolar interface change with individual and clustered necrotic keratinocytes (arrows) along the basal zone and in upper levels of the epidermis.

6.6 ICHTHYOSIS VULGARIS VS X-LINKED ICHTHYOSIS

	Ichthyosis Vulgaris	**X-Linked Ichthyosis**
Age	Typically begins in infancy and diminishes in severity by adulthood.	Presents in males at birth or in the first few weeks of life.
Location	Extensor surfaces of lower extremities and back most commonly affected. Typically spares flexural regions.	Initially generalized involvement of skin. Evolves to affecting anterior lower legs, predominantly, and also scalp, preauricular area, and neck. Palms, soles, and flexural surfaces are not involved.
Etiology	Inherited disorder (autosomal dominant) due to mutation in the gene encoding profilaggrin (*FLG*). Profilaggrin is the precursor of filaggrin, a crucial protein that promotes terminal differentiation of the epidermis and formation of the protective barrier of the stratum corneum.	Inherited disorder (recessive X-linked) caused by mutations or deletions in the *STS* gene that encodes steroid sulfatase enzyme. Cholesterol sulfate accumulates in the stratum corneum and interferes with proteases that are necessary for normal desquamation. This results in hyperkeratosis and impaired skin permeability.
Presentation	Xerosis and polygonal scales with hyperkeratosis of palms and soles and accentuation of normal skin creases. Scales often hyperpigmented, especially in people of color. May be associated with pruritus, atopic eczema, and keratosis pilaris.	Early presentation of diffuse mild erythema and scaling. Progresses to formation of polygonal, loosely adherent scales that become larger and desquamate. Later, the scales are replaced by dark, hyperpigmented, tightly adherent scales. May have extracutaneous manifestations including corneal opacities, cryptorchism, and neurologic abnormalities.
Histology	1. Hyperkeratosis that may be laminated or compacted (*Figs. 6.6.1-6.6.3*). 2. Epidermis is generally of normal thickness and has a preserved rete ridge architecture (*Figs. 6.6.1-6.6.3*). 3. Granular layer is diminished or absent (*Fig. 6.6.3*). 4. Follicular lumen distended by orthokeratin representing concomitant keratosis pilaris (*Figs. 6.6.1* and *6.6.2*). 5. Adnexal structures, in general, may be decreased in number and reduced in size.	1. Compact hyperkeratosis with epidermal acanthosis (*Figs. 6.6.4-6.6.6*). 2. Granular layer is normal, accentuated, or, rarely, absent (*Figs. 6.6.5* and *6.6.6*). 3. May have hyperkeratosis of follicular or eccrine duct orifices (*Figs. 6.6.5* and *6.6.6*).
Special studies	Genetic testing may be performed to confirm the diagnosis.	Diagnosis may be confirmed by biochemical or genetic analysis. Fluorescent in situ hybridization is used to identify female carriers.
Treatment	Bathing to remove scales and use of emollients and moisturizers is basis of treatment. Keratolytics, including urea, salicylic acid, glycolic acid, and lactic acid, may be used to exfoliate the scale.	Bathing to remove scales and use of emollients and moisturizers is basis of treatment. Keratolytics, including urea, salicylic acid, glycolic acid, and lactic acid, may be used to exfoliate the scale. Intermittent courses of topical or oral retinoids may be used in adults with severe disease.

(Continued)

	Ichthyosis Vulgaris	X-Linked Ichthyosis
Prognosis	No increased mortality. Patients may experience quality-of-life issues in severe cases, especially if there is concomitant atopic eczema.	Life-long disease that is not associated with increased morbidity or mortality, unless extracutaneous manifestations are present. Severe disease may be associated with reduced quality of life due to appearance of the skin.

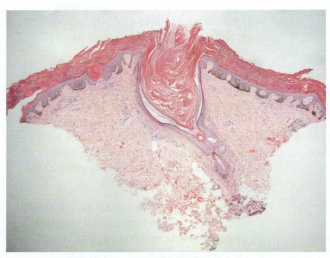

Figure 6.6.1 Ichthyosis vulgaris. Compact hyperkeratosis including involvement of follicular lumen representing concomitant keratosis pilaris. No appreciable acanthosis or inflammation.

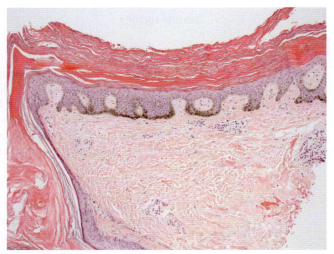

Figure 6.6.2 Ichthyosis vulgaris. Compact orthohyperkeratosis with an eosinophilic appearance.

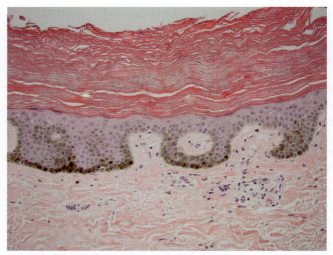

Figure 6.6.3 Ichthyosis vulgaris. Marked orthohyperkeratosis with a diminished granular layer.

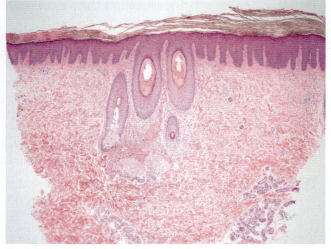

Figure 6.6.4 X-linked ichthyosis. Compact orthohyperkeratosis with mild acanthosis. There is hyperkeratosis of the follicular orifices. No appreciable inflammation.

6.6 Ichthyosis Vulgaris vs X-Linked Ichthyosis

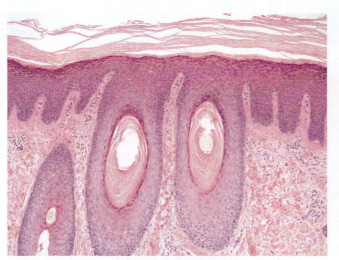

Figure 6.6.5 X-linked ichthyosis. Compact orthohyperkeratosis involving follicular orifices. The granular layer is present and mildly thickened.

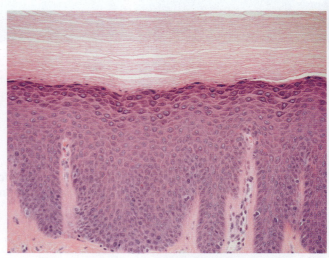

Figure 6.6.6 X-linked ichthyosis. Compact hyperkeratosis with mild epidermal acanthosis and accentuated granular layer.

6.7 SCLEREDEMA VS PRETIBIAL MYXEDEMA

	Scleredema	**Pretibial Myxedema**
Age	Any age.	Adults.
Location	Neck, shoulders, torso, and arms.	Bilateral pretibial region; less commonly, feet; rarely, upper extremities, upper back, neck.
Etiology	Unknown. Associations include infection, insulin-dependent diabetes, paraproteinemia, and medications.	Most commonly a manifestation of Graves disease, but may be seen in association with other thyroid disease. Thought to result from combination of immunologic, cellular, and mechanical processes that lead to deposition of glycosaminoglycans. Circulating thyroid-stimulating hormone (TSH) receptor antibodies bind with TSH receptor protein on fibroblasts initiating an inflammatory response and production of glycosaminoglycans. Trauma and dependency of the pretibial region are precipitating factors.
Presentation	Poorly delineated, indurated plaques with or without preceding erythema. Depending upon trigger, the onset may be abrupt (infection associated) or slow and progressive (paraproteinemia and diabetes associated).	Begins as waxy, yellow-brown, nonpitting, infiltrated plaques that become progressively indurated and have a peau d'orange appearance. Usually asymptomatic but may have pruritus or local discomfort.
Histology	1. Normal epidermis and stratum corneum *(Fig. 6.7.1)*. 2. Swollen collagen bundles in the reticular dermis with preserved fenestrations between fascicles *(Figs. 6.7.1-6.7.3)*. 3. Preserved adnexal structures *(Fig. 6.7.1)*. 4. Prominent mucin accumulation between collagen bundles *(Figs. 6.7.2-6.7.4)*.	1. Normal or acanthotic epidermis *(Fig. 6.7.5)*. 2. Copious mucin deposition in reticular dermis with sparing of papillary dermis *(Figs. 6.7.5-6.7.7)*. 3. Collagen bundles appear fragmented and frayed rather than swollen and thickened *(Figs. 6.7.5 and 6.7.6)*. 4. No appreciable stromal hypercellularity or inflammatory infiltrate.
Special studies	Colloidal iron, alcian blue, or toluidine blue stain to demonstrate mucin.	Colloidal iron, alcian blue, or toluidine blue stain to demonstrate mucin.
Treatment	Treatment is generally not needed for mild and transient cases. If more prolonged course with associated functional impairment, phototherapy, physical therapy, and immunosuppressants may be utilized.	Treatment is not necessary for mild forms. For more severe or progressive cases, high-potency topical corticosteroids or intralesional corticosteroids may be used. Normalization of thyroid function, smoking cessation, and weight loss may improve disease.
Prognosis	Variable course. Infection-associated cases typically show spontaneous resolution. Those associated with chronic disease may have a more protracted course accompanied by reduced mobility.	Variable. Mild forms may resolve spontaneously. Remission is less common with severe disease, despite treatment.

6.7 Scleredema vs Pretibial Myxedema

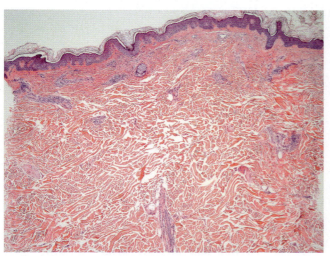

Figure 6.7.1 Scleredema. Normal epidermis and stratum corneum. The dermis is expanded by thickened eosinophilic collagen bundles. The cellularity of the dermis is relatively normal.

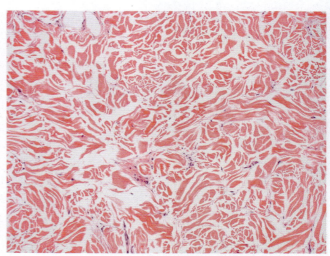

Figure 6.7.2 Scleredema. Thick collagen bundles in the reticular dermis that are separated by stringy basophilic material.

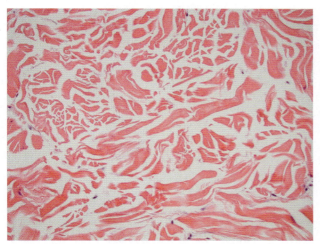

Figure 6.7.3 Scleredema. Thick, swollen collagen bundles with abnormal fenestrations and intervening mucin.

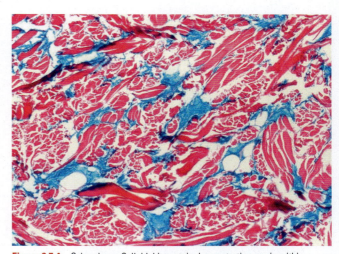

Figure 6.7.4 Scleredema. Colloidal iron stain demonstrating mucin within spaces between collagen bundles.

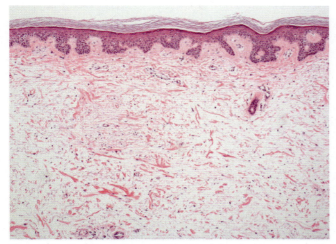

Figure 6.7.5 Pretibial myxedema. Mild hyperkeratosis and epidermal acanthosis overlying dermis with diffuse and abundant mucin deposition.

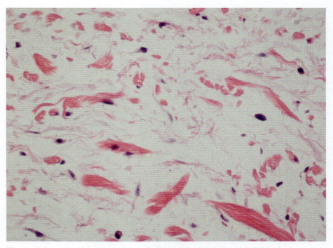

Figure 6.7.6 Pretibial myxedema. Collagen bundles in reticular dermis appear thin and fragmented. There is abundant, diffuse mucin with minimal cellularity including an occasional mast cell.

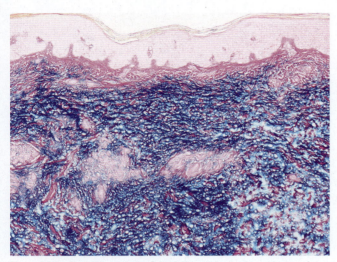

Figure 6.7.7 Pretibial myxedema. Colloidal iron stain showing copious mucin deposition throughout the reticular dermis.

6.8 SCLERODERMA VS SCLEREDEMA

	Scleroderma	Scleredema
Age	Children and middle-aged adults.	Any age.
Location	Dependent upon whether systemic or localized cutaneous form of disease. Systemic sclerosis is divided into limited cutaneous subtype involving fingers, hands, and face and diffuse cutaneous subtype involving the proximal upper and lower extremities and trunk, in addition to distal extremities. Morphea is localized scleroderma that may involve trunk, head and neck region, as well as extremities.	Neck, shoulders, torso, and arms.
Etiology	Etiology is unknown. Environmental factors are thought to be triggers in genetically susceptible individuals. Vascular injury causes endothelial activation and release of cytokines that stimulate collagen production. Activation of the immune system also plays a role with some subtypes associated with specific autoantibodies.	Unknown. Associations include infection, insulin-dependent diabetes, paraproteinemia, and medications.
Presentation	Pitting edema followed by progressive thickening of the skin and development of taut, waxy appearance. Changes begin distally and extend in a centripetal fashion. Indurated sclerotic plaques may have loss of hair and hyperpigmentation. May be associate with CREST syndrome (calcinosis, Raynaud phenomenon, esophageal dysmotility, sclerodactyly, telangiectasia) and nailfold capillary changes.	Poorly delineated indurated plaques with or without preceding erythema. Depending upon trigger, the onset may be abrupt (infection associated) or slow and progressive (paraproteinemia and diabetes associated).
Histology	1. Expansion of the dermis by swollen, eosinophilic collagen bundles that become fused and sclerotic with loss of intervening fenestrations. Note that there is no appreciable mucin deposition *(Figs. 6.8.1 and 6.8.2)*. 2. Patchy perivascular and perieccrine infiltrate of lymphocytes, plasma cells, and few eosinophils *(Figs. 6.8.2 and 6.8.3)*. 3. Loss of adipose tissue around adnexal structures; adnexal structures are entrapped by collagen and may be atrophic *(Fig. 6.8.3)*.	1. Normal epidermis and stratum corneum *(Fig. 6.8.4)*. 2. Swollen collagen bundles in the reticular dermis with preserved and widened fenestrations between fascicles *(Figs. 6.8.4-6.8.6)*. 3. Preserved adnexal structures and no appreciable inflammation *(Fig. 6.8.4)*. 4. Prominent mucin accumulation between collagen bundles *(Figs. 6.8.5-6.8.7)*.
Special studies	May perform serologies for autoantibodies. Anticentromere is associated with limited cutaneous systemic sclerosis, and anti-topoisomerase 1 (anti-Scl-70) is associated with diffuse cutaneous systemic sclerosis.	Colloidal iron, alcian blue, or toluidine blue stain to demonstrate mucin.

(Continued)

	Scleroderma	Scleredema
Treatment	Immune-modulating drugs including methotrexate, mycophenolate mofetil, and cyclophosphamide are first-line therapies. Phototherapy may be used for limited disease.	Treatment is generally not needed for mild and transient cases. If more prolonged course with associated functional impairment, phototherapy, physical therapy, and immunosuppressants may be utilized.
Prognosis	Dependent upon subtype and extent of skin and visceral involvement. May have significant morbidity from muscle atrophy, joint contractures, and skin ulceration. Renal and pulmonary involvement are associated with increased mortality.	Variable course. Infection-associated cases typically show spontaneous resolution. Those associated with chronic disease may have a more protracted course accompanied by reduced mobility.

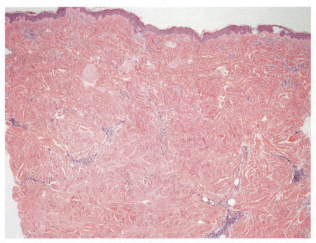

Figure 6.8.1 Scleroderma. At low magnification, the biopsy appears "squared off" due to expansion of the reticular dermis by thick, sclerotic collagen bundles. There is an inflammatory infiltrate around the eccrine units and deep vascular plexus.

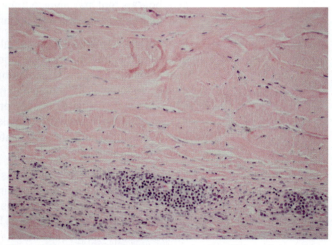

Figure 6.8.2 Scleroderma. Sclerotic collagen bundles with loss of intervening fenestrations making them appear smudgy and fused. No mucin accumulation between the collagen bundles. Infiltrate of lymphocytes and plasma cells is evident around the deep vessels.

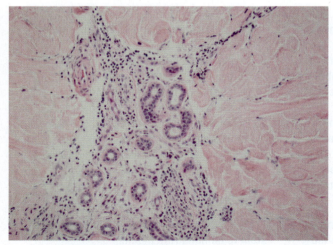

Figure 6.8.3 Scleroderma. Sclerotic collagen encroaches upon the eccrine unit that is associated with an infiltrate of lymphocytes and plasma cells.

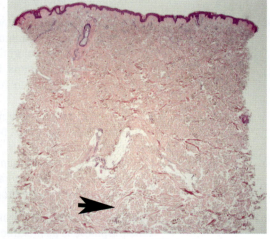

Figure 6.8.4 Scleredema. Dermis is expanded by swollen collagen bundles with increased space between the bundles (arrow).

6.8 Scleroderma vs Scleredema

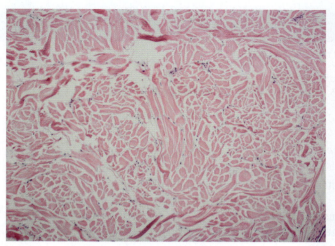

Figure 6.8.5 Scleredema. Thickened collagen bundles with widened fenestrations between the bundles.

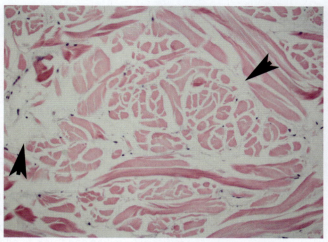

Figure 6.8.6 Scleredema. Stringy basophilic material (mucin) is evident in some of the spaces on H&E stain (arrows).

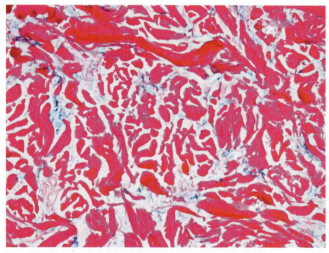

Figure 6.8.7 Scleredema. Colloidal iron stain demonstrating mucin between the swollen collagen bundles.

6.9 SCLERODERMA VS NEPHROGENIC SYSTEMIC FIBROSIS

	Scleroderma	**Nephrogenic Systemic Fibrosis**
Age	Children and middle-aged adults.	Wide age range, but predominantly in middle-aged adults.
Location	Dependent upon whether systemic or localized cutaneous form of disease. Systemic sclerosis is divided into limited cutaneous subtype involving fingers, hands, and face and diffuse cutaneous subtype involving the proximal upper and lower extremities and trunk, in addition to distal extremities. Morphea is localized scleroderma that may involve trunk, head and neck region, as well as extremities.	Begins symmetrically on lower extremities and spreads proximally to involve trunk and upper extremities. Head and neck region generally spared except for ocular sclera.
Etiology	Etiology is unknown. Environmental factors are thought to be triggers in genetically susceptible individuals. Vascular injury causes endothelial activation and release of cytokines that stimulate collagen production. Activation of the immune system also plays a role with some subtypes associated with specific autoantibodies.	Iatrogenic disease most commonly associated with the use of gadolinium-based contrast agents used for magnetic resonance imaging in individuals with renal insufficiency. Exact mechanism is unknown but postulated to involve decreased clearance of gadolinium due to renal dysfunction, binding of gadolinium to anions, deposition of the complexes in tissues, release of cytokines, and initiation of fibrosis.
Presentation	Pitting edema followed by progressive thickening of the skin and development of taut, waxy appearance. Changes begin distally and extend in a centripetal fashion. Indurated sclerotic plaques may have loss of hair and hyperpigmentation. May be associate with CREST syndrome (calcinosis, Raynaud phenomenon, esophageal dysmotility, sclerodactyly, telangiectasia) and nailfold capillary changes.	Erythematous, edematous papules or nodules that coalesce into indurated plaques. Plaques evolve into diffuse woody induration with hardening of the skin and a cobblestone appearance. May experience pruritus or burning sensation. Initial symptoms begin from 1 d to 10 y following exposure to gadolinium.
Histology	1. Expansion of the dermis by swollen, eosinophilic collagen bundles that become sclerotic with loss of intervening fenestrations. No increase in cellularity and no appreciable mucin deposition *(Figs. 6.9.1* and *6.9.3)*. 2. Patchy perivascular and perieccrine infiltrate of lymphocytes, plasma cells, and few eosinophils *(Fig. 6.9.2)*. 3. Loss of adipose tissue around adnexal structures; adnexal structures are entrapped by collagen and may be atrophic *(Fig. 6.9.2)*.	1. Dermis is expanded by fibrosis that often extends into septae of subcutis *(Fig. 6.9.4)*. 2. Collagen bundles are thickened and haphazardly arranged with preservation of intervening fenestrations *(Fig. 6.9.5)*. 3. Increased dermal cellularity imparted by bland, CD34-positive spindle cells between collagen bundles *(Fig. 6.9.6)*. 4. Mild mucin deposition between collagen bundles *(Fig. 6.9.7)*. 5. No appreciable inflammation.

	Scleroderma	Nephrogenic Systemic Fibrosis
Special studies	May perform serologies for autoantibodies. Anticentromere is associated with limited cutaneous systemic sclerosis, and anti-topoisomerase 1 (anti-Scl-70) is associated with diffuse cutaneous systemic sclerosis.	Spindle cells are CD34 positive. Colloidal iron, alcian blue, or toluidine blue stain to demonstrate mucin.
Treatment	Immune-modulating drugs including methotrexate, mycophenolate mofetil, and cyclophosphamide are first-line therapies. Phototherapy may be used for limited disease.	No proven effective therapy. Some patients have shown improvement with corticosteroids, psoralen and UVA (PUVA), intravenous immunoglobulins, retinoids, and extracorporeal photophoresis.
Prognosis	Dependent upon subtype and extent of skin and visceral involvement. May have significant morbidity from muscle atrophy, joint contractures, and skin ulceration. Renal and pulmonary involvement are associated with increased mortality.	Generally follows a progressive, unremitting, and chronic course. Subcutaneous involvement of fascia, joints, and muscle may lead to contractures and decreased range of motion with loss of ambulation. Involvement of visceral organs is associated with significant morbidity and possible mortality.

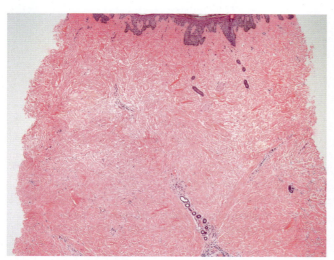

Figure 6.9.1 Scleroderma. Biopsy appears "squared off" due to expansion of the dermis by thick sclerotic collagen bundles.

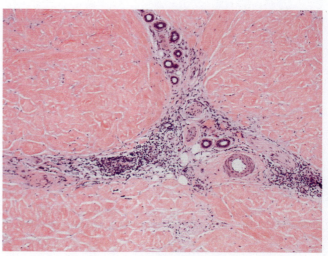

Figure 6.9.2 Scleroderma. Sclerotic collagen encroaches upon the eccrine unit that appears atrophic. Moderately dense infiltrate of lymphocytes and plasma cells surrounds the eccrine unit and vascular plexus in deep dermis.

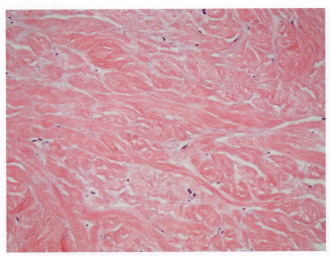

Figure 6.9.3 Scleroderma. Collagen bundles appear thick and smudgy with loss of normal intervening fenestrations. The dermis appears hypocellular with rare spindle cells and no mucin deposition.

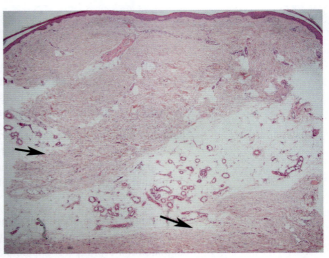

Figure 6.9.4 Nephrogenic systemic fibrosis. Low magnification showing expansion of deep dermis by thick collagen bundles that extend into subcutaneous septae (arrows).

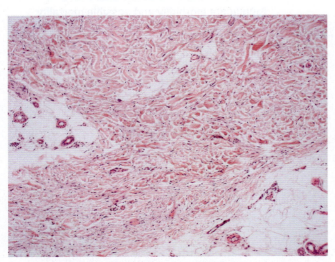

Figure 6.9.5 Nephrogenic systemic fibrosis. Thickened collagen bundles arranged in a haphazard fashion and accompanied by an increase in cellularity imparted by bland spindle cells.

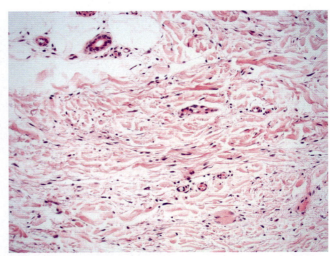

Figure 6.9.6 Nephrogenic systemic fibrosis. Spindle cells in the deep dermis associated with thickened collagen bundles and intervening stringy basophilic material (mucin).

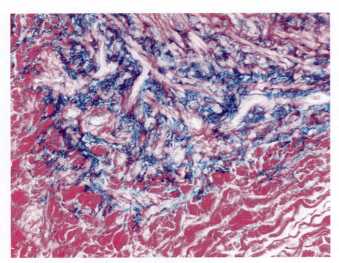

Figure 6.9.7 Nephrogenic systemic fibrosis. Colloidal stain demonstrating focal mucin deposition in area of thickened collagen bundles.

6.10 SCLEROMYXEDEMA VS PRETIBIAL MYXEDEMA

	Scleromyxedema	**Pretibial Myxedema**
Age	Adults, between the ages of 30 and 80 y.	Adults.
Location	Predilection for hands, forearms, thighs, upper torso, and head and neck region.	Bilateral pretibial region; less commonly, feet; rarely, upper extremities, upper back, neck.
Etiology	Unknown.	Most commonly a manifestation of Graves disease, but may be seen in association with other thyroid disease. Thought to result from combination of immunologic, cellular, and mechanical processes that lead to deposition of glycosaminoglycans. Circulating TSH receptor antibodies bind with TSH receptor protein on fibroblasts initiating an inflammatory response and production of glycosaminoglycans. Trauma and dependency of the pretibial region are precipitating factors.
Presentation	Multiple, waxy, firm papules with background of indurated, shiny skin. Papules often arranged in a linear fashion. Glabella may have thickening of skin with deep furrows ("leonine facies"). Deep induration of trunk or limbs gives the "Shar-Pei sign." Thickening of the proximal interphalangeal joints with adjacent depression ("doughnut sign"). Highly associated with monoclonal gammopathy.	Begins as waxy, yellow-brown, nonpitting, infiltrated plaques that become progressively indurated and have a peau d'orange appearance. Usually asymptomatic, but may have pruritus or local discomfort.
Histology	1. Epidermis has flattened rete ridge pattern *(Fig. 6.10.1)*. 2. Dermis is expanded by mildly thickened collagen bundles separated by mucin *(Figs. 6.10.1-6.10.4)*. 3. Increased cellularity in upper and mid-dermis comprised of irregular spindle and stellate fibroblasts *(Figs. 6.10.1-6.10.3)*.	1. Normal or acanthotic epidermis *(Fig. 6.10.5)*. 2. Copious mucin deposition in reticular dermis with sparing of papillary dermis *(Figs. 6.10.5-6.10.7)*. 3. Collagen bundles appear fragmented and frayed rather than thickened *(Figs. 6.10.5 and 6.10.6)*. 4. No appreciable stromal hypercellularity or inflammatory infiltrate *(Figs. 6.10.5 and 6.10.6)*.
Special studies	Colloidal iron, alcian blue, or toluidine blue stain to detect mucin. Serum protein electrophoresis to investigate possibility of monoclonal gammopathy.	Colloidal iron, alcian blue, or toluidine blue stain to demonstrate mucin.
Treatment	No proven effective therapies. Intravenous immunoglobulins, thalidomide or lenalidomide, and systemic corticosteroids show some benefit. Autologous stem cell transplantation has been used for severe and refractory cases.	Treatment is not necessary for mild forms. For more severe or progressive cases, high-potency topical corticosteroids or intralesional corticosteroids may be used. Normalization of thyroid function, smoking cessation, and weight loss may improve disease.

(Continued)

	Scleromyxedema	Pretibial Myxedema
Prognosis	Unpredictable but usually has a chronic and progressive course. Systemic involvement, especially of the nervous and cardiovascular systems, may lead to death.	Variable. Mild forms may resolve spontaneously. Remission is less common with severe disease, despite treatment.

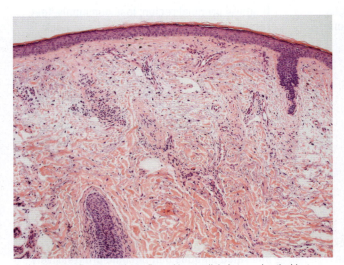

Figure 6.10.1 Scleromyxedema. Dermal hypercellularity associated with increased collagen, mucin deposition, and overlying flattened epidermis.

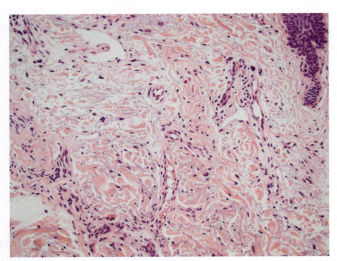

Figure 6.10.2 Scleromyxedema. Mildly thickened collagen bundles with intervening mucin and stromal hypercellularity.

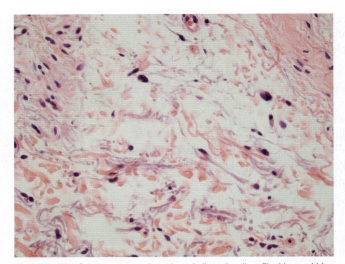

Figure 6.10.3 Scleromyxedema. Irregular spindle and stellate fibroblasts within the dermis.

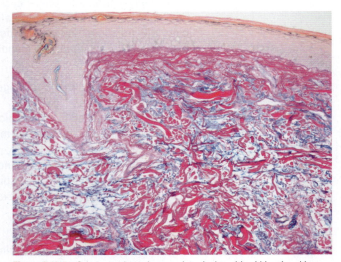

Figure 6.10.4 Scleromyxedema. Increased mucin deposition (thin stingy blue material) between collagen bundles demonstrated with colloidal iron stain.

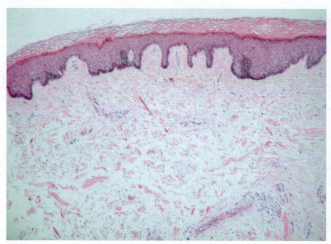

Figure 6.10.5 Pretibial myxedema. Epidermis is mildly acanthotic and hyperkeratotic. The dermis is expanded by significant mucin deposition making it appear pale.

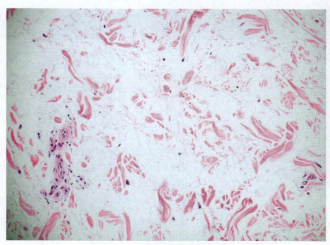

Figure 6.10.6 Pretibial myxedema. Collagen bundles in the dermis are fragmented and frayed, rather than thickened. Abundant mucin is evident, even on H&E stain, as stringy basophilic material between collagen. Note that the cellularity is not increased.

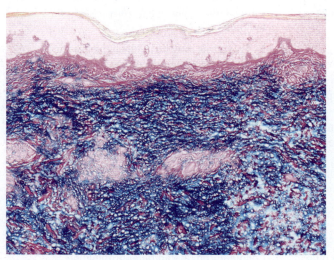

Figure 6.10.7 Pretibial myxedema. Colloidal iron stain demonstrates copious mucin deposition throughout the dermis.

6.11 FOCAL CUTANEOUS MUCINOSIS VS CUTANEOUS MYXOMA

	Focal Cutaneous Mucinosis	**Cutaneous Myxoma**
Age	Adults, typically between the ages of 30 and 60 y.	All ages, with peak incidence in the third and fourth decades of life.
Location	May occur anywhere but most commonly on the trunk or extremities, less commonly on head and neck.	Trunk, lower extremities, head and neck region. Those associated with Carney complex often located on eyelid, external auditory canal, and areola.
Etiology	Unknown. Thought to be a local reactive mucinosis.	Most frequently associated with the inherited disease Carney complex (autosomal dominant) with mutations in the protein kinase A type I-alpha regulatory subunit gene (*PRKAR1A*).
Presentation	Discrete, circumscribed, skin-colored to translucent papule measuring less than a centimeter in diameter. Generally asymptomatic.	Sharply circumscribed papule or nodule, usually measuring less than 1 cm, that is translucent or blue-gray. May be solitary or multiple.
Histology	1. Epidermis is generally normal or attenuated *(Figs. 6.11.1* and *6.11.2)*. 2. Discrete collection of mucin within reticular dermis with sparing of papillary dermis *(Figs. 6.11.1* and *6.11.2)*. 3. Collagen fibers are reduced in area of mucin collection but normal in other areas of the dermis *(Figs. 6.11.1-6.11.3)*. 4. Few bland spindle cells but no significant hypercellularity or inflammation *(Fig. 6.11.3)*.	1. Epidermis may be mildly hyperplastic forming a collarette or basaloid epithelial strands or islands *(Figs. 6.11.4* and *6.11.5)*. 2. Well-circumscribed lobular areas of myxoid stroma with mucin accumulation within the dermis *(Figs. 6.11.4-6.11.6)*. 3. Bland stellate and spindle cells within myxoid stroma with thin-walled, collapsed vascular structures *(Fig. 6.11.6)*. Rare mitotic figures. 4. Small collections of neutrophils within the myxoid stroma aid in differentiation from focal cutaneous mucinosis *(Fig. 6.11.7)*.
Special studies	Colloidal iron, alcian blue, or toluidine blue stain to demonstrate mucin.	Colloidal iron, alcian blue, or toluidine blue stain to demonstrate mucin. Genetic testing for mutations in *PRKAR1A*. Genetic counseling regarding potential for associated systemic manifestations of Carney complex, especially risk for neoplasia.
Treatment	Simple excision.	Simple excision is primary treatment modality. Recurrences may occur with incomplete excision.
Prognosis	Benign process, which, when solitary, is not associated with systemic conditions. Excision is curative and recurrence is generally not seen, even when incompletely removed.	Cutaneous myxomas are benign lesions with excellent prognosis but serve as a marker for Carney complex, especially those involving the eyelids, external auditory canal, and areola. Various endocrine and nonendocrine tumors are associated with Carney complex, notably including cardiac myxomas, psammomatous melanotic schwannoma, and large cell calcifying Sertoli tumor, which pose a risk for morbidity and mortality.

6.11 Focal Cutaneous Mucinosis vs Cutaneous Myxoma

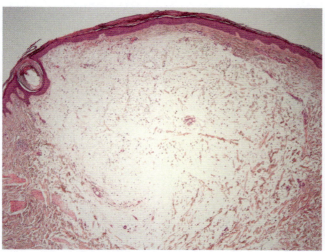

Figure 6.11.1 Focal cutaneous mucinosis. Discrete collection of mucin within the reticular dermis with normal overlying epidermis.

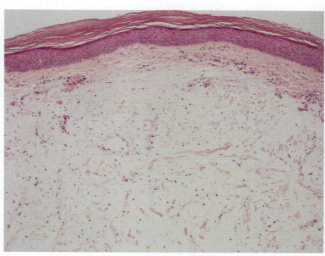

Figure 6.11.2 Focal cutaneous mucinosis. Collagen bundles are reduced in number within area of mucin accumulation. No significant hypercellularity, vascular proliferation, or inflammation.

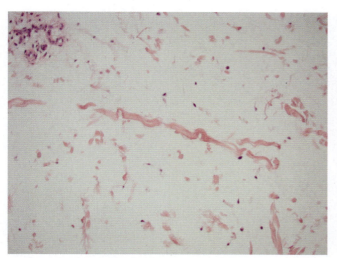

Figure 6.11.3 Focal cutaneous mucinosis. Few bland spindle cells are present within mucin. Collagen bundles are thin and reduced in number.

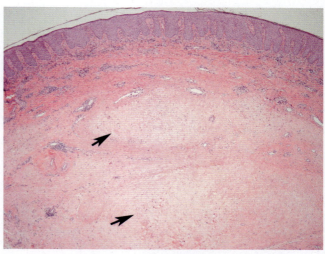

Figure 6.11.4 Cutaneous myxoma. Epidermal hyperplasia overlying lobular areas of myxoid stroma (arrows).

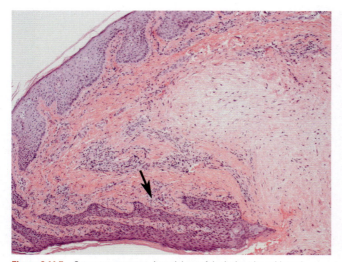

Figure 6.11.5 Cutaneous myxoma. At periphery of the lesion, the epidermal hyperplasia forms a collarette (arrow) around the myxoid stroma.

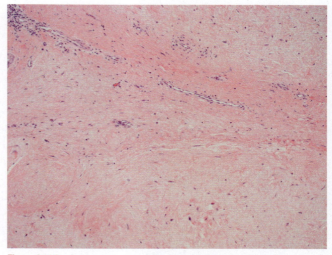

Figure 6.11.6 Cutaneous myxoma. Myxoid stroma is mildly cellular with stellate and spindle cells. Blood vessels are thin walled and collapsed.

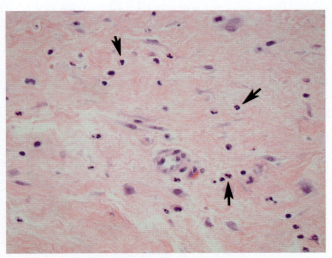

Figure 6.11.7 Cutaneous myxoma. The presence of small collections of neutrophils (arrows) within the myxoid stroma aids in differentiating cutaneous myxoma from other myxoid lesions, including focal cutaneous mucinosis.

6.12 FOCAL CUTANEOUS MUCINOSIS VS DIGITAL MUCOUS CYST

	Focal Cutaneous Mucinosis	**Digital Mucous Cyst**
Age	Adults, typically between the ages of 30 and 60 y.	Adults.
Location	May occur anywhere but most commonly on the trunk or extremities, less commonly on head and neck.	Most commonly on the hand, overlying the distal interphalangeal joint.
Etiology	Unknown. Thought to be a local reactive mucinosis.	Unknown. Thought to be a result of accumulation of mucin from the underlying joint space due to irritation or connective tissue degeneration.
Presentation	Discrete, circumscribed, skin-colored to translucent papule measuring less than a centimeter in diameter. Generally asymptomatic.	Translucent, firm, dome-shaped papule or nodule on the dorsal surface of the distal interphalangeal joint. Typically, slow growing and asymptomatic.
Histology	1. Epidermis is generally normal or attenuated *(Fig. 6.12.1)*. 2. Discrete collection of mucin within reticular dermis *(Figs. 6.12.1 and 6.12.4)*. 3. Few bland spindle cells but no hypercellularity *(Figs. 6.12.2 and 6.12.3)*. 4. Collagen fibers are reduced in area of mucin collection but normal in other areas of the dermis *(Figs. 6.12.2 and 6.12.3)*.	1. Epidermis is thinned and may have overlying hyperkeratosis and/or parakeratosis *(Fig. 6.12.5)*. 2. Loculated collections of mucin with scattered bland spindle cells *(Figs. 6.12.5-6.12.7)*. 3. Collections of mucin are surrounded by condensed collagen, but there is no cyst lining ("pseudocyst") *(Figs. 6.12.6 and 6.12.7)*. 4. Histologic features are identical to focal cutaneous mucinosis; therefore, distinction is primarily based on location.
Special studies	Colloidal iron, alcian blue, or toluidine blue stain to demonstrate mucin.	Colloidal iron, alcian blue, or toluidine blue stain to demonstrate mucin.
Treatment	Simple excision.	Observation for small lesions. Aspiration may be performed but has a high recurrence rate. Simple excision has a lower recurrence rate and is preferred for larger or symptomatic cases.
Prognosis	Benign process, which, when solitary, is not associated with systemic conditions. Excision is curative and recurrence is generally not seen, even when incompletely removed.	Benign lesion that may recur if not completely removed. May be associated with osteoarthritis of the involved joint.

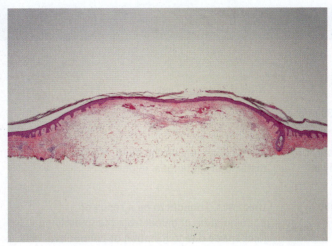

Figure 6.12.1 Focal cutaneous mucinosis. Shave biopsy of a low papule formed by a discrete collection of mucin within dermis. Overlying epidermis is attenuated at the summit of the papule.

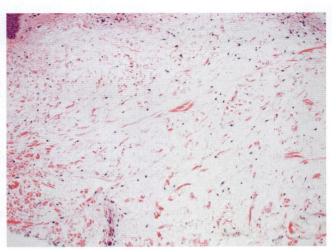

Figure 6.12.2 Focal cutaneous mucinosis. Collagen bundles are reduced in number and fragmented in the area of mucin accumulation. Low cellularity associated with mucin.

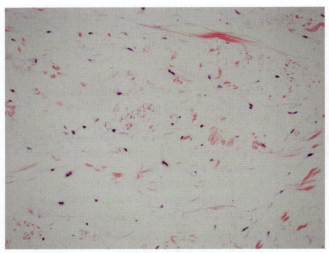

Figure 6.12.3 Focal cutaneous mucinosis. Higher magnification showing bland spindle cells floating in copious mucin.

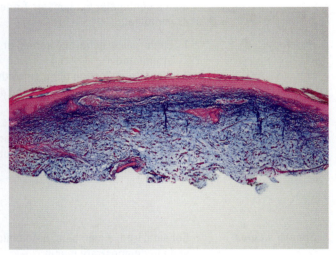

Figure 6.12.4 Focal cutaneous mucinosis. Colloidal iron stain demonstrating mucin.

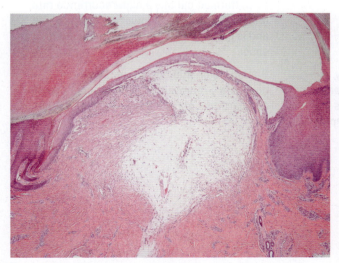

Figure 6.12.5 Digital mucous cyst. Acral skin characterized by thick stratum corneum. Central papule formed by discrete area of mucin accumulation with overlying thinned epidermis and parakeratosis.

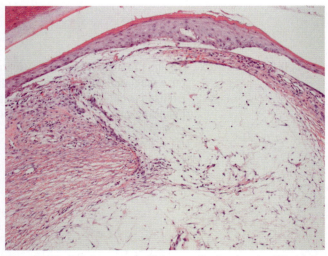

Figure 6.12.6 Digital mucous cyst. Higher magnification of mucin within dermis and reactive epidermal changes. Note that there is no epidermal lining and therefore not a true cyst ("pseudocyst").

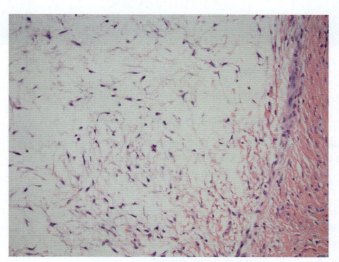

Figure 6.12.7 Digital mucous cyst. Bland spindle cells and thin collagen bundles within mucin collection.

6.13 CALCINOSIS CUTIS VS GOUTY TOPHUS

	Calcinosis Cutis	**Gouty Tophus**
Age	All ages.	Adults primarily, rarely in children.
Location	Any location. Location is dependent upon type of calcinosis cutis and presence of any associated disease.	Skin of ear and finger pulps. Deeper-seated lesions in subcutaneous tissue of first metatarsophalangeal joint, Achilles tendon, and olecranon bursa.
Etiology	Deposition of insoluble calcium salts in the skin. Classified as dystrophic, metastatic, idiopathic, iatrogenic, and calciphylaxis. Dystrophic occurs in the setting of tissue damage with normal serum calcium and phosphorus levels. Metastatic has an elevated calcium phosphate product. Idiopathic has no underlying tissue damage or abnormal serum levels of calcium and phosphorus. Iatrogenic is due to administration of calcium or phosphate-containing substances. Calciphylaxis is calcification of vessels, most commonly in the setting of renal disease with abnormal calcium phosphate product.	Deposition of monosodium urate crystals in the skin and subcutaneous tissue due to dysfunctional purine metabolism and long-standing hyperuricemia.
Presentation	Slow-growing white, firm papules, plaques, or nodules that may be tender. Lesions may ulcerate and appear chalky white on cut section.	Hard, white nodules that may discharge white crystalline material if traumatized. May have miliarial presentation with numerous grouped white papules. Lesions are typically asymptomatic.
Histology	1. Variably sized granular or nodular calcifications within dermis or subcutaneous tissues *(Figs. 6.13.1 and 6.13.2)*. 2. Calcium appears blue-purple on H&E stain and three dimensional in dermal spaces *(Figs. 6.13.1-6.13.3)*. 3. May be associated with histiocytes and foreign body–type giant cells *(Fig. 6.13.4)*.	1. Epidermis may show reactive change but is typically intact *(Fig. 6.13.5)*. 2. Circumscribed aggregates of pale, light eosinophilic to amphophilic deposits *(Figs. 6.13.5 and 6.13.6)*. 3. Deposits, on higher magnification, have a feathery, crystalline appearance with needle-like clefts *(Fig. 6.13.8)*. 4. Deposits are surrounded by histiocytes and multinucleate giant cells *(Figs. 6.13.7 and 6.13.8)*. 5. Water-soluble chemicals, such as formalin, dissolve gout crystals; therefore, specimen must be fixed in alcohol to preserve crystals.
Special studies	If not obvious on H&E stain, von Kossa stains calcium black. Calcium, phosphate, and protein levels for metastatic calcinosis cutis. Laboratory studies to investigate underlying disease in dystrophic forms.	Negative birefringence with polarization of scrapings or aspiration of tophus material.

	Calcinosis Cutis	**Gouty Tophus**
Treatment	Dependent on type of calcinosis. Dystrophic forms may require treatment of underlying disease to ameliorate the calcium deposition. Limited cutaneous involvement may be amenable to surgical excision or intralesional sodium thiosulfate. For extensive disease with inflammation, oral minocycline or colchicine may be used. Diltiazem is efficacious in extensive disease without inflammation.	Allopurinol, probenecid, or febuxostat as urate-lowering therapy along with colchicine to prevent flares. Surgical excision of tophus to reduce risk of compression and pain.
Prognosis	Dependent upon type of calcinosis.	Good prognosis with adequate therapy.

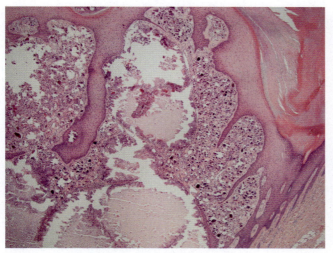

Figure 6.13.1 Calcinosis cutis. Aggregates of fine granular and coarse nodular crystalline material within the dermis.

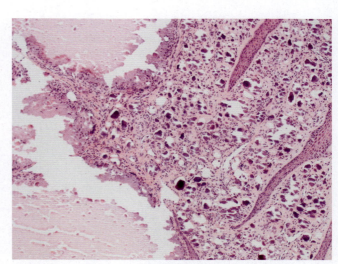

Figure 6.13.2 Calcinosis cutis. Dermal calcifications of varying size and shape that appear blue-purple on H&E-stained sections.

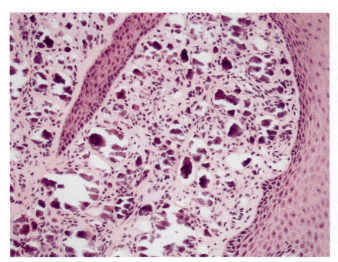

Figure 6.13.3 Calcinosis cutis. Coarse calcifications that appear three dimensional in dermal spaces.

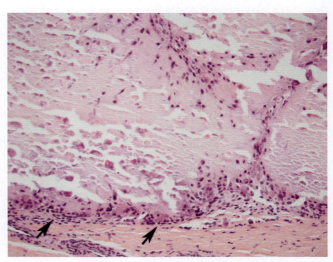

Figure 6.13.4 Calcinosis cutis. Finely granular calcifications surrounded by foreign-body giant cells (arrows).

6 Alterations of the Epidermis and Dermis

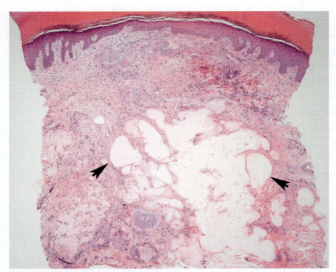

Figure 6.13.5 Gouty tophus. Circumscribed aggregates of pale crystalline material (arrows) surrounded by histiocytes and multinucleate giant cells.

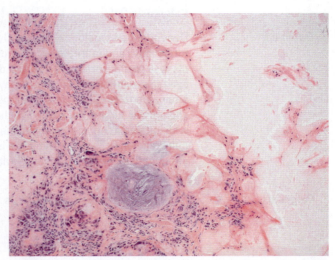

Figure 6.13.6 Gouty tophus. Pale eosinophilic aggregates of feathery crystalline material.

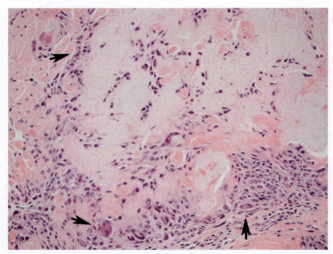

Figure 6.13.7 Gouty tophus. Crystals forming nodules surrounded by histiocytes and multinucleate giant cells (arrows).

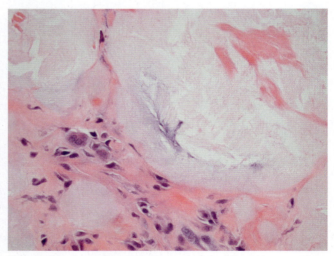

Figure 6.13.8 Gouty tophus. Deposits are pale eosinophilic and have a needle-like configuration. These features help distinguish from the granular/nodular blue-purple appearance of calcium in H&E-stained tissue sections.

6.14 GOUTY TOPHUS VS NODULAR AMYLOIDOSIS

	Gouty Tophus	**Nodular Amyloidosis**
Age	Adults primarily, rarely in children.	Adults.
Location	Skin of ear and finger pulps. Deeper-seated lesions in subcutaneous tissue of first metatarsophalangeal joint, Achilles tendon, and olecranon bursa.	Extremities, trunk, or head. Predilection for acral surfaces.
Etiology	Deposition of monosodium urate crystals in the skin and subcutaneous tissue due to dysfunctional purine metabolism and long-standing hyperuricemia.	Immunoglobulin-derived amyloid composed of either lambda or kappa light chains. Localized cutaneous deposition in the setting of plasma cell dyscrasia with clonal population of skin-homing plasma cells.
Presentation	Hard, white nodules that may discharge white crystalline material if traumatized. May have miliarial presentation with numerous grouped white papules. Lesions are typically asymptomatic.	Solitary or multiple, yellow-brown, waxy nodules or plaques. Lesions are generally asymptomatic. May be associated with Sjogren syndrome.
Histology	1. Normal epidermis and stratum corneum *(Fig. 6.14.1)*. 2. Circumscribed aggregates of feathery, amphophilic crystals surrounded by histiocytes and multinucleate giant cells *(Figs. 6.14.1 and 6.14.2)*. 3. Deposits, on higher magnification, have a feathery, crystalline appearance with needle-like clefts *(Figs. 6.14.3 and 6.14.4)*. 4. Water-soluble chemicals, such as formalin, dissolve gout crystals; therefore, specimen must be fixed in alcohol to preserve crystals.	1. Epidermis may be normal or atrophic. 2. Globules of pink amorphous material in the dermis *(Figs. 6.14.5-6.14.7)*. 3. Globules are separated by clefts and surrounded by aggregates of plasma cells. No appreciable histiocytic or multinucleate giant cell reaction *(Fig. 6.14.7)*. 4. Amorphous material stains with Congo red stain *(Fig. 6.14.8)*.
Special studies	Negative birefringence with polarization of scrapings or aspiration of tophus material.	Congo red stain (with green birefringence under polarized light), crystal violet stain revealing metachromatic staining, or yellow-green fluorescence with thioflavin T stain. Immunohistochemistry for kappa and lambda light chains or in situ hybridization.
Treatment	Allopurinol, probenecid, or febuxostat as urate-lowering therapy along with colchicine to prevent flares. Surgical excision of tophus to reduce risk of compression and pain.	Excision, curettage, or CO_2 laser ablation.
Prognosis	Good prognosis with adequate therapy.	Good prognosis. May recur if incompletely removed. Small risk of progression to systemic amyloidosis.

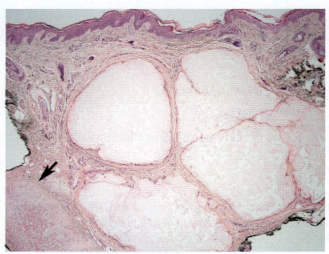

Figure 6.14.1 Gouty tophus. Gouty tophus of the ear, note auricular cartilage (arrow). Large aggregates of amorphous pale pink material in the dermis.

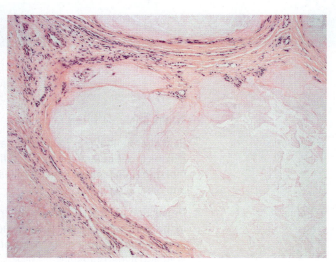

Figure 6.14.2 Gouty tophus. Gout crystals have been dissolved by formalin leaving amorphous light eosinophilic material with needle-shaped clefts.

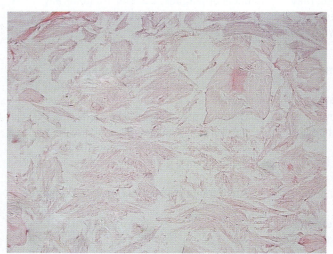

Figure 6.14.3 Gouty tophus. Acellular amorphous crystalline material with needle-like clefts.

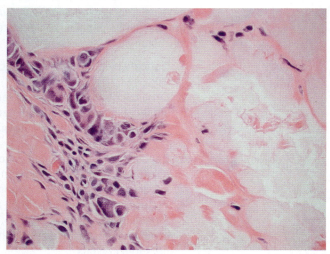

Figure 6.14.4 Gouty tophus. Histiocytes and multinucleate giant cells partially surround the amorphous material.

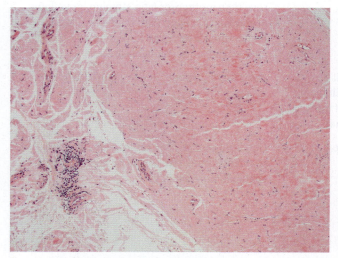

Figure 6.14.5 Nodular amyloidosis. Large nodular masses of bright eosinophilic amorphous material within dermis. The material appears smudgy with occasional fissures.

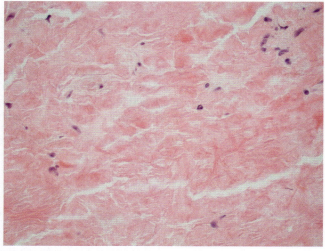

Figure 6.14.6 Nodular amyloidosis. Amyloid at higher magnification appears brightly eosinophilic and smudgy. There are intervening fissures but no needle-like clefts.

6.14 Gouty Tophus vs Nodular Amyloidosis

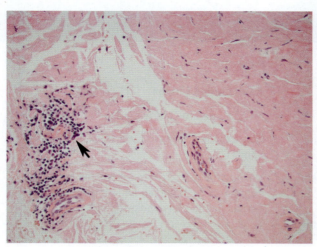

Figure 6.14.7 Nodular amyloidosis. Amyloid deposits are associated with infiltrate of plasma cells (arrow). As opposed to gout, histiocytes and giant cells are only rarely seen.

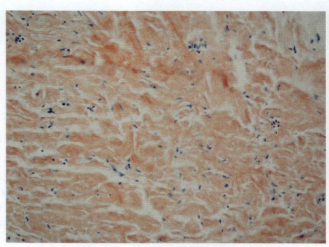

Figure 6.14.8 Nodular amyloidosis. Congo red positivity in amyloid. This produces apple-green birefringence with polarization.

6.15 NODULAR AMYLOIDOSIS VS ADULT COLLOID MILIUM

	Nodular Amyloidosis	**Adult Colloid Milium**
Age	Adults.	Middle-aged to elderly adults.
Location	Extremities, trunk, or head. Predilection for acral surfaces.	Sun-exposed areas of face, neck, dorsum of hands.
Etiology	Immunoglobulin-derived amyloid composed of either lambda or kappa light chains. Localized cutaneous deposition in the setting of plasma cell dyscrasia with clonal population of skin-homing plasma cells.	Unknown but thought to be caused by degeneration of elastin and collagen in the dermis due to sun exposure.
Presentation	Solitary or multiple, yellow-brown, waxy nodules or plaques. Lesions are generally asymptomatic. May be associated with Sjogren syndrome.	Dome-shaped, orange-yellow or skin-colored, firm, discrete papules. Papules develop slowly and are asymptomatic.
Histology	1. Epidermis may be normal or atrophic. 2. Globules of pink amorphous material in the dermis. Globules are separated by clefts and surrounded by plasma cells *(Figs. 6.15.1* and *6.15.2)*. 3. Amyloid is hypocellular and concentrates around blood vessels *(Fig. 6.15.3)*. 4. Amorphous material stains with Congo red stain *(Fig. 6.15.4)*.	1. Normal or atrophic epidermis *(Fig. 6.15.5)*. 2. Fissured, eosinophilic material in papillary dermis *(Figs. 6.15.5-6.15.7)*. 3. Grenz zone between material and epidermis, may contain elastic fibers *(Fig. 6.15.5)*. 4. Background of solar elastosis and sparse chronic inflammation. 5. Overlapping histologic features with amyloidosis, including histochemical staining pattern, but distinguished by clinical presentation.
Special studies	Congo red stain (with green birefringence under polarized light), crystal violet stain revealing metachromatic staining, or yellow-green fluorescence with thioflavin T stain. Immunohistochemistry for kappa and lambda light chains or in situ hybridization.	Material is PAS positive and weakly Congo red positive.
Treatment	Excision, curettage, or CO_2 laser ablation.	Ablation methods such as laser, cryotherapy, chemical peels, and dermabrasion have been used.
Prognosis	Good prognosis. May recur if incompletely removed. Small risk of progression to systemic amyloidosis.	Benign process with no disease association but may be marker of chronic sun damage.

6.15 Nodular Amyloidosis vs Adult Colloid Milium

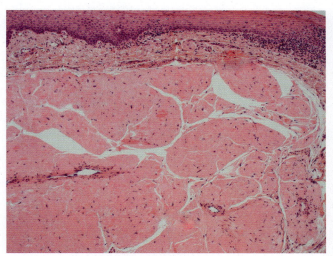

Figure 6.15.1 Nodular amyloidosis. Discrete aggregates of bright eosinophilic material within dermis. Note, clefting between the aggregates. Aggregates of plasma cells around aggregates.

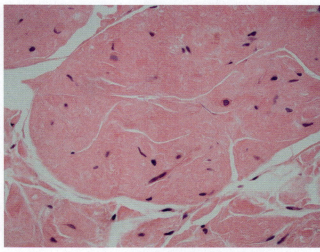

Figure 6.15.2 Nodular amyloidosis. Higher magnification demonstrating masses of smudgy eosinophilic material separated by clefts.

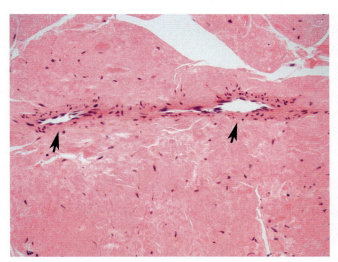

Figure 6.15.3 Nodular amyloidosis. Amyloid is hypocellular and typically concentrates around blood vessels (arrows).

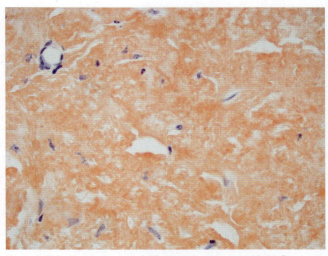

Figure 6.15.4 Nodular amyloidosis. Staining of nodular amyloid with Congo red stain.

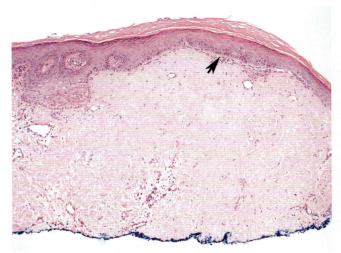

Figure 6.15.5 Adult colloid milium. Light eosinophilic material within the dermis separated from the epidermis by a thin grenz zone (arrow).

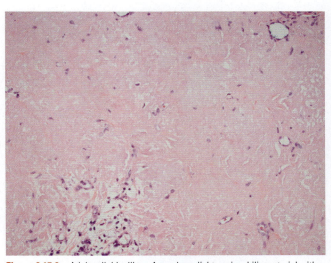

Figure 6.15.6 Adult colloid milium. Amorphous light eosinophilic material with subtle fissures and sparse chronic inflammation.

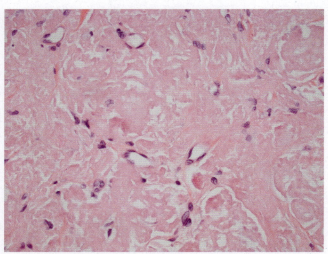

Figure 6.15.7 Adult colloid milium. Colloid milium has features similar to nodular amyloidosis, including staining with Congo red, crystal violet, and PAS, but papular configuration and association with solar elastosis are features that aid in distinction from amyloidosis.

6.16 PSEUDOXANTHOMA ELASTICUM VS SOLAR ELASTOSIS

	Pseudoxanthoma Elasticum	**Solar Elastosis**
Age	Children and young adults. Typically presenting in the second or third decades of life.	Adults.
Location	Lateral neck is characteristic location. Axillae, antecubital fossa, popliteal fossa, and groin also commonly involved.	Sun-exposed regions, especially face, neck, chest, dorsal hands, and legs.
Etiology	Autosomal recessive disorder due to mutations in the *ABCC6* gene encoding the cellular transmembrane transport protein ABCC6. Leads to reduced levels of inorganic pyrophosphate and ectopic mineralization of elastin-rich tissues.	Chronic exposure to ultraviolet radiation causes loss of integrity of dermal extracellular matrix, including collagen and elastin, through formation of reactive oxygen species and activation of matrix metalloproteinases.
Presentation	Yellow papules that coalesce into plaques. Skin is soft and lax, forming redundant folds with a "gooseflesh" or "plucked chicken" appearance. May have ocular involvement with retinal angioid streaks. Cardiovascular manifestations result in claudication, hypertension, myocardial infarction, and stroke.	Diffuse nodularity and yellowish discoloration of skin with fine to deep furrows. Combined with cysts and comedones on the periorbital region, it is referred to as Favre-Racouchot syndrome. Cutis rhomboidalis nuchae is solar elastosis with deep furrows in a rhomboid pattern involving the posterior neck.
Histology	1. Normal thickness of epidermis, although may have an undulating configuration due to loss of elasticity *(Figs. 6.16.1* and *6.16.2)*. 2. Distorted, fragmented, and clumped elastic fibers in mid-dermis *(Figs. 6.16.3* and *6.16.4)*. 3. Abnormal elastic fibers are coated with fine calcifications having a basophilic appearance *(Fig. 6.16.4)*.	1. Thinned epidermis with flattening of rete ridges *(Fig. 6.16.5)*. 2. Decreased dermal collagen with accumulation of amorphous, gray-blue masses of thickened and fragmented elastic fibers and collagen bundles *(Figs. 6.16.5-6.16.7)*.
Special studies	Verhoeff-Van Gieson stain for elastic fibers and von Kossa stain for calcification may be used to confirm the diagnosis. Genetic testing for pathogenic variants of *ABCC6*.	None.
Treatment	Surgical excision of lax skin if desired cosmetically. Genetic counseling with regular ophthalmology and cardiology assessments.	Preventative measures include sun avoidance and protection when in the sun. Photoaging may be treated with topical retinoids, antioxidants, and hydroxy acids. A variety of cosmetic procedures, including chemical peels, photodynamic therapy, laser resurfacing, injectable botulinum, and soft tissue fillers may reduce the cosmetic appearance of elastosis and other consequences of chronic sun exposure.

(Continued)

	Pseudoxanthoma Elasticum	**Solar Elastosis**
Prognosis	Dependent upon extent of extracutaneous organ involvement. Most patients have normal life span. Ocular involvement may be associated with visual impairment. Morbidity and mortality may be seen with cardiovascular involvement.	Solar elastosis and photoaging are benign but a marker of increased risk for sun-induced skin cancers, including squamous cell carcinoma, basal cell carcinoma, and melanoma.

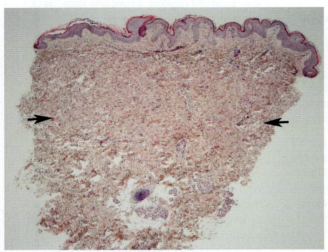

Figure 6.16.1 Pseudoxanthoma elasticum. Low magnification has appearance of relatively normal skin. Note, however, at the arrows subtle basophilia in the reticular dermis from clumped elastic fibers.

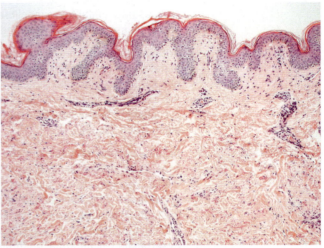

Figure 6.16.2 Pseudoxanthoma elasticum. The epidermis has a subtle undulating appearance due to loss of elasticity. There is an indistinct interface between the papillary dermis and abnormal elastic fibers in the reticular dermis.

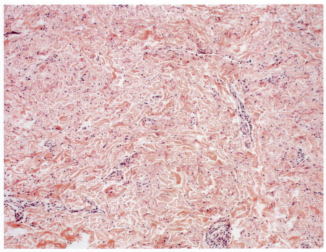

Figure 6.16.3 Pseudoxanthoma elasticum. Distorted, fragmented, and clumped elastic fibers in the mid-dermis. Note that the collagen bundles are normal.

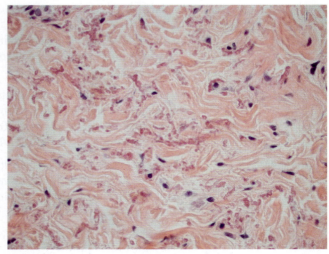

Figure 6.16.4 Pseudoxanthoma elasticum. Higher magnification of clumped elastic fibers showing fine calcification giving the fibers a basophilic appearance.

6.16 Pseudoxanthoma Elasticum vs Solar Elastosis

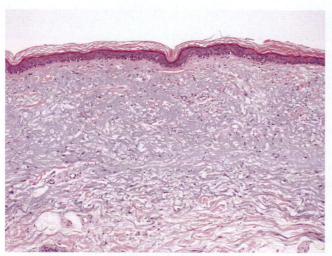

Figure 6.16.5 Solar elastosis. Thinned epidermis with flattened rete ridge pattern. The dermis has amorphous gray-blue mass of abnormal, degenerated collagen bundles and elastic fibers.

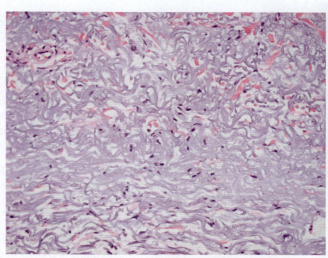

Figure 6.16.6 Solar elastosis. Few residual collagen bundles but most are degenerated creating the amorphous gray mass involving most of the superficial dermis.

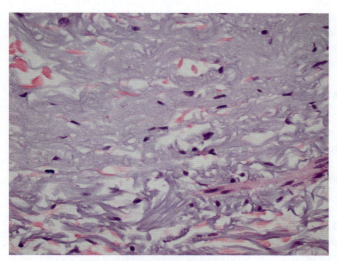

Figure 6.16.7 Solar elastosis. Higher magnification of abnormal, degenerated collagen bundles and elastic fibers. Note that there is no calcification.

6.17 PSEUDOXANTHOMA ELASTICUM VS MID-DERMAL ELASTOLYSIS

	Pseudoxanthoma Elasticum	**Mid-Dermal Elastolysis**
Age	Children and young adults. Typically presenting in the second or third decades of life.	Adults, primarily young woman.
Location	Lateral neck is characteristic location. Axillae, antecubital fossa, popliteal fossa, and groin also commonly involved.	Trunk and proximal upper extremities, predominately.
Etiology	Autosomal recessive disorder due to mutations in the *ABCC6* gene encoding the cellular transmembrane transport protein ABCC6. Leads to reduced levels of inorganic pyrophosphate and ectopic mineralization of elastin-rich tissues.	Unknown. Hypothesized that inflammatory or environmental factors trigger increased elastolytic activity and degradation of elastic fibers.
Presentation	Yellow papules that coalesce into plaques. Skin is soft and lax, forming redundant folds with a "gooseflesh" or "plucked chicken" appearance. May have ocular involvement with retinal angioid streaks. Cardiovascular manifestations result in claudication, hypertension, myocardial infarction, and stroke.	Asymptomatic, well-demarcated regions of fine wrinkling with perifollicular papular protrusions, peau d'orange appearance, and faint reticular erythema.
Histology	1. Epidermis of normal thickness but may have undulating appearance due to loss of elasticity *(Fig. 6.17.1)*. 2. Distorted, fragmented, and clumped elastic fibers in mid-dermis *(Figs. 6.17.1 and 6.17.2)*. 3. Abnormal elastic fibers are coated with fine calcifications that may be demonstrated by Verhoeff-Van Gieson and von Kossa stains *(Figs. 6.17.2-6.17.4)*.	1. Normal epidermis and stratum corneum. On H&E stain, skin has only subtle features with slight pallor of reticular dermis *(Fig. 6.17.5)*. 2. Selective loss of elastic fibers in mid-reticular dermis that is subtle on H&E-stained sections *(Figs. 6.17.6 and 6.17.7)*. No calcification of elastic fibers. 3. Decrease in elastic fibers in mid-dermis is best demonstrated with stain for elastic fibers *(Fig. 6.17.8)*. 4. Sparse lymphomononuclear infiltrate around vascular plexus *(Fig. 6.17.6)*. 5. Elastophagocytosis of elastic fibers by macrophages may be present.
Special studies	Verhoeff-Van Gieson stain for elastic fibers and von Kossa stain for calcification may be used to confirm the diagnosis. Genetic testing for pathogenic variants of *ABCC6*.	Verhoeff-Van Gieson stain to evaluate density of elastic fibers.
Treatment	Surgical excision of lax skin if desired cosmetically. Genetic counseling with regular ophthalmology and cardiology assessments.	No proven treatments. Topical tretinoin may be used to improve cosmesis but does not alter the course of the disease.

6.17 Pseudoxanthoma Elasticum vs Mid-Dermal Elastolysis

	Pseudoxanthoma Elasticum	**Mid-Dermal Elastolysis**
Prognosis	Dependent upon extent of extracutaneous organ involvement. Most patients have normal life span. Ocular involvement may be associated with visual impairment. Morbidity and mortality may be seen with cardiovascular involvement.	Benign, but persistent, condition that is not associated with systemic elastic fiber disease. Skin wrinkling may be of cosmetic concern.

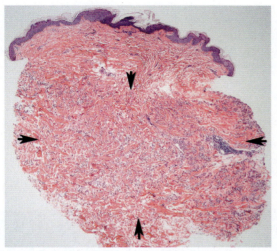

Figure 6.17.1 Pseudoxanthoma elasticum. Normal epidermis and superficial dermis with clumped basophilic fibers within mid-reticular dermis (arrows) but sparing the superficial dermis.

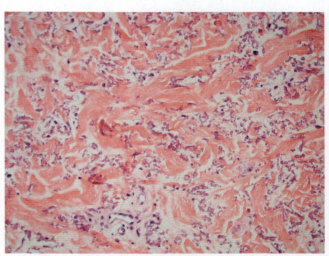

Figure 6.17.2 Pseudoxanthoma elasticum. Distorted, fragmented, and clumped elastic fibers coated with fine calcification.

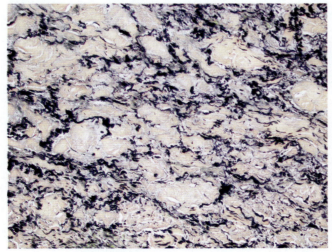

Figure 6.17.3 Pseudoxanthoma elasticum. Verhoeff-Van Gieson stain highlights the black distorted and fragmented elastic fibers.

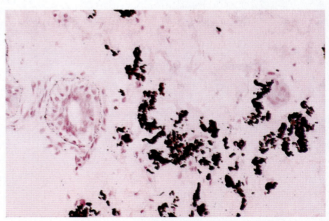

Figure 6.17.4 Pseudoxanthoma elasticum. Calcification of abnormal elastic fibers as demonstrated by von Kossa stain.

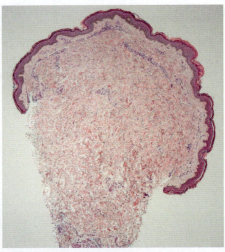

Figure 6.17.5 Mid-dermal elastolysis. Low magnification has the appearance of "normal skin" with unremarkable epidermis and stratum corneum. Mid-reticular dermis has subtle pallor with slight separation of collagen bundles.

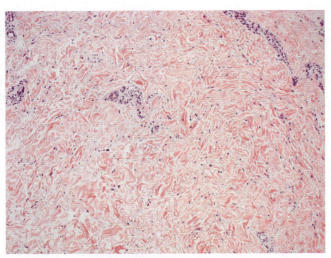

Figure 6.17.6 Mid-dermal elastolysis. Sparse perivascular lymphocytic infiltrate and subtle interstitial cellularity.

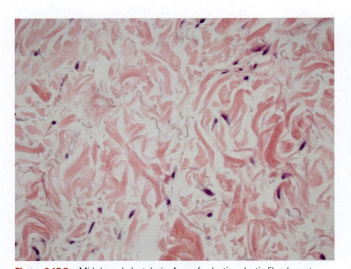

Figure 6.17.7 Mid-dermal elastolysis. Area of selective elastic fiber loss at higher magnification on H&E-stained section.

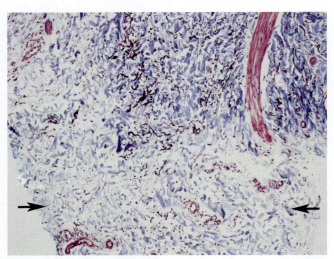

Figure 6.17.8 Mid-dermal elastolysis. Section prepared with Verhoeff-Van Gieson stain better illustrates the selective loss of elastic fibers within the mid-reticular dermis (arrows). Note that elastic fibers in other areas of the dermis are not clumped or calcified.

6.18 HYPERTROPHIC SCAR VS KELOID

	Hypertrophic Scar	**Keloid**
Age	Adults, highest incidence in the second to third decades.	Adults, highest incidence in the second to third decades.
Location	Any site, but typically over extensor joints or areas of excess tension such as shoulders, neck, sternum, knees, and ankles.	Anterior chest, shoulder, upper arms, face, and earlobes.
Etiology	Dysregulation of wound healing after insult to deep dermis. This may occur in any of the three phases of healing that include the inflammatory, proliferative, and remodeling phases.	Dysregulation of wound healing after insult to deep dermis. This may occur in any of the three phases of healing that include the inflammatory, proliferative, and remodeling phases.
Presentation	Firm raised plaque, often linear, or nodule within the site of injury that develops within 4-8 w of injury. Typically, has a rapid growth phase for up to 6 mo then gradually regresses over years. May be pruritic.	Firm, bosselated plaque or nodule that extends beyond the site of injury and may appear years after injury. May occur spontaneously, in the absence of known injury. Persistent with no spontaneous regression. May be painful.
Histology	1. Epidermis has flattened rete ridge pattern and reparative changes *(Fig. 6.18.1)*. 2. Superficial dermis has fine, well-organized, wavy collagen bundles oriented parallel to the epidermis with perpendicular small vessels *(Fig. 6.18.1)*. 3. Whorled nodules of spindle-shaped myofibroblasts with small vessels, erythrocyte extravasation, and mucopolysaccharides *(Figs. 6.18.2 and 6.18.3)*.	1. Epidermis has flattened rete ridge pattern and reparative changes *(Figs. 6.18.4 and 6.18.5)*. 2. Disorganized, hypereosinophilic collagen bundles (keloidal fibers) *(Figs. 6.18.5 and 6.18.6)*. 3. No distinct nodules or excess of spindle-shaped myofibroblasts *(Figs. 6.18.5 and 6.18.6)*. 4. Poor vascularization with occasional dilated blood vessels *(Fig. 6.18.5)*.
Special studies	None.	None.
Treatment	Techniques are directed at prophylaxis, especially in those prone to form hypertrophic scars, as well as treatment. Methods for prophylaxis include compression therapy, silicone gel sheeting, and flavonoids. Avoidance of tension on the wound is important. Scar revision is efficacious to treat. Intralesional corticosteroids, along with cryotherapy and laser therapy, are alternatives.	Techniques are directed at prophylaxis, especially in those prone to form keloids, in addition to treatment. Methods for prophylaxis include pressure therapy, silicone gel sheeting, and flavonoids. Intralesional corticosteroids are first-line therapy. Fluorouracil injection, with or without corticosteroids, shows efficacy. Cryotherapy, radiotherapy, and laser therapy are effective treatments. Given high rate of recurrence, surgical excision is discouraged unless combined with adjuvant therapy.
Prognosis	Benign condition but may have cosmetic consequences affecting quality of life. Hypertrophic scars over joints may cause pain and contractures. Low recurrence rate after excision of original scar.	Benign condition but may have cosmetic consequences affecting quality of life. High recurrence rate following excision.

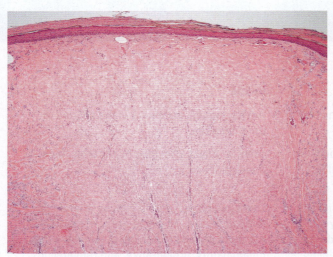

Figure 6.18.1 Hypertrophic scar. Flattened epidermis with reparative changes. The superficial dermis has collagen bundles oriented parallel to the epidermis.

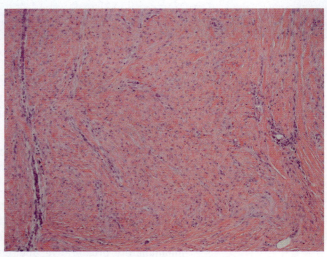

Figure 6.18.2 Hypertrophic scar. Deeper in the dermis, there are whorled nodules of spindle-shaped myofibroblasts.

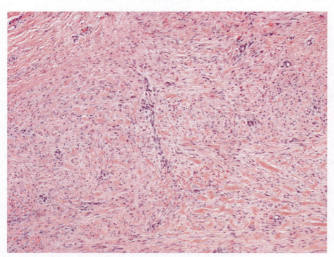

Figure 6.18.3 Hypertrophic scar. Whorled nodule of spindle-shaped myofibroblasts, small capillaries, erythrocyte extravasation, and mild accumulation of mucopolysaccharides between thickened collagen bundles.

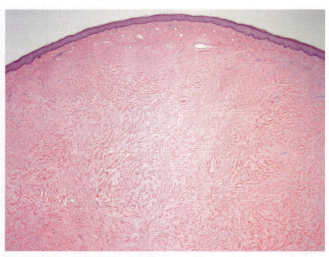

Figure 6.18.4 Keloid. Epidermis is flattened and has reparative change. Dermis is expanded by disorganized, thickened collagen bundles. Note that there is no distinct whorled nodules.

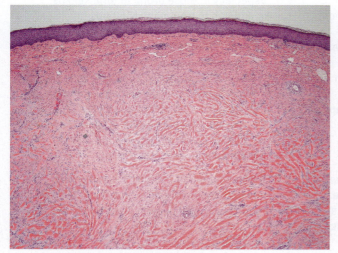

Figure 6.18.5 Keloid. Flattened epidermis overlying dermis containing thick, hypereosinophilic collagen bundles (keloidal fibers). Poor vascularity within the area of repair with few dilated vessels around the periphery.

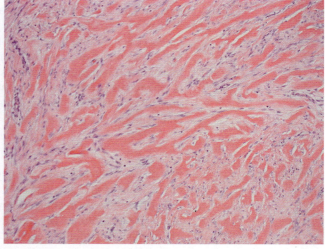

Figure 6.18.6 Keloid. Thick, smudgy, hypereosinophilic keloidal fibers.

6.19 TATTOO VS TUMORAL MELANOSIS

	Tattoo	**Tumoral Melanosis**
Age	Any age, but typically young adults.	Any age, but typically adults.
Location	Any location.	Any location.
Etiology	Introduction of ink or other insoluble pigment into the dermis. Most are ornamental, but some may be accidently traumatically implanted, such as graphite tattoo.	Generally seen in the context of regressed melanoma or melanoma treated with immunotherapy. Represents melanin pigment left behind within the dermis.
Presentation	Ornamental tattoos typically have design and may be multicolored. Traumatic tattoos are generally black and irregular.	Brown, black, blue, or purple macules, papules, or nodules. May be irregular in shape and have heterogeneous pigmentation.
Histology	1. Normal epidermis and stratum corneum *(Figs. 6.19.1* and *6.19.2)*. 2. Granular pigment is present in macrophages that localize around blood vessels and eccrine units *(Figs. 6.19.1-6.19.4)*. 3. Ornamental tattoos have uniform, refractile pigment granules of varying color, but not commonly brown *(Fig. 6.19.4)*. 4. Traumatic tattoos often have larger deposits that are variable in size and shape.	1. Epidermis may be atrophic or hyperplastic *(Figs. 6.19.5* and *6.19.6)*. 2. Absence of melanocytes along the dermal-epidermal junction. 3. Dense band of heavily pigmented melanophages within the superficial dermis *(Figs. 6.19.5* and *6.19.6)*. Melanophages have uniform, coarse, brown melanin granules *(Fig. 6.19.7)*. 4. Superficial dermis has edema, mild fibroplasia, variable lymphocytic inflammation, and reactive vessels *(Figs. 6.19.6* and *6.19.7)*.
Special studies	None.	Fontana-Masson stain to confirm pigment as melanin. Melanocyte markers (SOX10, MART1/Melan A, HMB45) to detect any melanocytic proliferation.
Treatment	Treatment is not necessary unless associated with complications such as infection, hypersensitivity reaction, or neoplasia. Unwanted tattoos may be removed with laser therapy, requiring multiple sessions, or excision leaving scar.	Excision to exclude melanocytic proliferation.
Prognosis	Benign condition desired for decorative effects. Complications include infections, allergic reactions, and tumor induction. Lichenoid hypersensitivity reactions are commonly seen with red tattoo pigment. Cutaneous diseases, including sarcoidosis, may localize in tattoos.	Frequently a consequence of the regression of melanoma. Evaluation for metastatic melanoma is indicated.

6 Alterations of the Epidermis and Dermis

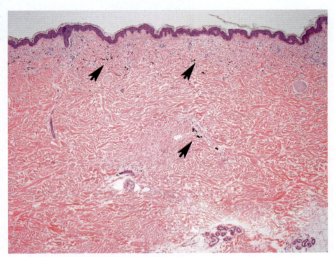

Figure 6.19.1 Tattoo. Normal epidermis and stratum corneum. Within the dermis, there are black granular pigment granules within macrophages (arrows). Macrophages localize in the vicinity of the vascular plexus.

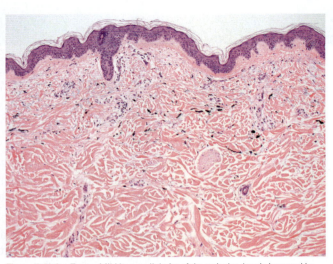

Figure 6.19.2 Tattoo. Mild hypercellularity of the reticular dermis imparted by pigment containing macrophages and reactive vessels.

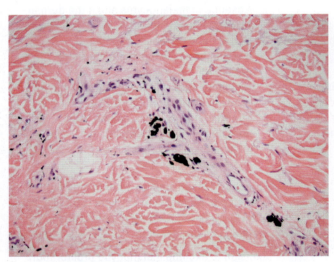

Figure 6.19.3 Tattoo. Heavy laden macrophages with uniform black pigment granules around blood vessel.

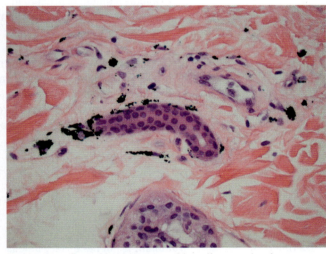

Figure 6.19.4 Tattoo. Macrophages containing uniform granules of exogenous black and blue pigments. Pigment is accentuated around vessels and eccrine duct.

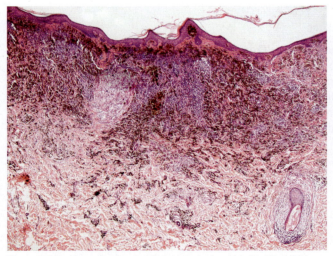

Figure 6.19.5 Tumoral melanosis. Mildly hyperplastic epidermis with underlying dense band of macrophages containing abundant melanin pigment (melanophages). Melanophages do not localize around vessels but fill superficial dermis.

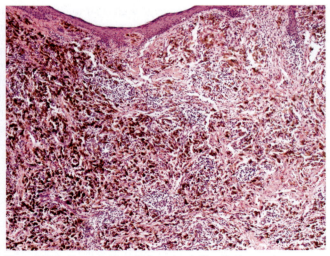

Figure 6.19.6 Tumoral melanosis. Dense band of heavily pigmented melanophages with admixed aggregates of lymphocytes. Note that overlying epidermis has lack of junctional melanocytes.

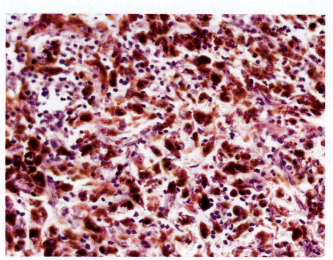

Figure 6.19.7 Tumoral melanosis. Melanophages characterized by relatively uniform, brown, coarse melanin granules. There are admixed lymphocytes.

6.20 EXOGENOUS OCHRONOSIS VS MINOCYCLINE-INDUCED HYPERPIGMENTATION

	Exogenous Ochronosis	**Minocycline-Induced Hyperpigmentation**
Age	Any age, but typically adults.	Any age.
Location	Hydroquinone-induced ochronosis localizes to sites of application, most commonly face, neck, ears, back, and extensor surfaces of extremities.	Depends upon the type. Type I affects face in areas of prior inflammation and/or scarring; type II involves previously normal skin, classically pretibial area and forearms; and type III is more diffuse involvement of sun-exposed regions.
Etiology	Phenolic compounds enzymatically inhibit homogentisate dioxygenase leading to accumulation of homogentisic acid in collagen of the skin. Homogentisic acid polymerizes and forms pigment deposits in the skin. Hydroquinone, used as lightening agent, is the most common cause, but it has also been associated with use of phenol, resorcinol, oral antimalarials, picric acid, and quinine.	Hemosiderin or iron chelate of minocycline depositing in scars (type I). Minocycline metabolite-protein complex chelated with iron and calcium (type II) depositing in dermis. Type III is thought to be due to sun-induced basal zone melanization.
Presentation	Blue-gray-black macules and patches that may be accompanied by erythema. On the face, "caviar-like" papules may be present.	Ill-defined blue-gray patches, which, in some cases, are within preexisting scar (types I and II). Diffuse muddy brown patches in sun-exposed areas (type III).
Histology	1. Normal epidermis and stratum corneum *(Fig. 6.20.1)*. 2. Yellow-brown curvilinear "banana-shaped" fibers within superficial dermis *(Figs. 6.20.1-6.20.3)*. 3. Fragmented collagen fibers and pigment deposits lying free in dermis or within macrophages *(Fig. 6.20.3)*.	1. Epidermis in type I may show flattening and reparative change. Normal epidermis in type II *(Fig. 6.20.4)*. Increased basal layer melanin in type III with underlying melanophages. 2. Brown-black and yellow-brown pigment granules deposited on elastic fibers and within macrophages and dermal dendrocytes around vessels and eccrine units *(Figs. 6.20.4-6.20.6)*. 3. Type I often associated with scar and reparative changes. 4. Pigment typically positive with both Perl iron and Fontana-Masson stains *(Figs. 6.20.7 and 6.20.8)*.
Special studies	None.	Pigment granules stain with Fontana-Masson and Perl iron stains (types I and II).
Treatment	Cessation of offending agent is necessary to prevent further pigmentation. Dermabrasion, chemical peels, and laser therapy have been used to treat the hyperpigmentation. Topical treatments, including low-potency corticosteroids and retinoic acid, have been utilized but show mixed results.	Slow resolution over months to years with discontinuation of minocycline. Avoidance of sun exposure, especially in type III. Q-switched laser may be utilized to decrease hyperpigmentation.

6.20 Exogenous Ochronosis vs Minocycline-Induced Hyperpigmentation

	Exogenous Ochronosis	Minocycline-Induced Hyperpigmentation
Prognosis	Exogenous ochronosis does not have the systemic manifestations of alkaptonuria-associated ochronosis. However, the hyperpigmentation may be of cosmetic concern and interfere with quality of life.	No systemic effects but may cause cosmetic concern.

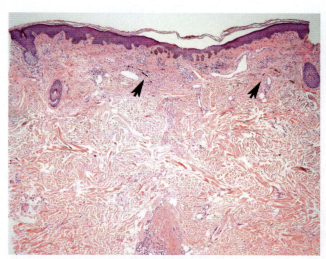

Figure 6.20.1 Exogenous ochronosis. Normal epidermis and stratum corneum with yellow-brown curvilinear pigment deposits and fragmented collagen fibers within superficial dermis (arrows).

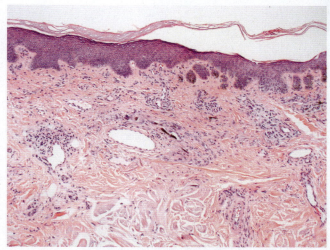

Figure 6.20.2 Exogenous ochronosis. Yellow-brown curvilinear fibers within macrophages and lying free within the dermis. Vessels show reactive change.

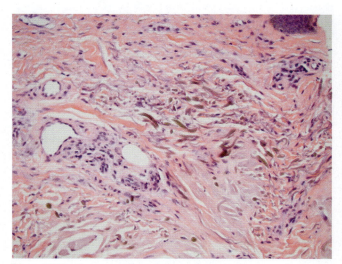

Figure 6.20.3 Exogenous ochronosis. Banana-shaped yellow-brown fibers within the dermis.

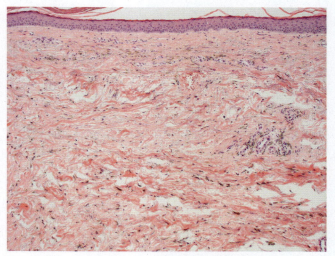

Figure 6.20.4 Minocycline-induced hyperpigmentation. Example of type II with relatively normal epidermis overlying dermis with diffuse interstitial deposition of pigment.

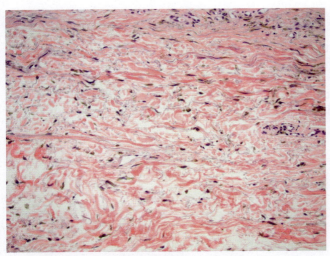

Figure 6.20.5 Minocycline-induced hyperpigmentation. Brown-black and yellow-brown pigment granules deposited on elastic fibers and within macrophages and dermal dendrocytes around vessels and eccrine units.

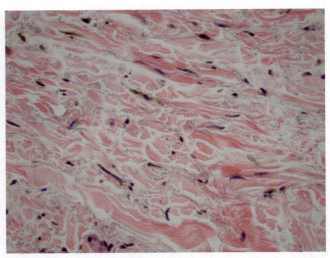

Figure 6.20.6 Minocycline-induced hyperpigmentation. Pigment appears yellow-brown to brown-black and refractile. Present in macrophages, within dendrocytes, and on elastic fibers.

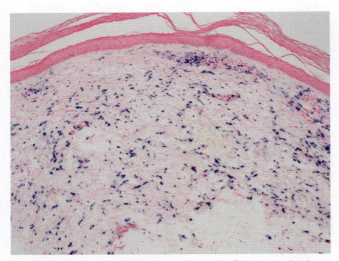

Figure 6.20.7 Minocycline-induced hyperpigmentation. Pigment granules show staining with Perl iron stain.

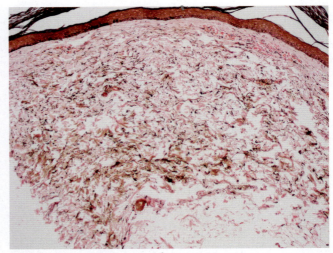

Figure 6.20.8 Minocycline-induced hyperpigmentation. Pigment granules show staining with Fontana-Masson stain.

SUGGESTED READINGS

Chapter 6.1

Alikhan A, Felsten LM, Daly M, Petronic-Rosic V. Vitiligo: a comprehensive overview part I. Introduction, epidemiology, quality of life, diagnosis, differential diagnosis, associations, histopathology, etiology, and work-up. *J Am Acad Dermatol.* 2011;65(3):473-491.

Faria AR, Tarlé RG, Dellatorre G, Mira MT, de Castro CCS. Vitiligo–Part 2–classification, histopathology and treatment. *An Bras Dermatol.* 2014;89(5):784-790.

Iannella G, Greco A, Didona D, et al. Vitiligo: pathogenesis, clinical variants and treatment approaches. *Autoimmun Rev.* 2016;15(4):335-4343.

Kumar S, Singh A, Prasad RR. Role of histopathology in vitiligo. *J Indian Med Assoc.* 2011;109(9):657-658, 665.

Saleem MD, Oussedik E, Picardo M, Schoch JJ. Acquired disorders with hypopigmentation: a clinical approach to diagnosis and treatment. *J Am Acad Dermatol.* 2019;80(5):1233-1250.e10.

Vachiramon V, Thadanipon K. Postinflammatory hypopigmentation. *Clin Exp Dermatol.* 2011;36(7):708-714.

Chapter 6.2

Elmariah S, Kim B, Berger T, Chisolm S, Kwatra SG, Mollanazar N, Yosipovitch G. Practical approaches for diagnosis and management of prurigo nodularis: United States expert panel consensus. *J Am Acad Dermatol.* 2021;84(3):747-760.

Gupta G, Hohman MH, Kwan E. *Chondrodermatitis nodularis helicis.* In: *StatPearls.* StatPearls Publishing; 2022.

Huang AH, Williams KA, Kwatra SG. Prurigo nodularis: epidemiology and clinical features. *J Am Acad Dermatol.* 2020;83(6):1559-1565.

Thompson L D R. Chondrodermatitis nodularis helicis. *Ear Nose Throat J.* 2007;86(12):734-735.

Vázquez-López F, Gómez-Vila B, Vázquez-Losada B, Palacios García L, Vivanco-Allende B, Gómez de Castro C. Chondrodermatitis nodularis helicis in the 21st century: demographic trends from a gender and age perspective. A single university hospital retrospective histopathological register study of 215 patients in Asturias, North Spain (2000-2017). *J Eur Acad Dermatol Venereol.* 2021;35(8):e506-e507.

Williams KA, Huang AH, Belzberg M, Kwatra SG. Prurigo nodularis: pathogenesis and management. *J Am Acad Dermatol.* 2020;83(6):1567-1575.

Chapters 6.3-6.4

Davis M D P, Weenig RH, Camilleri MJ. Confluent and reticulate papillomatosis (Gougerot-Carteaud syndrome): a minocycline-responsive dermatosis without evidence for yeast in pathogenesis. A study of 39 patients and a proposal of diagnostic criteria. *Br J Dermatol.* 2006;154(2):287-293.

Higgins SP, Freemark M, Prose NS. Acanthosis nigricans: a practical approach to evaluation and management. *Dermatol Online J.* 2008;14(9):2.

Kutlubay Z, Engin B, Bairamov O, Tüzün Y. Acanthosis nigricans: a fold (intertriginous) dermatosis. *Clin Dermatol.* 2015;33(4):466-470.

Lin Q, Zhang D, Ma W. Granular parakeratosis: a case report. *Clin Cosmet Investig Dermatol.* 2022;15:1367-1370.

Lucero R, Horowitz D. *Granular parakeratosis.* In: *StatPearls.* StatPearls Publishing; 2022.

Tamraz H, Raffoul M, Kurban M, Kibbi A-G, Abbas O. Confluent and reticulated papillomatosis: clinical and histopathological study of 10 cases from Lebanon. *J Eur Acad Dermatol Venereol.* 2013;27(1):e119-e123.

Chapter 6.5

Biswas A. Cornoid lamellation revisited: apropos of porokeratosis with emphasis on unusual clinicopathological variants. *Am J Dermatopathol.* 2015;37(2):145-155.

Palleschi GM, Torchia D. Porokeratosis of Mibelli and superficial disseminated porokeratosis. *J Cutan Pathol.* 2008;35(2):253-255.

Prieto VG, Casal M, McNutt NS. Lichen planus-like keratosis. A clinical and histological reexamination. *Am J Surg Pathol.* 1993;17(3):259-263.

Sertznig P, von Felbert V, Megahed M. Porokeratosis: present concepts. *J Eur Acad Dermatol Venereol.* 2012;26(4):404-412.

Vincek V. Lichen planus-like keratosis: clinicopathological evaluation of 1366 cases. *Int J Dermatol.* 2019;58(7):830-833.

Chapter 6.6

Crane JS, Paller AS. *X-Linked Ichthyosis.* In: *StatPearls.* StatPearls Publishing; 2022.

Okulicz JF, Schwartz RA. Hereditary and acquired ichthyosis vulgaris. *Int J Dermatol.* 2003;42(2):95-98.

Takeichi T, Akiyama M. Inherited ichthyosis: non-syndromic forms. *J Dermatol.* 2016;43(3):242-51.

Thyssen JP, Godoy-Gijon E, Elias PM. Ichthyosis vulgaris: the filaggrin mutation disease. *Br J Dermatol.* 2013;168(6):1155-1566.

Chapters 6.7-6.12

Beers WH, Ince A, Moore TL. Scleredema adultorum of Buschke: a case report and review of the literature. *Semin Arthritis Rheum.* 2006;35(6):355-359.

Cárdenas-Gonzalez RE, Ruelas MEH, Candiani JO. Lichen myxedematosus: a rare group of cutaneous mucinosis. *An Bras Dermatol.* 2019;94(4):462-469.

Cowper SE. Nephrogenic systemic fibrosis: an overview. *J Am Coll Radiol.* 2008;5(1):23-28.

Fernandez-Flores A, Gatica-Torres M, Ruelas-Villavicencio AL, Saeb-Lima M. Morphological clues in the diagnosis of sclerodermiform dermatitis. *Am J Dermatopathol.* 2014;36(6):449-464.

Ferreli C, Gasparini G, Parodi A, Cozzani E, Rongioletti F, Atzori L. Cutaneous manifestations of scleroderma and scleroderma-like disorders: a comprehensive review. *Clin Rev Allergy Immunol.* 2017;53(3):306-336.

Fett N. Scleroderma—nomenclature, etiology, pathogenesis, prognosis, and treatments: facts and controversies. *Clin Dermatol.* 2013;31(4):432-437.

Girardi M, Kay J, Elston DM, Leboit PE, Abu-Alfa A, Cowper SE. Nephrogenic systemic fibrosis: clinicopathological definition and workup recommendations. *J Am Acad Dermatol.* 2011;65(6):1095-1106.e7.

Haber R, Bachour J, El Gemayel M. Scleromyxedema treatment: a systematic review and update. *Int J Dermatol.* 2020;59(10):1191-1201.

Hummers LK. Scleromyxedema. *Curr Opin Rheumatol.* 2014;26(6):658-662.

Jackson EM, English JCIII. Diffuse cutaneous mucinoses. *Dermatol Clin.* 2002;20(3):493-501.

Leblebici C. A case of cutaneous focal mucinosis with follicular induction. *Am J Dermatopathol.* 2018;40(1):72-73.

Li K, Barankin B. Digital mucous cysts. *J Cutan Med Surg.* 2010;14(5):199-206.

Meyers AL, Fallahi AKM. *Digital Mucous Cyst.* In: StatPearls. StatPearls Publishing; 2022.

Raboudi A, Litaiem N. *Scleredema.* In: StatPearls. StatPearls Publishing; 2022.

Rongioletti F, Ferreli C, Atzori L, Bottoni U, Soda G. Scleroderma with an update about clinico-pathological correlation. *G Ital Dermatol Venereol.* 2018;153(2):208-215.

Rongioletti F, Rebora A. Cutaneous mucinoses: microscopic criteria for diagnosis. *Am J Dermatopathol.* 2001;23(3):257-267.

Rongioletti F. New and emerging conditions of acquired cutaneous mucinoses in adults. *J Eur Acad Dermatol Venereol.* 2022;36(7):1016-1024.

Takemura N, Fujii N, Tanaka T. Cutaneous focal mucinosis: a case report. *J Dermatol.* 2005;32(12):1051-1054.

Truhan AP, Roenigk HHJr. The cutaneous mucinoses. *J Am Acad Dermatol.* 1986;14:1-18.

Chapters 6.13-6.15

Borowicz J, Gillespie M, Miller R. Cutaneous amyloidosis. *Skinmed.* 2011;9(2):96-100; quiz 101.

Chen SL, Chen JR, Yang SW. Painless gouty tophus in the nasal bridge: a case report and literature review. *Medicine (Baltimore).* 2019;98(11):e14850.

Chhana A, Dalbeth N. The gouty tophus: a review. *Curr Rheumatol Rep.* 2015;17(3):19.

Fernandez-Flores A. Calcinosis cutis: critical review. *Acta Dermatovenerol Croat.* 2011;19(1):43-50.

Kumar P. Calcinosis Cutis. *Indian Pediatr.* 2017;54(3):253.

Mehregan D, Hooten J. Adult colloid milium: a case report and literature review. *Int J Dermatol.* 2011;50(12):1531-1534.

Molina-Ruiz AM, Cerroni L, Kutzner H, Requena L. Cutaneous deposits. *Am J Dermatopathol.* 2014;36:1-48.

Reiter N, El-Shabrawi L, Leinweber B, Berghold A, Aberer E. Calcinosis cutis: part I. Diagnostic pathway. *J Am Acad Dermatol.* 2011;65:1-12; quiz 13-4.

Siadat AH, Mokhtari F. Colloid milium. *Adv Biomed Res.* 2013;2:28.

Weidner T, Illing T, Elsner P. Primary localized cutaneous amyloidosis: a systematic treatment review. *Am J Clin Dermatol.* 2017;18(5):629-642.

Chapters 6.16-6.17

Bergen AA, Plomp AS, Hu X, de Jong PT, Gorgels TG. ABCC6 and pseudoxanthoma elasticum. *Pflugers Arch.* 2007;453(5):685-691.

Brokamp G, Mori M, Faith EF. Pseudoxanthoma elasticum. *JAMA Dermatol.* 2022;158(1):100.

Hardin J, Dupuis E, Haber RM. Mid-dermal elastolysis: a female-centric disease; case report and updated review of the literature. *Int J Womens Dermatol.* 2015;1(3):126-130.

Marconi B, Bobyr I, Campanati A, et al. Pseudoxanthoma elasticum and skin: clinical manifestations, histopathology, pathomechanism, perspectives of treatment. *Intractable Rare Dis Res.* 2015;4(3):113-122.

Rao BK, Endzweig CH, Kagen MH, Kriegel D, Freeman RG. Wrinkling due to mid-dermal elastolysis: two cases and literature review. *J Cutan Med Surg.* 2000;4(1):40-44.

Chapter 6.18

Del Toro D, Dedhia R, Tollefson TT. Advances in scar management: prevention and management of hypertrophic scars and keloids. *Curr Opin Otolaryngol Head Neck Surg.* 2016;24(4):322-329.

Elsaie ML. Update on management of keloid and hypertrophic scars: a systemic review. *J Cosmet Dermatol.* 2021;20(9):2729-2738.

Lee JY, Yang CC, Chao SC, Wong TW. Histopathological differential diagnosis of keloid and hypertrophic scar. *Am J Dermatopathol.* 2004;26(5):379-384.

Limandjaja GC, Niessen FB, Scheper RJ, Gibbs S. The keloid disorder: heterogeneity, histopathology, mechanisms and models. *Front Cell Dev Biol.* 2020;8:360.

Chapter 6.19

Jurgens A, Guru S, Guo R, Brewer J, Bridges A, Jakub J, Comfere N. Tumoral melanosis in the setting of targeted immunotherapy for metastatic melanoma-a single institutional experience and literature review. *Am J Dermatopathol.* 2021;43(1):9-14.

Staser K, Chen D, Solus J, et al. Extensive tumoral melanosis associated with ipilimumab-treated melanoma. *Br J Dermatol.* 2016;175(2):391-393.

Torre-Castro J, Nájera L, Suárez D, et al. Histopathology of dermatologic complications of tattoos. *Am J Dermatopathol.* 2022;44(9):632-649.

Chapter 6.20

Bhattar PA, Zawar VP, Godse KV, Patil SP, Nadkarni NJ, Gautam MM. Exogenous ochronosis. *Indian J Dermatol*. 2015;60(6):537-543.

Geria AN, Tajirian AL, Kihiczak G, Schwartz RA. Minocycline-induced skin pigmentation: an update. *Acta Dermatovenerol Croat*. 2009;17(2):123-126.

Ishack S, Lipner SR. Exogenous ochronosis associated with hydroquinone: a systematic review. *Int J Dermatol*. 2022;61(6):675-684.

Simmons BJ, Griffith RD, Bray FN, Falto-Aizpurua LA, Nouri K. Exogenous ochronosis: a comprehensive review of the diagnosis, epidemiology, causes, and treatments. *Am J Clin Dermatol*. 2015;16(3):205-212.

Wang RF, Ko D, Friedman BJ, Lim HW, Mohammad TF. Disorders of hyperpigmentation. Part I. Pathogenesis and clinical features of common pigmentary disorders. *J Am Acad Dermatol*. 2023;88(2):271-288.

7
Infectious Diseases and Infestations of the Skin

- **7.1** Bullous Impetigo vs Staphylococcal Scalded Skin Syndrome
- **7.2** Dermatophytosis vs Erythrasma
- **7.3** Bullous Dermatophytosis vs Dyshidrotic Dermatitis
- **7.4** Tinea Versicolor vs Dermatophytosis
- **7.5** Dermatophytosis vs Cutaneous Candidiasis
- **7.6** Cryptococcosis vs Blastomycosis
- **7.7** Coccidioidomycosis vs Blastomycosis
- **7.8** Chromomycosis vs Phaeohyphomycosis
- **7.9** Mucormycosis vs Aspergillosis
- **7.10** Histoplasmosis vs Leishmaniasis
- **7.11** Majocchi Granuloma vs Pityrosporum Folliculitis
- **7.12** Herpes Simplex Infection vs Pemphigus Vulgaris
- **7.13** Varicella-Zoster Virus Infection vs Benign Familial Pemphigus (Hailey-Hailey Disease)
- **7.14** Molluscum Contagiosum vs Verruca Vulgaris
- **7.15** Condyloma Acuminatum vs Epidermolytic Acanthoma
- **7.16** Leprosy vs Sarcoidosis
- **7.17** Atypical Mycobacterium vs Erythema Nodosum
- **7.18** Nocardiosis vs Actinomycosis
- **7.19** Secondary Syphilis vs Lupus Erythematosus
- **7.20** Secondary Syphilis (Condyloma Lata) vs Psoriasis
- **7.21** Scabies vs Demodicosis
- **7.22** Myiasis vs Tungiasis

7.1 BULLOUS IMPETIGO VS STAPHYLOCOCCAL SCALDED SKIN SYNDROME

	Bullous Impetigo	**Staphylococcal Scalded Skin Syndrome**
Age	Any age but primarily infants and young children, less than 2 y of age.	Children, predominately under the age of 6 y. Less commonly seen in adults.
Location	Any location but frequently trunk and intertriginous areas, including neck, axillae, groin, inframammary crease, and gluteal cleft.	Face and intertriginous regions including neck, axillae, and groin. No mucosal involvement.
Etiology	Local infection by *Staphylococcus aureus* that produces exfoliative toxin A. The exfoliative toxin targets desmoglein-1, the desmosomal cadherin that mediates cell-to-cell adhesion and is important in the maintenance of epidermal integrity.	Exotoxin-producing strains of *S aureus* produce exfoliative toxins that target desmoglein-1, a cell-to-cell adhesion protein found in the superficial epidermis. As opposed to bullous impetigo, the infection occurs at a remote site such as the oral cavity, nasopharynx, or umbilicus. The toxins spread hematogenously to act upon the skin, causing formation of a blister cavity in the superficial epidermis.
Presentation	Well-demarcated clusters of small vesicles that progress to flaccid bullae that have clear fluid. The blisters commonly erode, leaving collarettes of scale and a thin yellow-brown crust. Nikolsky sign (gentle pressure on vesicle causing desquamation) is negative. No systemic involvement.	Tender, diffuse erythema that rapidly progresses to flaccid, fragile bullae with superficial desquamation. Positive Nikolsky sign (desquamation of skin with gentle pressure at edge of bullae) is present. Usually associated with fever, malaise, and fatigue. Blisters heal without scarring.
Histology	1. A basket-weave orthokeratotic stratum corneum indicative of an acute process *(Figs. 7.1.1* and *7.1.2)*. 2. Subcorneal acantholysis within the granular layer with formation of a vesicle containing neutrophils *(Figs. 7.1.2* and *7.1.3)*. 3. Tissue Gram stain reveals gram-positive cocci within the vesicle *(Fig. 7.1.4)*. This is opposed to staphylococcal scalded skin syndrome in which the vesicle is sterile and tissue Gram stain is negative.	1. A basket-weave orthokeratotic stratum corneum indicative of an acute process *(Figs. 7.1.5* and *7.1.6)*. 2. Subcorneal acantholysis with intraepidermal cleavage in the granular layer *(Figs. 7.1.6* and *7.1.7)*. 3. Scant neutrophilic inflammation associated with the acantholysis *(Fig. 7.1.6)*. 4. No bacteria present with the vesicle cavity with tissue Gram stain, as opposed to bullous impetigo.
Special studies	Tissue Gram stain to identify bacteria. Microbiologic culture may be performed for confirmation and to detect resistant strains.	
Treatment	If limited disease, topical mupirocin is first-line treatment. For more extensive or nonresponsive disease, systemic antibiotics may be necessary. Antibiotic selection is based upon sensitivities established from cultures.	Intravenous antistaphylococcal antibiotics such as nafcillin, oxacillin, or flucloxacillin. Clarithromycin or cefazolin may be utilized in cases of penicillin allergy. Vancomycin is indicated if methicillin resistance is detected. Supportive measures including wound care, nutritional support, and maintenance of fluid balance are imperative.

(continued)

	Bullous Impetigo	Staphylococcal Scalded Skin Syndrome
Prognosis	Generally a self-limited condition that resolves in 2-3 w without treatment and within 10 d if treated. Typically, there are no sequelae.	Most cases resolve without sequelae in 2-3 w with appropriate therapy. Morbidity and mortality are increased with extensive skin involvement, fluid and electrolyte imbalance, and sepsis. Mortality is greater in adults due to presence of comorbidities.

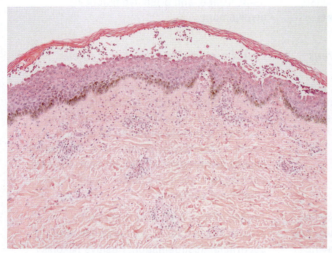

Figure 7.1.1 Bullous impetigo. A basket-weave orthokeratotic stratum corneum with subcorneal vesicle formation. There is a moderately dense mixed inflammatory infiltrate in the superficial dermis.

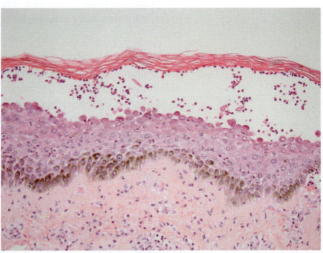

Figure 7.1.2 Bullous impetigo. Subcorneal vesicle formed by acantholysis within the granular layer. Neutrophils are present in the vesicle cavity.

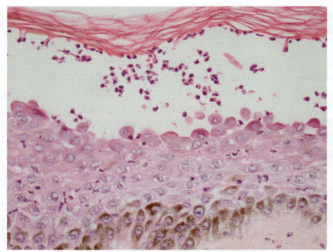

Figure 7.1.3 Bullous impetigo. Acantholytic cells that are rounded up and dissociated from each other forming subcorneal split.

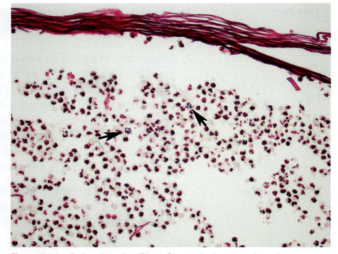

Figure 7.1.4 Bullous impetigo. Tissue Gram stain demonstrating a few gram-positive cocci (arrows) within the vesicle in association with neutrophils.

7.1 Bullous Impetigo vs Staphylococcal Scalded Skin Syndrome

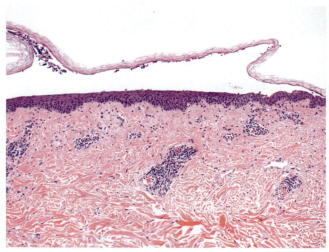

Figure 7.1.5 Staphylococcal scalded skin syndrome. A basket-weave orthokeratotic stratum corneum overlying the subcorneal vesicle. A vesicle formed by acantholysis within the granular layer with few acantholytic cells and rare neutrophils within the vesicle cavity.

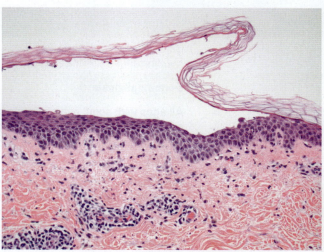

Figure 7.1.6 Staphylococcal scalded skin syndrome. The subcorneal vesicle is similar to that seen in bullous impetigo, but there is less inflammation and no bacteria present.

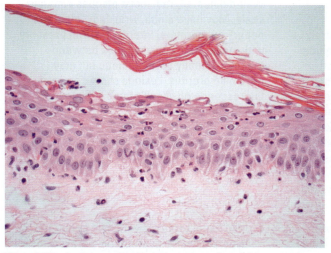

Figure 7.1.7 Staphylococcal scalded skin syndrome. Superficial acantholysis forming a subcorneal vesicle with scant inflammation.

7.2 DERMATOPHYTOSIS VS ERYTHRASMA

	Dermatophytosis	**Erythrasma**
Age	All ages with some clinical forms showing age predilection (such as tinea capitis in children; tinea cruris and tinea unguium in adults).	Adults, rare in children.
Location	Any location. Clinical forms are divided into those affecting glabrous skin (tinea corporis, tinea cruris, tinea faciei), acral skin (tinea manus, tinea pedis), skin rich in terminal hair follicles (tinea capitis, tinea barbae), and nails (tinea unguium).	Predilection for areas of moisture and occlusion, especially toe webs, axillae, and groin.
Etiology	Superficial fungal infection caused by *Trichophyton*, *Microsporum*, and *Epidermophyton* genera.	Superficial bacterial infection caused by the gram-positive, non–spore-forming bacillus *Corynebacterium minutissimum*.
Presentation	Variable and dependent upon clinical form. Tinea corporis, tinea cruris, and tinea faciei are characterized by a sharply demarcated red-pink erythematous annular patch or plaque with scale and a raised edge. Some lesions may have pustules or vesicles. Tinea manus and tinea pedis typically are not as well demarcated and present as dry, erythematous, scaly skin that may become vesicular. Tinea capitis and tinea barbae form annular patches and plaques with folliculocentric pustules. Tinea unguium causes thickening, dystrophy, and discoloration of nails.	Well-delineated, red, moist plaques with fine scale. May have a fine, wrinkled, "cigarette paper" appearance. Interdigital form presents with macerated, scaly plaques between the toes. Usually asymptomatic but may have mild pruritus. Lesions show coral red fluorescence on Wood's lamp examination due to coproporphyrin III.
Histology	1. Hyperkeratosis and parakeratosis with aggregates of neutrophils *(Figs. 7.2.1 and 7.2.2)*. 2. Mild epidermal hyperplasia and reactive changes *(Fig. 7.2.1)*. 3. Nonpigmented hyphae on longitudinal section and cross section present in the stratum corneum on H&E stain *(Fig. 7.2.3)* and best seen with **PAS** or **GMS** stain *(Fig. 7.2.4)*. Hyphae are larger than the bacilli of erythrasma. 4. Patchy, sparse chronic inflammation in superficial dermis *(Fig. 7.2.1)*.	1. Mild hyperkeratosis with mild epidermal hyperplasia. No appreciable parakeratosis or intracorneal inflammation *(Fig. 7.2.5)*. 2. Thin, delicate, bacillary organisms may be evident within the stratum corneum on H&E-stained sections *(Fig. 7.2.6)*. Bacilli are thinner than dermatophyte hyphae *(Fig. 7.2.7)*. 3. Tissue Gram stain may be used to show gram-positive bacilli within the stratum corneum. 4. Sparse lymphomononuclear infiltrate in the superficial dermis.
Special studies	PAS or GMS stain to identify the fungus. KOH preparation to identify fungi in scrapings. Culture may be performed to confirm and speciate the fungus.	Wood's lamp examination used clinically. Tissue Gram stain to detect bacteria and assess morphology. PAS or GMS stains may highlight organisms but also used to morphologically exclude the fungus.

	Dermatophytosis	**Erythrasma**
Treatment	Topical antifungal agents, including azoles, allylamines, tolnaftate, ciclopirox, and butenafine, may be used for localized infection. A widespread infection may require oral antifungal therapy including terbinafine, itraconazole, fluconazole, or griseofulvin.	Topical clindamycin or erythromycin are first-line therapies for localized disease. Oral clindamycin or erythromycin may be necessary for more extensive or diffuse cutaneous involvement. Prevention involves techniques to minimize skin occlusion and moisture.
Prognosis	A superficial infection typically responds to adequate therapy, but recurrences are common. Onychomycosis and deep-seated follicular-based infections may be refractory and generally require oral antifungal therapy. A widespread infection is often associated with immunodeficiency.	Generally excellent in healthy individuals. Typically responds well to topical and oral therapies but often recurs if skin occlusion and moisture persist. Complications, including abscess formation, cellulitis, and endocarditis, may occur in immunocompromised patients.

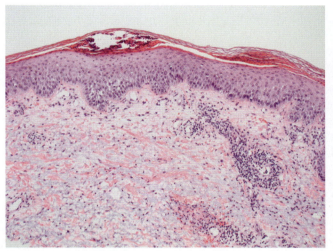

Figure 7.2.1 Dermatophytosis. Example of tinea corporis with mild reactive epidermal hyperplasia, foci of parakeratosis, and entrapped neutrophils. A sparse, patchy inflammatory infiltrate in the dermis.

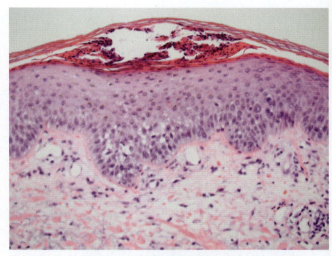

Figure 7.2.2 Dermatophytosis. Slight epidermal spongiosis with mounded parakeratosis and aggregate of neutrophils.

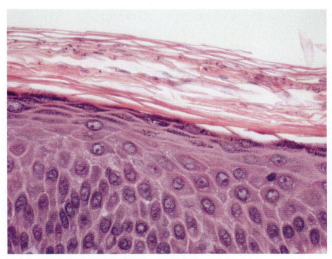

Figure 7.2.3 Dermatophytosis. Nonpigmented hyphae in stratum corneum seen on longitudinal section and cross section.

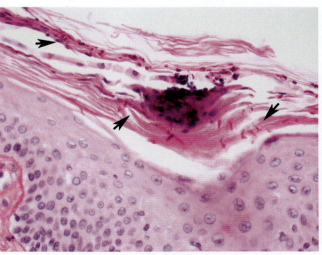

Figure 7.2.4 Dermatophytosis. PAS stain demonstrates hyphae within the stratum corneum (arrows).

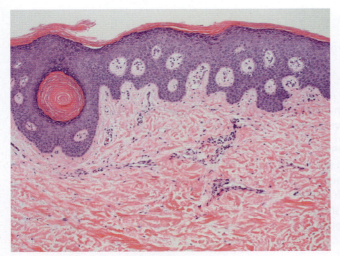

Figure 7.2.5 Erythrasma. Mild epidermal hyperplasia with compact hyperkeratosis and minimal dermal inflammation.

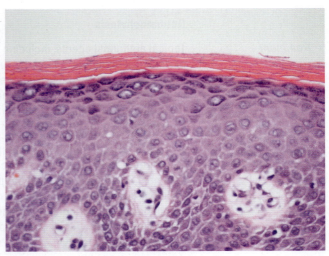

Figure 7.2.6 Erythrasma. Thin, delicate bacillary organisms within the compact stratum corneum.

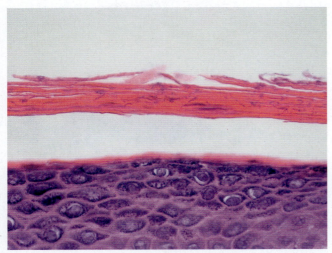

Figure 7.2.7 Erythrasma. Higher magnification of bacillary organisms that are thinner and more delicate than fungal hyphae of dermatophytosis.

7.3 BULLOUS DERMATOPHYTOSIS VS DYSHIDROTIC DERMATITIS

	Bullous Dermatophytosis	**Dyshidrotic Dermatitis**
Age	All ages.	Any age with peak incidence in middle-aged individuals.
Location	Feet most commonly involved.	Palms and soles.
Etiology	Most often caused by *Trichophyton rubrum* or *Trichophyton mentagrophytes/Trichophyton interdigitale*. Blister formation is thought to represent a secondary delayed hypersensitivity reaction triggered by dermatophyte antigens.	Unknown but close association with atopy. May be triggered by metal (nickel, cobalt) exposure, warm weather, fungal infection, and psychological stress.
Presentation	Unilateral, erythematous, annular, scaly plaques that evolve to vesicles and bullae. Vesicles and bullae rupture leaving a collarette of scale and heal without scarring. Unilateral disease and associated interdigital skin maceration are diagnostic clues. The lesions are often pruritic and tender.	Symmetric, intensely pruritic, deep-seated vesicles ("tapioca-like") on lateral aspects of fingers and toes. May progress to bullae.
Histology	1. Orthohyperkeratosis with intracorneal neutrophils *(Fig. 7.3.1)*. 2. The epidermis has elongated rete ridges with reactive changes and formation of vesicle containing edema and neutrophils *(Figs. 7.3.1* and *7.3.2)*. 3. Nonpigmented hyphae on longitudinal section and cross section present in the stratum corneum on an H&E-stained section *(Fig. 7.3.3)* and best seen with PAS *(Fig. 7.3.4)* or GMS stain. 4. A sparse superficial mixed inflammatory infiltrate with lymphocytes and neutrophils.	1. Prominent epidermal spongiosis with formation of large, discrete intraepidermal vesicles *(Figs. 7.3.5* and *7.3.6)*. 2. Exocytosis of lymphocytes in areas of spongiosis; neutrophils not present unless eroded or with a bacterial superinfection *(Fig. 7.3.7)*. 3. A superficial perivascular lymphohistiocytic infiltrate with occasional eosinophils *(Figs. 7.3.5* and *7.3.6)*.
Special studies	PAS or GMS stain to detect fungal organisms. KOH preparation performed on skin scrapings. Culture may be performed to confirm and speciate the fungus.	PAS stain to exclude a fungal infection.
Treatment	Topical or systemic antifungal agents depending on the extent of involvement, duration of disease, and comorbidities. Topical antifungal agents, including azoles, allylamines, tolnaftate, ciclopirox, butenafine, may be used for localized infection. A widespread infection may require oral antifungal therapy including terbinafine, itraconazole, fluconazole, or griseofulvin.	High-potency topical steroids with soaks and cold compresses are first-line therapy. Calcineurin inhibitors may be used in mild to moderate cases. Systemic corticosteroids may be necessary in severe disease. Avoidance of triggers.
Prognosis	Infection typically responds with adequate therapy. Maceration may lead to a bacterial superinfection.	Although episodes typically resolve within a month, it is a chronic condition with frequent recurrences.

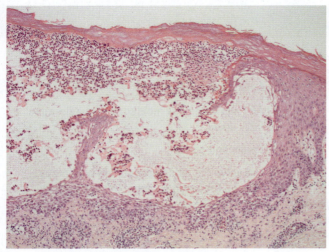

Figure 7.3.1 Bullous dermatophytosis. Acral skin with mild hyperkeratosis and intraepidermal pustule with intracorneal neutrophils.

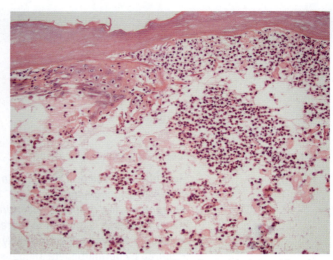

Figure 7.3.2 Bullous dermatophytosis. A pustule containing neutrophils and degenerated keratinocytes.

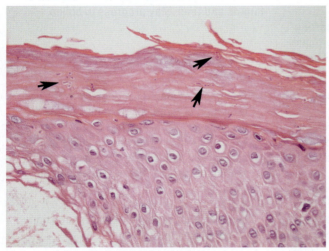

Figure 7.3.3 Bullous dermatophytosis. Nonpigmented hyphae present within the stratum corneum on an H&E-stained section (arrows).

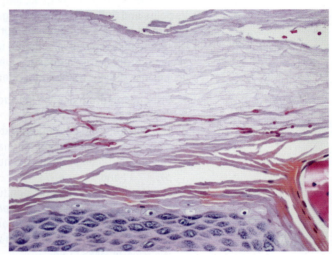

Figure 7.3.4 Bullous dermatophytosis. Fungal hyphae highlighted within the stratum corneum with PAS stain.

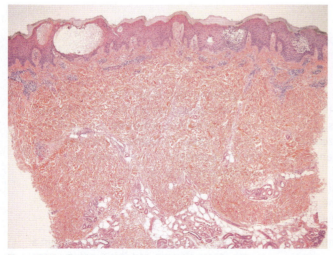

Figure 7.3.5 Dyshidrotic dermatitis. Acral skin with large, discrete spongiotic intraepidermal vesicles. A sparse mixed inflammatory infiltrate within the superficial dermis.

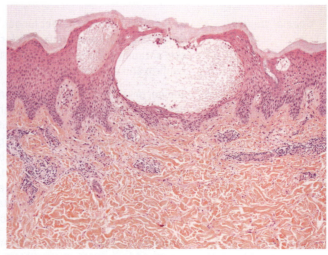

Figure 7.3.6 Dyshidrotic dermatitis. Discrete spongiotic vesicles within the epidermis.

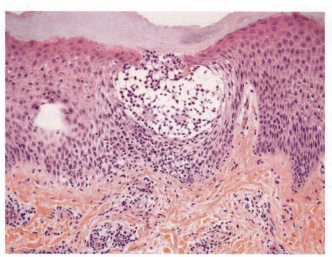

Figure 7.3.7 Dyshidrotic dermatitis. Spongiotic vesicle associated with lymphocytic, rather than neutrophilic, exocytosis.

7.4 TINEA VERSICOLOR VS DERMATOPHYTOSIS

	Tinea Versicolor	**Dermatophytosis**
Age	Any age but most commonly in adolescents and young adults.	All ages with some clinical forms showing age predilection (such as tinea capitis in children; tinea cruris and tinea unguium in adults).
Location	Chest, back, abdomen, neck, and proximal extremities.	Any location. Clinical forms are divided into those affecting glabrous skin (tinea corporis, tinea cruris, tinea faciei), acral skin (tinea manus, tinea pedis), skin rich in terminal hair follicles (tinea capitis, tinea barbae), and nails (tinea unguium).
Etiology	Fungi from the genus *Malassezia*, most commonly *Malassezia globosa* but also *Malassezia furfur* and *Malassezia sympodialis*.	A superficial fungal infection caused *Trichophyton*, *Microsporum*, and *Epidermophyton* genera.
Presentation	Hypo- or hyperpigmented macules, patches, or thin plaques with fine scales. Hyperhidrosis, heat and humidity, and use of topical oils may potentiate the development of the disease.	Variable and dependent upon clinical form. Tinea corporis, tinea cruris, and tinea faciei are characterized by a sharply demarcated red-pink erythematous annular patch or plaque with scale and a raised edge. Some lesions may have pustules or vesicles. Tinea manus and tinea pedis typically are not as well demarcated and present as dry, erythematous, scaly skin that may become vesicular. Tinea capitis and tinea barbae form annular patches and plaques with folliculocentric pustules. Tinea unguium causes thickening, dystrophy, and discoloration of nails.
Histology	1. Subtle laminated or basket-weave hyperkeratosis *(Figs. 7.4.1* and *7.4.2)*. 2. Aggregates of round spores and short curved hyphae in the stratum corneum ("spaghetti/ziti and meatballs"), best seen with PAS or GMS stain *(Figs. 7.4.2-7.4.4)*. 3. Epidermis appears relatively unremarkable *(Figs. 7.4.1* and *7.4.2)*. 4. As opposed to dermatophytosis, no significant inflammation within the epidermis or dermis *(Fig. 7.4.1)*.	1. Hyperkeratosis and parakeratosis with aggregates of neutrophils *(Figs. 7.4.5* and *7.4.6)*. 2. Mild epidermal hyperplasia and reactive changes *(Figs. 7.4.5* and *7.4.6)*. 3. Nonpigmented hyphae on longitudinal section and cross section present in stratum corneum and best seen with PAS or GMS stain *(Fig. 7.4.7)*. Hyphae on cross section are tubular and should not be misinterpreted as spores. 4. Patchy, sparse chronic inflammation in the superficial dermis.
Special studies	PAS or GMS stain to detect fungi and examine morphology. KOH preparation may be performed from skin scraping. Examination of lesions with Wood's lamp may show yellow-green fluorescence.	PAS or GMS stain to identify the fungus. KOH preparation to identify fungi in scrapings. Culture may be performed to confirm and speciate the fungus.

7.4 Tinea Versicolor vs Dermatophytosis

	Tinea Versicolor	**Dermatophytosis**
Treatment	Topical agents including azole antifungals, selenium sulfide, and zinc pyrithione, are effective in most cases. Severe or recalcitrant disease may require systemic therapy with oral itraconazole or fluconazole.	Topical antifungal agents, including azoles, allylamines, tolnaftate, ciclopirox, butenafine, may be used for localized infection. A widespread infection may require oral antifungal therapy including terbinafine, itraconazole, fluconazole, or griseofulvin.
Prognosis	Good response to therapy in most cases. Recurrences may occur particularly in immunocompromised individuals. Hypo- and hyperpigmentation may persist long after eradication of the fungal organisms.	A superficial infection typically responds to adequate therapy but recurrences are common. Onychomycosis and deep-seated follicular-based infections may be refractory and generally require oral antifungal therapy. A widespread infection is often associated with immunodeficiency.

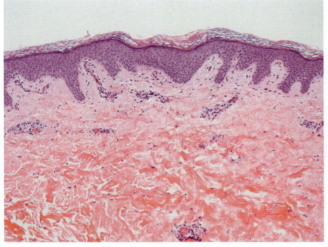

Figure 7.4.1 Tinea versicolor. Relatively normal appearing epidermis with an overlying basket-weave orthokeratotic stratum corneum. Minimal inflammation in the dermis.

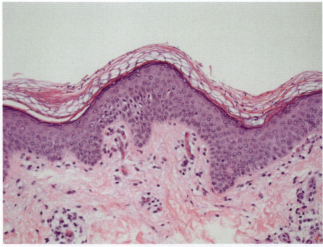

Figure 7.4.2 Tinea versicolor. Higher magnification reveals short hyphae and spores ("spaghetti/ziti and meatballs") in the stratum corneum.

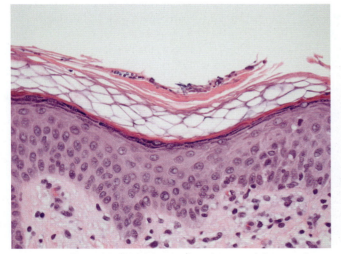

Figure 7.4.3 Tinea versicolor. Aggregates of round spores and short curved hyphae in the stratum corneum. Note that there is no appreciable parakeratosis or neutrophilic inflammation as typically seen in dermatophytosis.

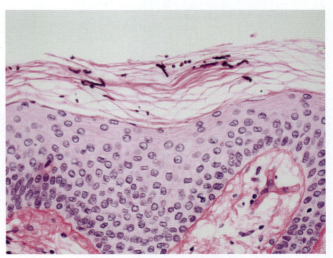

Figure 7.4.4 Tinea versicolor. PAS stain showing short hyphae and spores.

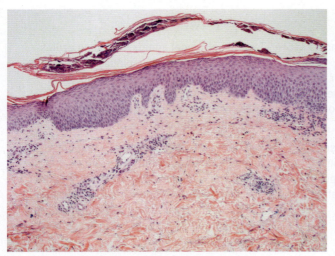

Figure 7.4.5 Dermatophytosis. Mild reactive epidermal hyperplasia with overlying parakeratosis and a patchy inflammatory infiltrate in the dermis.

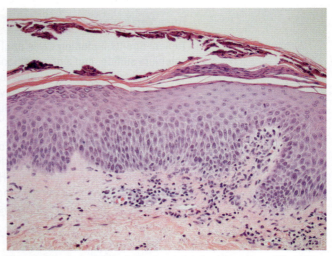

Figure 7.4.6 Dermatophytosis. Degenerated neutrophils and basophilic debris associated with parakeratosis.

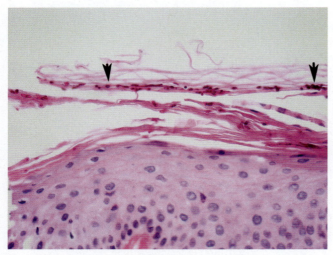

Figure 7.4.7 Dermatophytosis. PAS stain demonstrating hyphal forms within the stratum corneum. Note that hyphae on cross section are tubular (arrows) and should not be misinterpreted as spores.

7.5 DERMATOPHYTOSIS VS CUTANEOUS CANDIDIASIS

	Dermatophytosis	**Cutaneous Candidiasis**
Age	All ages with some clinical forms showing age predilection (such as tinea capitis in children; tinea cruris and tinea unguium in adults).	All ages.
Location	Any location. Clinical forms are divided into those affecting glabrous skin (tinea corporis, tinea cruris, tinea faciei), acral skin (tinea manus, tinea pedis), skin rich in terminal hair follicles (tinea capitis, tinea barbae), and nails (tinea unguium).	All regions of the body but especially intertriginous areas including axillae, genitocrural folds, inframammary crease, interdigital regions, and oral commissure.
Etiology	Superficial fungal infection caused by fungi of the *Trichophyton*, *Microsporum*, and *Epidermophyton* genera.	Various species of *Candida* but most commonly *Candida albicans*.
Presentation	Variable and dependent upon clinical form. Tinea corporis, cruris, and faciei are characterized by a sharply demarcated red-pink erythematous annular patch or plaque with scale and a raised edge. Some lesions may have pustules or vesicles. Tinea manus and tinea pedis typically are not as well demarcated and present as dry, erythematous, scaly skin that may become vesicular. Tinea capitis and tinea barbae form annular patches and plaques with folliculocentric pustules. Tinea unguium causes thickening, dystrophy, and discoloration of nails.	Moist beefy red patches and plaques studded with vesicles, pustules, and crusted erosions. Satellite papules and pustules are often present. Skin may be macerated and fissured. Frequently triggered by heat and moisture.
Histology	1. Hyperkeratosis and parakeratosis with aggregates of neutrophils *(Figs. 7.5.1 and 7.5.2)*. 2. Mild epidermal hyperplasia and reactive changes *(Figs. 7.5.1 and 7.5.2)*. 3. Nonpigmented hyphae on longitudinal section and cross section present in stratum corneum and best seen with PAS or GMS stain *(Fig. 7.5.3)*. Hyphae on cross section are tubular and should not be misinterpreted as spores. 4. Patchy, mixed inflammation in the superficial dermis *(Fig. 7.5.1)*.	1. Hyperkeratosis and parakeratosis with aggregates of neutrophils within the stratum corneum *(Figs. 7.5.4 and 7.5.5)*. 2. The epidermis may be hyperplastic and have mild edema and exocytosis of neutrophils *(Figs. 7.5.4 and 7.5.5)*. 3. Fungal organisms including yeast, hyphae, and pseudohyphae are present within the stratum corneum and may be seen on H&E-stained sections *(Figs. 7.5.5 and 7.5.6)*. 4. Fungi are best illustrated with PAS or GMS stain *(Fig. 7.5.7)*. The identification of yeast and pseudohyphae aid in distinguishing it from dermatophytosis. Pseudohyphae consist of chains with constriction between cellular elements, while hyphae are tubular with parallel sides and no constrictions. 5. Mild dermal superficial perivascular inflammation.

(continued)

	Dermatophytosis	**Cutaneous Candidiasis**
Special studies	PAS or GMS stain to identify the fungus. KOH preparation to identify fungi in scrapings. Culture may be performed to confirm and speciate the fungus.	PAS or GMS stain to detect fungi. Culture may be performed to confirm infection and speciate the fungus. KOH preparation of skin scraping may be performed.
Treatment	Topical antifungal agents, including azoles, allylamines, tolnaftate, ciclopirox, butenafine, may be used for localized infection. A widespread infection may require oral antifungal therapy including terbinafine, itraconazole, fluconazole, or griseofulvin.	Topical azole antifungals for localized cases. Oral antifungal agents may be necessary for widespread or resistant infections.
Prognosis	A superficial infection typically responds to adequate therapy but recurrences are common. Onychomycosis and deep-seated follicular-based infections may be refractory and generally require oral antifungal therapy. A widespread infection is often associated with immunodeficiency.	Superficial cutaneous infections generally respond well to therapy and do not generally progress to disseminated, systemic candidiasis.

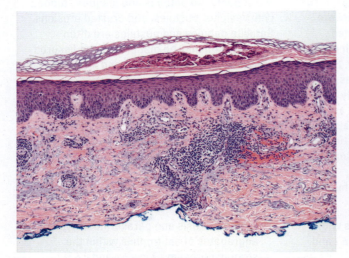

Figure 7.5.1 Dermatophytosis. Mild epidermal hyperplasia with mounds of parakeratosis, intracorneal neutrophils, and moderate dermal inflammation.

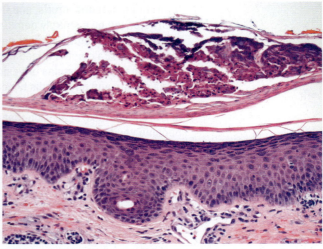

Figure 7.5.2 Dermatophytosis. Parakeratosis with entrapped neutrophils.

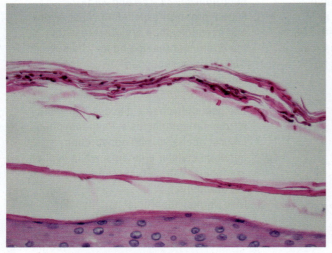

Figure 7.5.3 Dermatophytosis. PAS stain revealing fungal hyphae consisting of tubular structures seen longitudinally and on cross section.

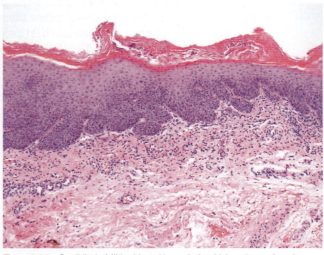

Figure 7.5.4 Candidiasis. Mild epidermal hyperplasia with hyperkeratosis and parakeratosis with neutrophils. A mild dermal inflammatory infiltrate.

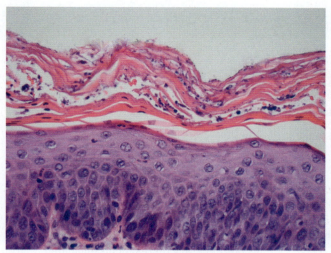

Figure 7.5.5 Candidiasis. The stratum corneum has a ragged appearance with hyperkeratosis, parakeratosis, and entrapped neutrophils. Fungal forms evident in the stratum corneum.

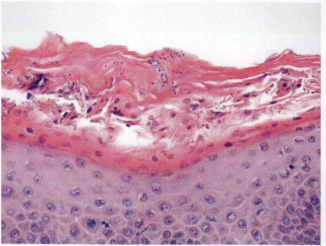

Figure 7.5.6 Candidiasis. Fungal organisms, including hyphae, pseudohyphae, and spores, evident within the stratum corneum on an H&E-stained section.

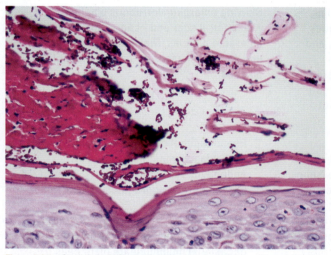

Figure 7.5.7 Candidiasis. PAS stain illustrates fungal morphology with pseudohyphae (consisting of chains with intervening constrictions), hyphae (tubular structure with parallel sides and no constrictions), and spores.

7.6 CRYPTOCOCCOSIS VS BLASTOMYCOSIS

	Cryptococcosis	Blastomycosis
Age	Any age but typically middle-aged adults.	All ages may be affected.
Location	Any location including head and neck region, extremities, and trunk.	Any site.
Etiology	Infection with fungi of the genus *Cryptococcus*, including *Cryptococcus neoformans* and *Cryptococcus gattii*. Infection may be localized to the skin or represent secondary involvement of the skin in disseminated or systemic disease.	Infection caused by *Blastomyces dermatitidis* that is endemic in the Ohio River and Mississippi River valleys, Midwestern United States, and areas bordering the Great Lakes and St. Lawrence Riverway. Cutaneous lesions generally represent disseminated infection following inhalation of fungal conidia. A minority of cases represent direct inoculation of the skin.
Presentation	A wide variety of presentations including papules and nodules, violaceous plaques, ulcers, pustules, cellulitis, abscesses, and draining sinuses. Umbilicated papules resembling molluscum contagiosum are common in patients with HIV. Solid-organ transplant recipients often present with cellulitis.	Slowing enlarging verrucous plaques with central scar and heaped up edges or ulcerated plaques. May develop pustules and microabscesses at the periphery of the plaques.
Histology	1. Epidermis may be hyperplastic or ulcerated *(Fig. 7.6.1)*. 2. Dermal inflammatory infiltrate consisting of aggregates and sheets of histiocytes *(Fig. 7.6.2)*. 3. Pleomorphic yeast forms that vary in size (from 5 to 10 µm) and shape seen on H&E stain *(Figs. 7.6.2* and *7.6.3)* and PAS *(Fig. 7.6.4)* or GMS *(Fig. 7.6.5)* stains. 4. Yeast have gelatinous capsule that stains red with mucicarmine *(Fig. 7.6.6)*. 5. *C. neoformans* shows staining with Fontana-Masson melanin stain *(Fig. 7.6.7)*.	1. Pseudoepitheliomatous epidermal hyperplasia with complex and an endophytic rete ridge pattern *(Fig. 7.6.8)*. 2. Intraepidermal aggregates of neutrophils forming pustules *(Fig. 7.6.9)*. 3. A dense mixed inflammatory infiltrate with loose, noncaseating granulomas and occasional multinucleate giant cells *(Figs. 7.6.8* and *7.6.10)*. 4. Organisms may be evident on H&E-stained sections *(Fig. 7.6.11)* and better illustrated with GMS stain. Fungi consist of yeast that are uniform in size (7-15 µm) and shape and have a thick, refractile wall and a central nucleus. Identification of broad-based budding is helpful for distinguishing it from other yeast *(Fig. 7.6.12)*.
Special studies	PAS or GMS stain to confirm the presence of the fungus. Mucicarmine stain to identify the capsule. Fontana-Masson stain to confirm the species as *C. neoformans*. Cryptococcal antigen test on pleural fluid, CSF, urine, or serum.	PAS or GMS stain to identify yeast in tissue sections. Culture may be performed to confirm diagnosis.

7.6 Cryptococcosis vs Blastomycosis

	Cryptococcosis	**Blastomycosis**
Treatment	Systemic antifungal therapy with amphotericin B, flucytosine, or fluconazole is indicated. Choice of antifungal agent, dose, and duration of therapy is dependent upon fungal burden and immunocompetency of the individual.	Treatment depends upon extent of disease, organ involvement, and immune status of the individual. Therapy options include amphotericin B or azole antifungal agent, typically itraconazole.
Prognosis	Isolated skin lesions in immunocompetent patients have a good prognosis. The majority of lesions occur as a result of disseminated disease with pulmonary and central nervous system involvement that has a worse prognosis. Underlying immunocompromised state, including HIV, solid-organ transplantation, and long-term corticosteroid use, also contributes to increased morbidity and mortality.	Overall low mortality rate. Increased morbidity and mortality in immunocompromised patients and in individuals who develop central nervous system involvement or acute respiratory distress syndrome.

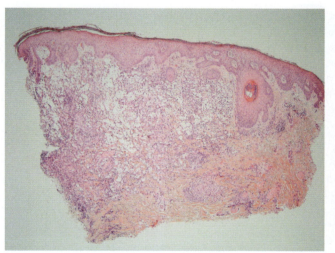

Figure 7.6.1 Cryptococcosis. Moderately irregular epidermal hyperplasia with a dense granulomatous dermal inflammatory infiltrate.

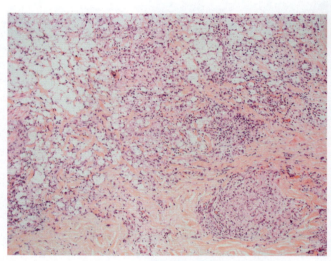

Figure 7.6.2 Cryptococcosis. Sheets of histiocytes with spaces containing refractile yeast forms.

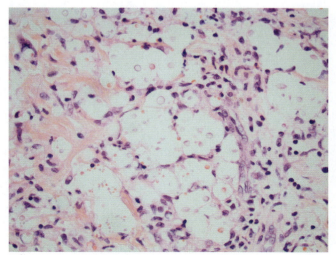

Figure 7.6.3 Cryptococcosis. Pleomorphic yeast forms that vary considerably in size and shape.

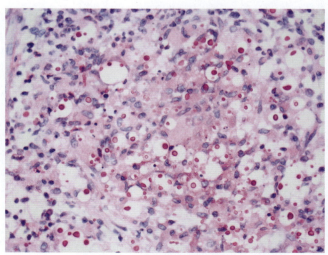

Figure 7.6.4 Cryptococcosis. PAS stain highlights yeast forms and shows variation in size.

7 Infectious Diseases and Infestations of the Skin

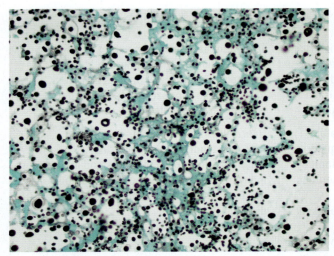

Figure 7.6.5 Cryptococcosis. GMS stain revealing numerous yeast forms associated with granulomatous inflammation.

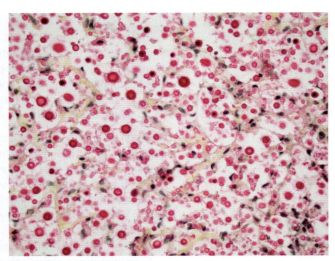

Figure 7.6.6 Cryptococcosis. Mucicarmine stain illustrates the gelatinous capsule surrounding yeast forms.

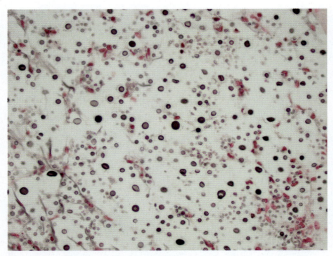

Figure 7.6.7 Cryptococcosis. Fontana-Masson stain positivity confirming *C. neoformans*.

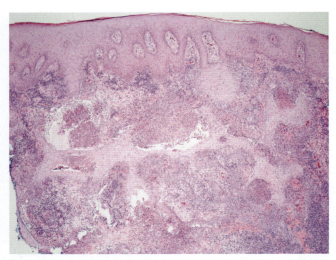

Figure 7.6.8 Blastomycosis. Pseudoepitheliomatous epidermal hyperplasia with dense mixed inflammation.

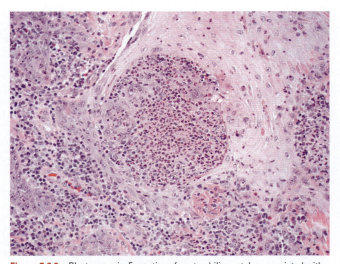

Figure 7.6.9 Blastomycosis. Formation of neutrophilic pustules associated with pseudoepitheliomatous epidermal hyperplasia.

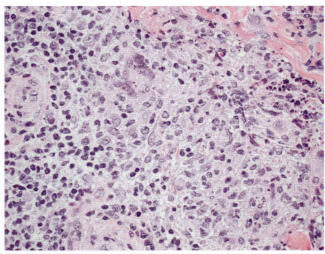

Figure 7.6.10 Blastomycosis. Ill-defined, loose, noncaseating granulomas with occasional multinucleate giant cells.

7.6 Cryptococcosis vs Blastomycosis

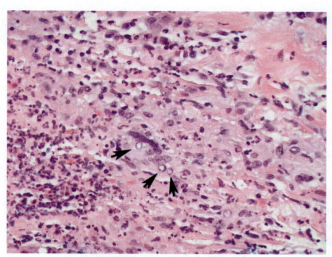

Figure 7.6.11 Blastomycosis. Yeast that are uniform in size and have thick, refractile walls (arrows).

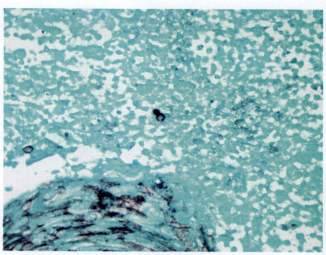

Figure 7.6.12 Blastomycosis. GMS stain reveals broad-based budding characteristic of blastomycosis.

7.7 COCCIDIOIDOMYCOSIS VS BLASTOMYCOSIS

	Coccidioidomycosis	**Blastomycosis**
Age	All ages.	All ages may be affected.
Location	Any location but commonly on face with less frequent involvement of extremities and trunk.	Any site.
Etiology	Infection by dimorphic fungi *Coccidioides immitis* and *Coccidioides posadasii* that are endemic to southwestern United States, California, Northern Mexico, and South America. Infection is typically by inhalation of arthroconidia and dissemination to the skin. Primary cutaneous infection by direct inoculation is rare.	Infection caused by *B. dermatitidis* that is endemic in the Ohio River and Mississippi River valleys, Midwestern United States, and areas bordering the Great Lakes and St. Lawrence Riverway. Cutaneous lesions generally represent disseminated infection following inhalation of fungal conidia. A minority of cases represent direct inoculation of the skin.
Presentation	Highly variable presentation but typically verrucous plaques or ulcerative nodules. Pustules and abscess formation may be present. Lymphangitic spread in a "sporotrichoid" pattern may be seen.	Slowing enlarging verrucous plaques with central scar and heaped up edges or ulcerated plaques. May develop pustules and microabscesses at the periphery of the plaques.
Histology	1. Pseudoepitheliomatous epidermal hyperplasia with dense dermal inflammation *(Fig. 7.7.1)*. 2. Dense mixed inflammation with granuloma and microabscess formation *(Fig. 7.7.2)*. 3. Fungal organisms consist of large, 10-80 μm, spherules that are uniform in size and shape and have a refractile wall. The spherules are much larger than the yeast of blastomycosis and have internal endospores *(Fig. 7.7.3)*. 4. Spherules are easily seen on H&E-stained sections, but their presence may be confirmed with PAS or GMS stain *(Fig. 7.7.4)*.	1. Pseudoepitheliomatous epidermal hyperplasia with complex and an endophytic rete ridge pattern *(Fig. 7.7.5)*. 2. Intraepidermal aggregates of neutrophils forming microabscesses *(Fig. 7.7.6)*. 3. A dense mixed inflammatory infiltrate with loose aggregates of histiocytes and occasional multinucleate giant cells *(Fig. 7.7.7)*. 4. Organisms may be evident on H&E-stained sections *(Fig. 7.7.8)* and better illustrated with GMS stain *(Fig. 7.7.9)*. Fungi consist of yeast that are relatively uniform in size (7-15 μm) and shape and have a thick, refractile wall and central nucleus. Identification of broad-based budding is helpful for distinguishing it from other yeast *(Fig. 7.7.10)*.
Special studies	PAS or GMS stains to detect and confirm the presence of fungal organisms in tissue sections. Culture may be performed but diagnosis is commonly made serologically.	PAS or GMS stain to identify yeast in tissue sections. Culture may be performed to confirm diagnosis.
Treatment	Amphotericin B and azole antifungal agents.	Treatment depends upon extent of disease, organ involvement, and immune status of the individual. Therapy options include amphotericin B or azole antifungal agent, typically itraconazole.

	Coccidioidomycosis	Blastomycosis
Prognosis	Relapses may occur following therapy and some individuals may require antifungal therapy indefinitely. Higher morbidity and mortality in immunocompromised patients, elderly, and with extensive systemic involvement.	Overall low mortality rate. Increased morbidity and mortality in immunocompromised patients and in individuals who develop central nervous system involvement or acute respiratory distress syndrome.

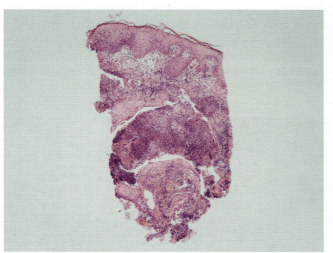

Figure 7.7.1 Coccidioidomycosis. Pseudoepitheliomatous epidermal hyperplasia with dense dermal inflammation.

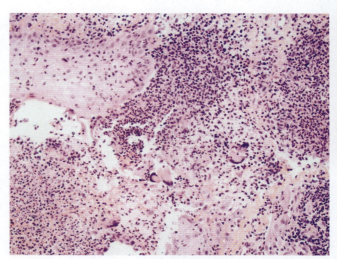

Figure 7.7.2 Coccidioidomycosis. Loose granulomas and microabscess formation with occasional multinucleate giant cells.

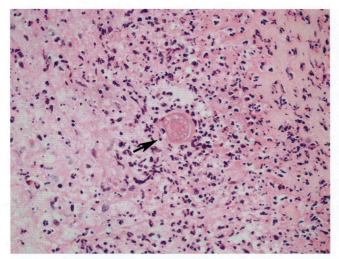

Figure 7.7.3 Coccidioidomycosis. Organisms are typically evident on H&E-stained sections and consist of a large spherule with internal endospores (arrow).

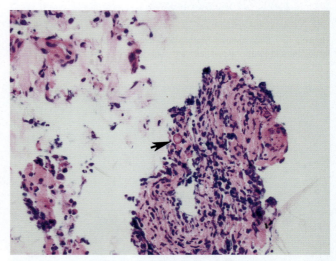

Figure 7.7.4 Coccidioidomycosis. PAS stain demonstrating spherule (arrow) with internal endospores.

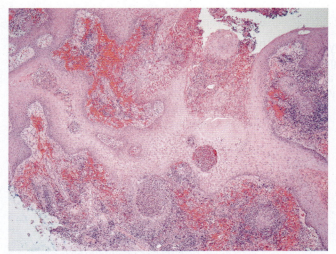

Figure 7.7.5 Blastomycosis. Pseudoepitheliomatous epidermal hyperplasia with dense inflammation.

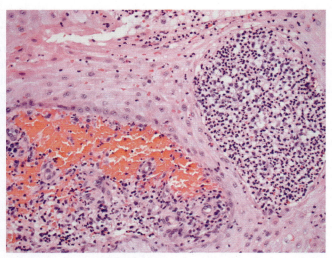

Figure 7.7.6 Blastomycosis. Conspicuous microabscess formation in association with pseudoepitheliomatous epidermal hyperplasia.

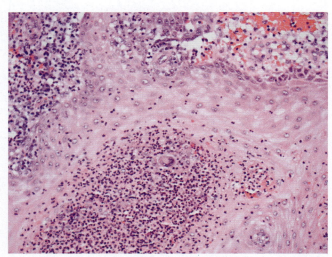

Figure 7.7.7 Blastomycosis. Microabscess formation with loose aggregates of histiocytes and occasional multinucleate giant cells.

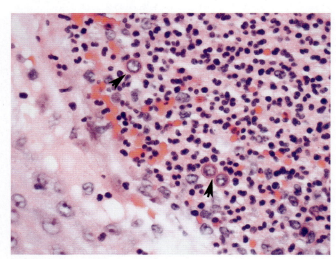

Figure 7.7.8 Blastomycosis. Yeast on H&E-stained sections are uniform and have thick, refractile walls (arrows).

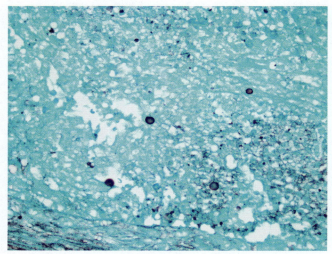

Figure 7.7.9 Blastomycosis. GMS stain showing relatively uniform yeast forms that are smaller than the spherule of coccidioidomycosis and lack endospores.

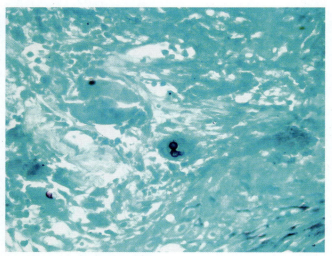

Figure 7.7.10 Blastomycosis. GMS stain demonstrating broad-base budding characteristic of blastomycosis.

7.8 CHROMOMYCOSIS VS PHAEOHYPHOMYCOSIS

	Chromomycosis	**Phaeohyphomycosis**
Age	Any age but most frequently seen in adults.	All ages but most commonly in adults.
Location	Any location but most commonly extremities, particularly feet, knees, lower legs, and hands.	Any site but typically extremities including feet, hands, forearms, and lower legs.
Etiology	Infection by pigmented fungi of the family of dematiaceous fungi including species from the *Fonsecaea*, *Cladophialophora*, *Phialophora*, *Rhinocladiella*, and *Exophiala* genera. The fungi reside in soil or on plant matter, and cutaneous infection is a result of direct inoculation.	Cutaneous and subcutaneous infection by various species of pigmented, dematiaceous fungi including those from *Bipolaris*, *Cladophialophora*, *Alternaria*, *Cladosporium*, *Exophiala*, *Fonsecaea*, *Phialophora*, *Rhinocladiella*, and *Wangiella* genera.
Presentation	Lesions slowly evolve from initial erythematous macules through various morphologies including nodular, verrucous, cauliflower-like tumorous, cicatricial, and plaque. Some lesions may have superficial black dots or "cayenne pepper" appearance. New satellite lesions may develop locally. Tenderness and pruritus are common complaints.	Generally solitary lesions that are cystic, nodular, or verrucous. Occur at the site of trauma often with implantation of plant material or wood debris. May have multiple lesions in a sporotricoid pattern.
Histology	1. Pseudoepitheliomatous epidermal hyperplasia with intraepidermal microabscesses and an extensive crust *(Fig. 7.8.1)*. 2. Dense mixed dermal inflammation with microabscesses and multinucleate giant cells *(Figs. 7.8.2 and 7.8.3)*. 3. Pigmented, round spores (Medlar bodies, muriform cells, "copper pennies") in groups within multinucleate giant cells or free within inflammation *(Figs. 7.8.3 and 7.8.4)*. Note that no hyphae are present.	1. Pseudoepitheliomatous epidermal hyperplasia with dense inflammation may be present. The histiocytic inflammation often forms a discrete nodule or cyst containing neutrophils *(Fig. 7.8.5)*. 2. A dense mixed inflammatory infiltrate with histiocytes, multinucleate giant cells, and neutrophils within the dermis *(Fig. 7.8.6)*. 3. Pigmented fungi with heterogeneous morphology including yeast forms, septate hyphae, and pseudohyphae *(Fig. 7.8.7)*. The presence of hyphae aids in distinction from chromomycosis. 4. Although evident on H&E-stained sections due to pigment, PAS or GMS stain may aid in the examination of morphology *(Fig. 7.8.8)*. 5. Portion of plant material may be present *(Fig. 7.8.9)*.
Special studies	Fungi are generally easily identified in tissue sections due to pigmentation but PAS or GMS stains may be used to detect and confirm the presence of organisms. Culture may be performed to confirm and speciate fungus.	Fungi are typically easy to detect in tissue sections due to the melanin pigment in the cell walls, but PAS or GMS stain can be used to visual the fungi. Culture to confirm and speciate the fungus, if desired.

(continued)

	Chromomycosis	**Phaeohyphomycosis**
Treatment	Localized disease may be treated with local excision. Oral antifungal agents, including itraconazole and terbinafine, may be used for more extensive disease.	Surgical excision for localized cutaneous disease. More extensive or deep-seated lesions may require systemic antifungal agents such as itraconazole, voriconazole, terbinafine, or amphotericin B.
Prognosis	Excellent prognosis for localized lesions. Extensive and progressive disease may lead to complications such as lymphedema due to scarring, secondary bacterial infection, and malignant transformation to squamous cell carcinoma.	Localized cutaneous disease has a good prognosis. A disseminated infection, generally only seen in immunocompromised individuals, has a high rate of mortality especially with pulmonary and central nervous system involvement.

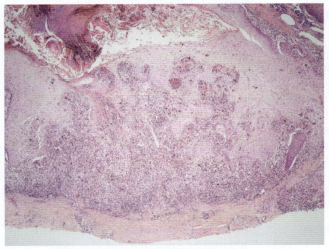

Figure 7.8.1 Chromomycosis. Pseudoepitheliomatous epidermal hyperplasia with an overlying crust and dense mixed inflammation.

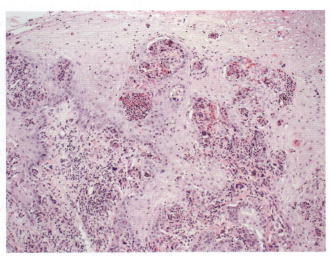

Figure 7.8.2 Chromomycosis. Neutrophilic microabscesses and loose granulomas associated with irregular epidermal hyperplasia and reactive changes.

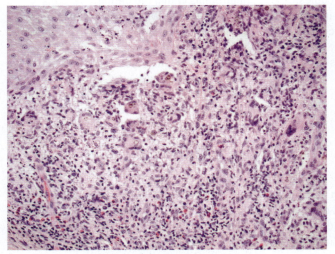

Figure 7.8.3 Chromomycosis. Mixed inflammation with neutrophilic microabscesses, ill-defined granulomas, and multinucleate giant cells. Pigmented organisms present within histiocytes and giant cells.

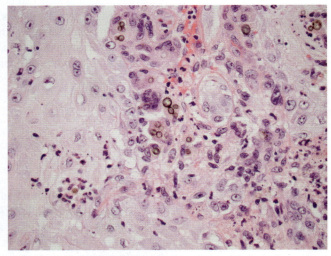

Figure 7.8.4 Chromomycosis. Pigmented, round spores (Medlar bodies, muriform cells, "copper pennies") in groups within multinucleate giant cells and free within inflammation.

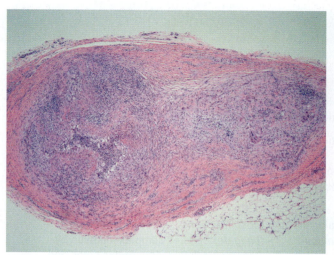

Figure 7.8.5 Phaeohyphomycosis. A discrete nodule formed by histiocytic inflammation and microabscess formation and surrounded by condensed collagen.

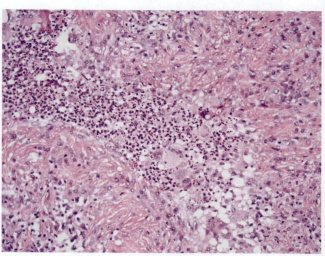

Figure 7.8.6 Phaeohyphomycosis. A dense mixed inflammatory infiltrate with histiocytes, multinucleate giant cells, and neutrophils.

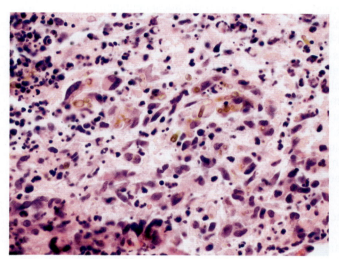

Figure 7.8.7 Phaeohyphomycosis. Pigmented fungi with heterogeneous morphology including yeast forms, septate hyphae, and pseudohyphae.

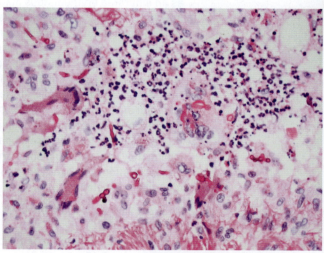

Figure 7.8.8 Phaeohyphomycosis. PAS stain highlights variable morphology, including hyphae, aiding in distinction from chromomycosis.

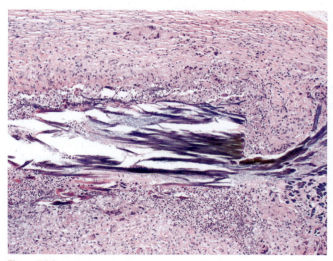

Figure 7.8.9 Phaeohyphomycosis. Plant material is often evident in association with dematiaceous fungi.

7.9 MUCORMYCOSIS VS ASPERGILLOSIS

	Mucormycosis	**Aspergillosis**
Age	All ages, most commonly middle-aged adults.	All ages.
Location	Any site, but most commonly extremities in primary cutaneous mucormycosis. Secondary cutaneous disease is often due to rhinocerebral infection and involves the periorbital skin and oral mucosa.	Any location. Primary cutaneous infections usually occur at sites of trauma, burns, or catheters.
Etiology	Infection by fungi in the order Mucorales that includes *Rhizopus*, *Mucor*, and *Rhizomucor* genera.	Most infections caused by *Aspergillus fumigatus* species complex followed by *Aspergillus flavus*, *Aspergillus niger*, and *Aspergillus terreus*.
Presentation	Primary cutaneous mucormycosis begins as an indurated erythematous plaque that becomes necrotic and develops eschar. Other presentations include ecthyma-like cellulitis, nodules, and ulcers. Lesions are often associated with trauma and open wounds. A secondary cutaneous involvement results from rhinocerebral or disseminated infection and, when involving the sinuses, may present with periorbital cellulitis. Predisposing factors include hematologic malignancy, stem cell and solid-organ transplantation, iron overload, and poorly controlled diabetes mellitus.	A primary cutaneous infection typically occurs by traumatic inoculation or in open wounds. A secondary cutaneous involvement occurs from hematogenous spread or contiguous extension. Lesions consist of erythematous papules, plaques, or nodules that become necrotic and ulcerated. Hemorrhagic bullae may also be present. A disseminated disease is often associated with hematological malignancy, burns, transplantation, or other immunocompromised state.
Histology	1. The epidermis may be intact or necrotic *(Fig. 7.9.1)*. 2. Broad, irregularly branched hyphae, measuring 5-15 μm in diameter, which have rare septations are present in the dermis *(Fig. 7.9.2)*. Note that the hyphae of *Aspergillus* are narrow, have regular branching, and have multiple septations. 3. PAS and GMS stains show broad, irregular hyphae with rare septae *(Figs. 7.9.3 and 7.9.4)*. 4. Like *Aspergillus*, members of Mucorales are angioinvasive and may be found within thrombosed vessels *(Fig. 7.9.5)*.	1. The epidermis may be unremarkable or necrotic and ulcerated *(Fig. 7.9.6)*. 2. Perivascular inflammation with neutrophils *(Fig. 7.9.7)*. 3. Narrow (3-6 μm in diameter), septate hyphae with regular, 45° angle branching present within vessels and the dermis *(Fig. 7.9.8)*. Notably, hyphae of Mucorales are broad with irregular branching and rare septae. 4. PAS and GMS stains highlight fungal hyphae *(Figs. 7.9.9 and 7.9.10)*.
Special studies	PAS or GMS stain to highlight fungal organisms. Culture on Sabouraud and potato dextrose agar media to confirm.	PAS or GMS stain to detect the fungus in tissue sections. Culture to confirm. Ancillary tests for invasive *Aspergillus* include serum galactomannan antigen, serum 1,3-β-D-glucan, and polymerase chain reaction (PCR) assays.

7.9 Mucormycosis vs Aspergillosis

	Mucormycosis	**Aspergillosis**
Treatment	Surgical debridement and antifungal therapy with amphotericin B or azole antifungal agents depending upon the susceptibility profile. Members of Mucorales are not susceptible to voriconazole. Treatment of underlying predisposing conditions, such as diabetes mellitus, is important.	Dependent upon the immune status, comorbidities, and susceptibility. First-line therapy for invasive *Aspergillus* is typically voriconazole with other azole antifungal agents and amphotericin B as second-line therapy. Debridement is recommended for primary infections of the skin associated with burns or open wounds.
Prognosis	Mortality for primary localized cutaneous mucormycosis ranges from 4%-10%, while it is much higher, up to 83%, for disseminated disease. Risk factors for increased mortality risk include uncontrolled diabetes mellitus, metabolic acidosis, renal failure, and extensive disseminated disease.	Prognosis for a primary cutaneous infection is much better than that for a secondary cutaneous or disseminated invasive disease, which has a high mortality. Survival is lower with a disseminated disease, cerebral involvement, severe neutropenia, and use of glucocorticoids.

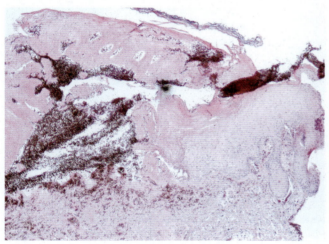

Figure 7.9.1 Mucormycosis. Epidermal necrosis and hemorrhage due to vascular occlusion by fungi.

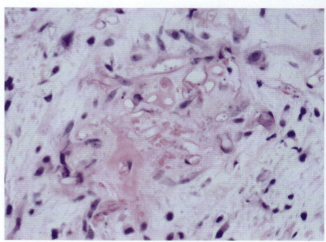

Figure 7.9.2 Mucormycosis. Broad, irregularly branched hyphae that have rare septations.

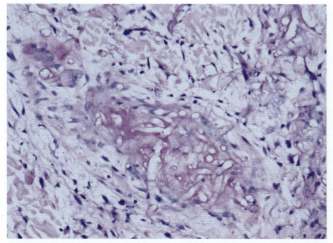

Figure 7.9.3 Mucormycosis. PAS stain highlights broad, irregularly branched, nonseptate hyphae.

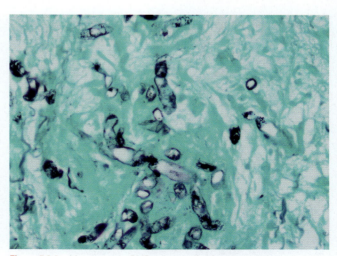

Figure 7.9.4 Mucormycosis. GMS stain revealing fungal morphology.

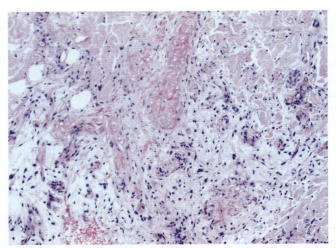

Figure 7.9.5 Mucormycosis. Broad, nonseptate hyphae within thrombosed vessels.

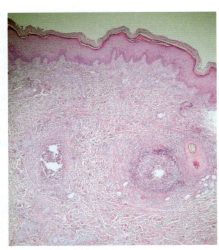

Figure 7.9.6 Aspergillosis. Relatively normal epidermis dermis with neutrophilic inflammation surrounding dilated and thrombosed vessels.

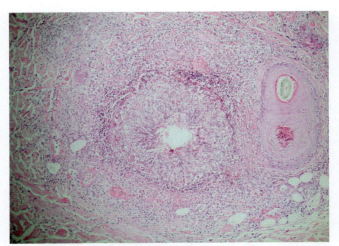

Figure 7.9.7 Aspergillosis. A dilated vessel distended by a thrombus and fungal hyphae.

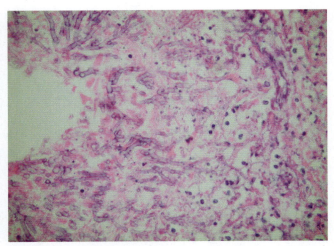

Figure 7.9.8 Aspergillosis. Narrow, branching, septate hyphae on an H&E-stained section.

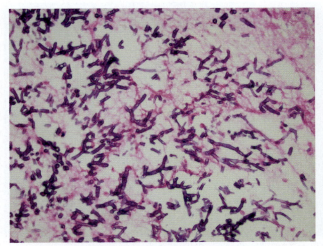

Figure 7.9.9 Aspergillosis. PAS stain highlights narrow hyphae with regular, 45° branching and septae.

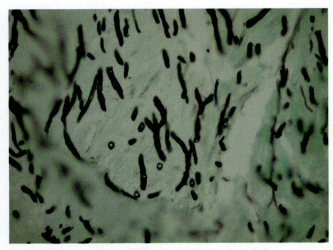

Figure 7.9.10 Aspergillosis. GMS stain revealing fungal morphology.

7.10 HISTOPLASMOSIS VS LEISHMANIASIS

	Histoplasmosis	**Leishmaniasis**
Age	All ages, but most frequently seen in adults.	Any age.
Location	Any location.	Exposed areas of skin, especially extremities and head and neck region.
Etiology	Infection by the fungus *Histoplasma capsulatum*. Cutaneous involvement is generally secondary to a primary pulmonary infection. A primary cutaneous infection from a direct inoculation is rare. The fungus is found in soil contaminated with bird and bat feces. It is endemic to tropical and temperate regions including Mississippi River and Ohio River valleys.	Infection by protozoa of the genus *Leishmania* that is transmitted by the sand fly vector. Species differ geographically and, accordingly, cutaneous leishmaniasis is generally classified as Old World and New World.
Presentation	A wide spectrum of manifestations including erythematous plaques, crusted papules and nodules, verrucous plaques, abscesses, and ulcers. Umbilicated papules and nodules more common in individuals with HIV. May be associated with fever, weight loss, and fatigue.	A wide variety of clinical manifestations that is somewhat dependent upon the species. A localized form typically begins as an erythematous papule that enlarges into a plaque or nodule with central ulceration. The lesions may appear furuncular, verrucous, zosteriform, psoriasiform, sporotrichoid, or eczematous. Lesions heal with scarring that may be extensive.
Histology	1. The epidermis is normal or shows reactive hyperplasia *(Fig. 7.10.1)*. 2. Granulomatous inflammation with a variable lymphocytic infiltrate *(Fig. 7.10.2)*. 3. Multiple, small, round-oval yeast forms measuring between 2-4 µm within histiocytes *(Fig. 7.10.3)*. Organisms are more uniformly distributed within the histiocytes than leishmaniasis and often have a surrounding halo. 4. GMS stain helps to confirm, and highlights the obligate intracellular yeast forms *(Fig. 7.10.4)*.	1. Epidermal ulceration with an overlying fibrinous exudate *(Fig. 7.10.5)*. 2. A dense inflammatory infiltrate composed of lymphocytes, neutrophils, histiocytes, and numerous plasma cells. Ill-defined granulomas may be present *(Fig. 7.10.6)*. 3. Intracellular organisms consist of amastigotes that measure 2-4 µm *(Fig. 7.10.7)*. Organisms often align along the outer rim of intracytoplasmic vacuoles, forming the "marquee sign" *(Fig. 7.10.8)*. 4. Giemsa stain is helpful in confirming the diagnosis with identification of kinetoplasts *(Fig. 7.10.9)*. This, and the absence of staining with GMS, aids in distinguishing it from histoplasmosis.
Special studies	Intracellular organisms stain with PAS and GMS stains. Additional testing for disseminated histoplasmosis includes immunodiffusion, complement fixation, and urine or serum antigen tests.	Giemsa stain to identify organisms. GMS, PAS, AFB, and tissue Gram stains to exclude other intracellular organisms. Confirmation by culture but requires specialized media, PCR, and fluorescent antibody tests.

(continued)

	Histoplasmosis	**Leishmaniasis**
Treatment	Itraconazole is used for localized or mild disease. Amphotericin B is necessary for a widely disseminated or severe infection.	Treatment is dependent on the species, the extent of infection (complicated vs uncomplicated), and whether mucosal or visceral disease is present. Antimonial drugs are considered first-line treatment. Sodium stibogluconate and meglumine antimoniate are available in the United States only from the U.S. Food and Drug Administration. Other drugs that have been used for treatment include azoles, miltefosine, amphotericin, and pentamidine. Local therapy may be used for uncomplicated cases, while systemic therapy is used in complicated infections.
Prognosis	Dependent upon the extent of disease and the adequacy of treatment. If untreated, disseminated histoplasmosis is fatal but early and adequate therapy reduces mortality risk. Complications of visceral involvement include acute respiratory distress syndrome, pericarditis, adrenal insufficiency, and meningitis.	Some infections resolve without treatment but incur scarring. Long-term treatment necessary to eradicate the infection. Does not pose a threat to life but may lead to debilitating scar formation, stigmatization, psychological distress, and decreased quality of life.

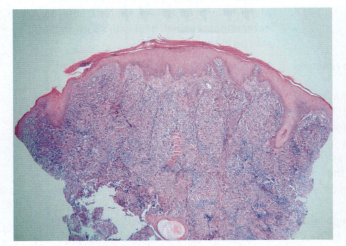

Figure 7.10.1 Histoplasmosis. Reactive epidermal hyperplasia with dense granulomatous inflammation.

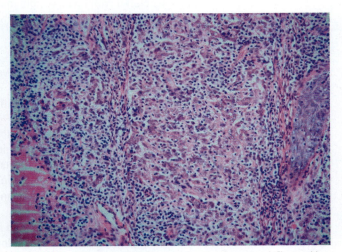

Figure 7.10.2 Histoplasmosis. A lymphohistiocytic inflammatory infiltrate with formation of loose granulomas.

7.10 Histoplasmosis vs Leishmaniasis

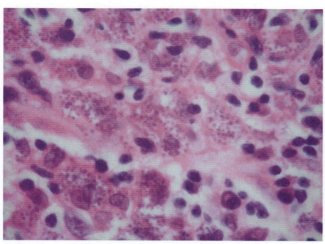

Figure 7.10.3 Histoplasmosis. Numerous, small, round yeast forms within histiocytes. Yeasts are relatively uniformly distributed within histiocytes and surrounded by a halo.

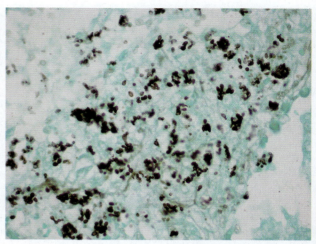

Figure 7.10.4 Histoplasmosis. GMS stain demonstrating small intracellular yeast forms.

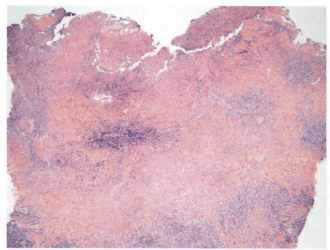

Figure 7.10.5 Leishmaniasis. Epidermal ulceration with dense dermal inflammation.

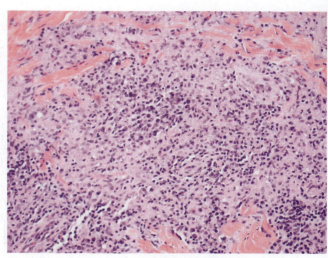

Figure 7.10.6 Leishmaniasis. A mixed inflammatory infiltrate with numerous plasma cells and formation of ill-defined granulomas.

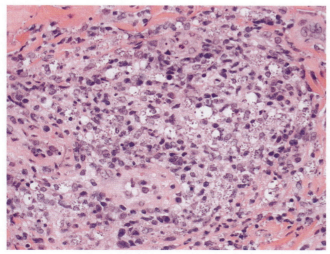

Figure 7.10.7 Leishmaniasis. Intracellular organisms consist of amastigotes that are similar in size to histoplasmosis but have kinetoplasts.

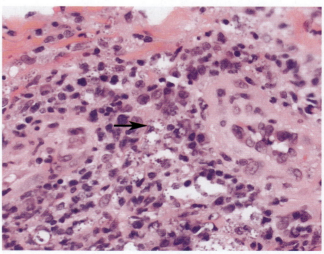

Figure 7.10.8 Leishmaniasis. Organisms often arranged along the outer rim of intracytoplasmic vacuoles forming the "marquee sign" (arrow).

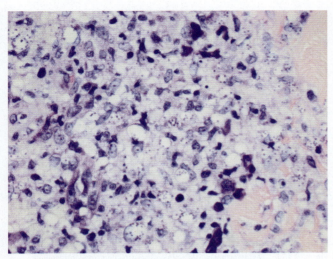
Figure 7.10.9 Leishmaniasis. Giemsa stain highlights organisms and demonstrates kinetoplasts.

7.11 MAJOCCHI GRANULOMA VS PITYROSPORUM FOLLICULITIS

	Majocchi Granuloma	**Pityrosporum Folliculitis**
Age	All ages but predominately in young and middle-aged adults.	Adolescents and young adults.
Location	Extremities primarily; most frequently on legs.	Trunk, especially upper chest, back, upper arms, and shoulders. Face, typically forehead, chin, and hairline, sparing central face.
Etiology	Deep follicular or dermal infection typically by the dermatophytic fungi of the *Trichophyton*, *Epidermophyton*, and *Microsporum* species. The most frequent cause is anthropophilic *T. rubrum*. In immunocompetent individuals, infection is often associated with penetrating injury or occlusion of hair follicles. Also occurs in the setting of immunocompromise or after use of topical steroids on undiagnosed superficial dermatophytosis.	Folliculitis due to species of *Malassezia* species (including *M. furfur*, *M. globosa*, *M. sympodialis*, and *M. restricta*) that are lipophilic yeasts present on the skin as a component of normal flora.
Presentation	An erythematous, scaly nodule or plaque studded with follicular papules and pustules. In immunocompromised individuals, the lesions tend to be nodular and indurated.	Monomorphic, small, 2-3 mm, folliculocentric papules and pustules. Papules often pruritic and worsen with use of antibiotics. Predisposing factors include heat and increased sweating, high sebum production, antibiotic use, corticosteroids, and immunosuppression.
Histology	1. Reactive epidermal hyperplasia with neutrophilic inflammation involving follicular units *(Figs. 7.11.1* and *7.11.2)*. 2. The follicular lumen is distended by keratin and parakeratotic debris *(Fig. 7.11.2)*. 3. Fungal organisms (hyphae) are present within the follicular lumen *(Fig. 7.11.2)*. The hair shaft shows features of trichomalacia. 4. Fungi are present within hair shafts (endothrix) as best seen with PAS stain *(Fig. 7.11.3)*. 5. A deep dermal, perifollicular inflammatory infiltrate of neutrophils, lymphocytes, and histiocytes forming loose granulomas *(Fig. 7.11.1)*.	1. Dilated, distorted, and disrupted hair follicles. The lumen is distended by inspissated sebum, keratin, and debris *(Fig. 7.11.4)*. 2. Neutrophilic inflammation extends into the follicular epithelium and is present within the surrounding dermis *(Fig. 7.11.5)*. 3. Small budding yeast forms are evident within the lumen *(Fig. 7.11.6)*. 4. PAS stain demonstrates yeast forms within the lumen and the surrounding inflammatory infiltrate *(Figs. 7.11.7* and *7.11.8)*. Note that there are no hyphae and no involvement of hair shafts by the fungal organisms.
Special studies	PAS or GMS stain to highlight fungal organisms. Microbiologic culture for confirmation and speciation.	PAS or GMS stain to demonstrate fungal organisms. Tissue Gram stain often performed to exclude bacterial folliculitis.

(continued)

	Majocchi Granuloma	**Pityrosporum Folliculitis**
Treatment	Oral antifungal agents are usually necessary given the deep dermal and follicular nature of the infection. These include terbinafine, itraconazole, and griseofulvin.	Topical treatments include ketoconazole shampoo or cream and selenium sulfide shampoo. Oral therapy with fluconazole or itraconazole may also be utilized.
Prognosis	Infection generally responds well to appropriate therapy. Recurrences frequently seen if source of dermatophytosis, such as nails or feet, is not treated. Continued immunosuppression can also lead to an increased rate of relapse. Resolution of infection may be followed by postinflammatory pigmentary changes, scarring, and alopecia.	Typically responds well to appropriate therapy; however, recurrences are frequently seen, especially if the predisposing factors are not resolved.

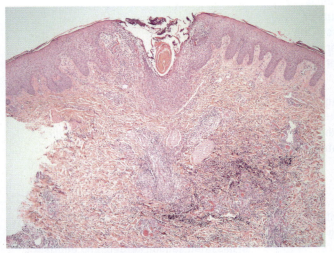

Figure 7.11.1 Majocchi granuloma. Reactive epidermal hyperplasia with neutrophilic inflammation involving superficial and deep follicular units.

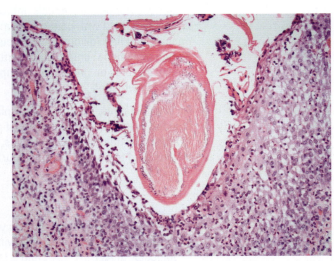

Figure 7.11.2 Majocchi granuloma. Neutrophilic inflammation and edema of follicular epithelium. Fungal hyphae are evident on H&E stain within the hair shaft that shows features of trichomalacia.

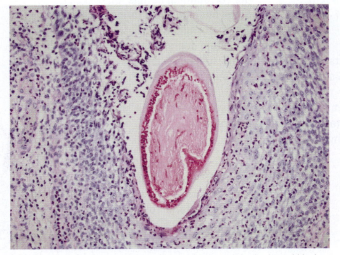

Figure 7.11.3 Majocchi granuloma. PAS stain demonstrating hyphae within the hair shaft.

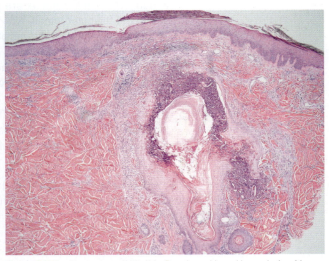

Figure 7.11.4 Pityrosporum folliculitis. Reactive epidermal hyperplasia with parakeratosis overlying the distorted and inflamed hair follicle.

7.11 Majocchi Granuloma vs Pityrosporum Folliculitis

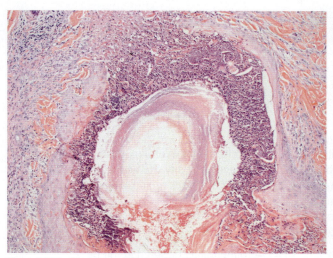

Figure 7.11.5 Pityrosporum folliculitis. The follicular lumen distended by keratinous debris and inspissated sebum. Neutrophilic inflammation with disruption of the follicular epithelium.

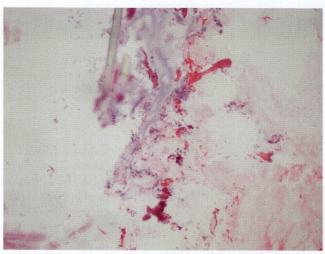

Figure 7.11.6 Pityrosporum folliculitis. Small budding yeast forms evident on H&E-stained sections within the follicular lumen. Note that hyphal forms are not present.

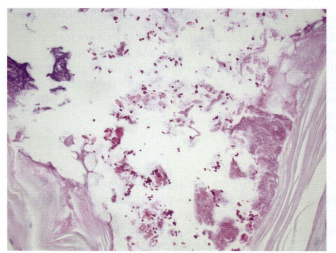

Figure 7.11.7 Pityrosporum folliculitis. PAS stain highlights budding yeast within the follicular lumen.

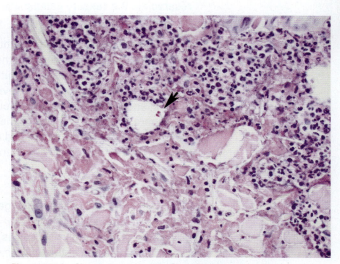

Figure 7.11.8 Pityrosporum folliculitis. Since *Pityrosporum* species are commensals, the finding of yeast forms outside of the follicle (arrow) supports the diagnosis of pityrosporum folliculitis.

7.12 HERPES SIMPLEX INFECTION VS PEMPHIGUS VULGARIS

	Herpes Simplex Infection	**Pemphigus Vulgaris**
Age	All ages.	Adults, generally between ages of 45 and 65 y.
Location	Herpes simplex virus 1 (HSV1) primarily involves facial skin and oral mucosa, but other sites on trunk and extremities may be affected. Genital skin involvement is most commonly due to herpes simplex virus 2 (HSV2) but HSV1 may also be implicated.	Typically begins in oral mucosa. Skin lesions can develop at any site with a predilection for head and neck region, axillae, and upper trunk.
Etiology	Infection by HSV1 or HSV2 is acquired through direct exposure of skin or mucous membranes to secretions of an infected individual. The virus establishes latent reservoir in the sensory ganglia and then can be intermittently reactivated.	Autoantibodies targeted at the Ca^{2+}-dependent cadherin desmoglein 3 and, to a lesser degree, desmoglein 1. Binding of the antibodies disrupts the integrity of the desmosomes responsible for cell-cell adhesion with resultant vesicle formation.
Presentation	Grouped vesicles on an erythematous base that progress to vesiculopustules that then ulcerate and become crusted. Genital lesions may present with painful ulcers, fever, dysuria, and lymphadenopathy. Recurrences are generally less severe and of shorter duration than primary infection and often heralded by pruritus, tingling, or burning sensation.	Flaccid vesicles and bullae that are fragile and become eroded and crusted. Nikolsky sign (induction of vesicle when mechanical pressure is applied to perilesional skin) present.
Histology	1. An intraepidermal vesicle with acantholysis and ballooning degeneration of the epidermal keratinocytes *(Figs. 7.12.1 and 7.12.2)*. Acantholysis involves the mid–stratum spinosum of the epidermis, not just at the suprabasal level. 2. The epidermis may be eroded and ulcerated with an overlying crust. 3. Acantholytic keratinocytes show viral cytopathic changes including multinucleation, molding of nuclei, and margination of chromatin *(Figs. 7.12.2 and 7.12.3)*. Intranuclear inclusions (Cowdry type A) may be present. 4. Dermal edema and a mixed inflammatory infiltrate with neutrophils and nuclear debris.	1. Suprabasal acantholysis with formation of an intraepidermal (suprabasal) vesicle *(Figs. 7.12.4 and 7.12.5)*. 2. The superficial epidermis forming the roof of the vesicle is intact. Note that the acantholytic cells do not have multinucleation or inclusions *(Figs. 7.12.4 and 7.12.5)*. 3. Basal keratinocytes retained along the basement membrane zone resembling "tombstones" *(Fig. 7.12.6)*. 4. A sparse superficial perivascular inflammatory infiltrate that includes eosinophils *(Figs. 7.12.4 and 7.12.5)*.
Special studies	Confirmation with PCR, culture, or direct fluorescent antibody testing.	Direct immunofluorescence shows intercellular deposition of IgG and/or C3. Serology detecting serum antibodies to desmoglein 3.

	Herpes Simplex Infection	Pemphigus Vulgaris
Treatment	Antiviral therapy with acyclovir, famciclovir, or valacyclovir.	Systemic corticosteroids to rapidly slow disease progression. Other immunosuppressive agents, such as rituximab, azathioprine, mycophenolate mofetil, and cyclophosphamide, are typically utilized for a steroid-sparing effect.
Prognosis	Lifelong condition but typically not life-threatening. Risk for more severe complications or dissemination in infants, persons with HIV/AIDS, organ transplantation, malignancy, and immunosuppression.	Severe disease with potential for significant morbidity and mortality. Without treatment, often fatal within 5 years of onset of disease. Morbidity from infection, fluid and electrolyte disturbances, and medication-related complications.

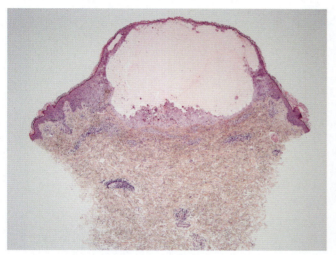

Figure 7.12.1 Herpes simplex infection. An intraepidermal vesicle formed by acantholysis involving the mid–stratum spinosum. The vesicle contains serum and has an intact roof.

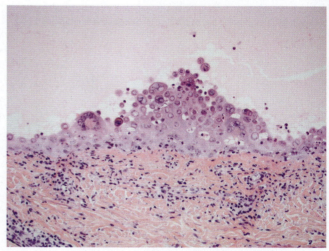

Figure 7.12.2 Herpes simplex infection. Acantholytic cells within the vesicle that are rounded up and dissociated from one another. Note nuclear changes including multinucleation, molding, and margination of chromatin.

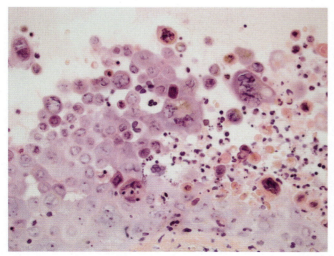

Figure 7.12.3 Herpes simplex infection. Characteristic herpetic viral cytopathic changes including multinucleation, molding of nuclei, margination of chromatin, and intranuclear inclusions.

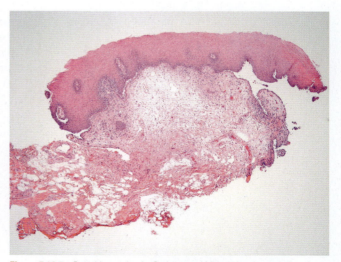

Figure 7.12.4 Pemphigus vulgaris. Oral mucosal biopsy showing suprabasal acantholysis forming a vesicle.

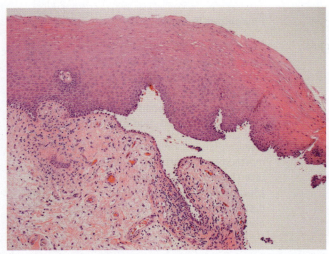

Figure 7.12.5 Pemphigus vulgaris. Acantholysis limited to the suprabasal layer with an intact epithelium forming the vesicle roof. Note that the epithelial cells mature in an orderly fashion and do not have multinucleation or inclusions.

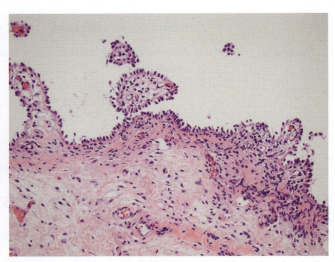

Figure 7.12.6 Pemphigus vulgaris. The floor of the vesicle consists of retained basal cells in a "tombstone" pattern.

7.13 VARICELLA-ZOSTER VIRUS INFECTION VS BENIGN FAMILIAL PEMPHIGUS (HAILEY-HAILEY DISEASE)

	Varicella-Zoster Virus (VZV) Infection	Benign Familial Pemphigus (Hailey-Hailey Disease)
Age	Adults, typically middle-aged to elderly, greater than 50 y of age.	Adults, onset typically between 20 and 40 y of age.
Location	Thoracic trunk is most common location but face (trigeminal nerve) and lumbosacral region also frequently involved.	Symmetric intertriginous regions including axillae, groin, perianal region, and lateral neck. Oral mucosa generally not involved.
Etiology	Reactivation of VZV after a latent period in peripheral ganglia following a primary varicella (chickenpox) infection.	Mutation of the *ATP2C1* gene on chromosome 3 that encodes proteins of calcium ATPase on the Golgi apparatus. This results in failure of calcium transport, leading to loss of desmosomal integrity and acantholysis.
Presentation	Painful, unilateral eruption of grouped vesicles or bullae in a dermatomal distribution. Vesicles typically become pustular and ulcerate. Often preceded by a prodrome of pruritus, tingling, and hyperesthesia. Triggers for reactivation include immunosuppression, malignancy, infection, stress, and trauma.	Fragile vesicles on an erythematous base that are easily disrupted and become crusted. The lesions are generally moist and may be foul-smelling due to secondary impetiginization. Nikolsky sign is negative.
Histology	1. An intraepidermal vesicle with acantholysis and ballooning degeneration of the epidermal keratinocytes *(Fig. 7.13.1)*. 2. The epidermis is eroded and ulcerated with an overlying crust *(Fig. 7.13.1)*. 3. Acantholytic keratinocytes show viral cytopathic changes including multinucleation, molding of nuclei, and margination of chromatin. Intranuclear inclusions (Cowdry type A) may be present *(Fig. 7.13.2)*. 4. Acantholysis and viral cytopathic changes may involve follicular units *(Fig. 7.13.3)*. 5. Dermal edema and a mixed inflammatory infiltrate with neutrophils and nuclear debris *(Fig. 7.13.1)*.	1. Epidermal hyperplasia with hyperkeratosis and parakeratosis with crust formation *(Figs. 7.13.4 and 7.13.5)*. 2. Suprabasal acantholysis with florid acantholysis throughout upper levels of the epidermis ("dilapidated brick wall") *(Figs. 7.13.4-7.13.6)*. This is similar to herpes virus/varicella zoster infection; however, the acantholytic cells do not show multinucleation or inclusions. 3. A sparse superficial perivascular lymphocytic infiltrate.
Special studies	Confirmation with PCR, culture, direct fluorescent antibody, and serology.	None.
Treatment	Antiviral treatment with acyclovir, famciclovir, or valacyclovir.	Reduction of exacerbating factors such as friction from clothing, sweating, and a secondary infection is key to control of the disease. First-line therapies include a combination of topical antibiotics and intermittent topical corticosteroids or topical calcineurin inhibitors. Botulinum toxin injections efficacious in some cases to reduce sweating.

(continued)

	Varicella-Zoster Virus (VZV) Infection	**Benign Familial Pemphigus (Hailey-Hailey Disease)**
Prognosis	Complications include postherpetic neuralgia and vasculopathy. Specific dermatomal involvement may lead to other ocular, otic, and neurologic complications. A disseminated disease is typically only seen in immunocompromised individuals but may be life-threatening.	A chronic disease with a relapsing and remitting course.

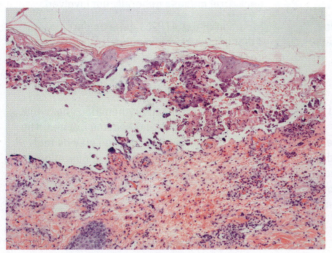

Figure 7.13.1 Herpes simplex infection. An intraepidermal vesicle, formed by acantholysis and ballooning degeneration of keratinocytes, with epidermal erosion and dense mixed inflammation.

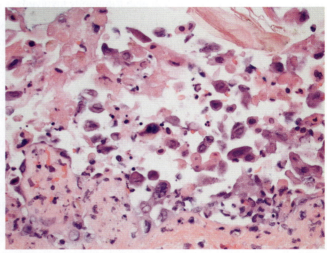

Figure 7.13.2 Herpes simplex infection. Acantholytic cells show herpetic viral cytopathic changes with multinucleation, molding of nuclei, and margination of chromatin.

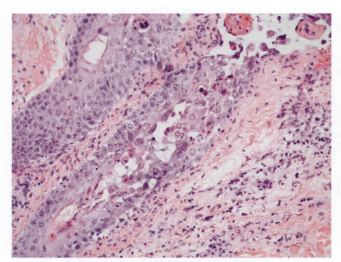

Figure 7.13.3 Herpes simplex infection. Acantholysis and viral cytopathic changes involve the epithelium of follicular units.

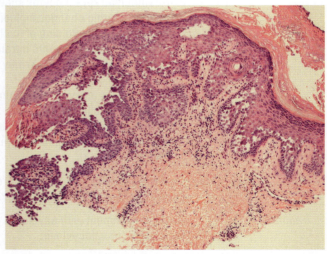

Figure 7.13.4 Benign familial pemphigus (Hailey-Hailey disease). Epidermal hyperplasia with hyperkeratosis and acantholysis.

7.13 Varicella-Zoster Virus Infection vs Benign Familial Pemphigus (Hailey-Hailey Disease)

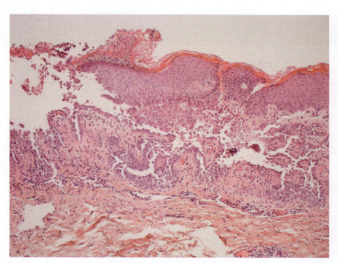

Figure 7.13.5 Benign familial pemphigus (Hailey-Hailey disease). Acantholysis involves much of the stratum spinosum creating a "dilapidated brick wall" appearance.

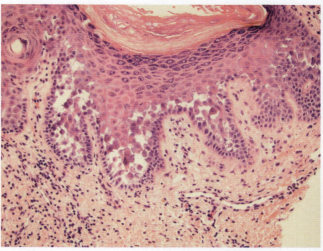

Figure 7.13.6 Benign familial pemphigus (Hailey-Hailey disease). Acantholytic cells are rounded up and dissociated from each other. Note that multinucleation and nuclear inclusions are not present.

7.14 MOLLUSCUM CONTAGIOSUM VS VERRUCA VULGARIS

	Molluscum Contagiosum	**Verruca Vulgaris**
Age	Predominately seen in children, most commonly between the ages of 2 and 5 y, and sexually active adolescents and young adults; less frequently seen in older adults.	Any age but most common in children and young adults.
Location	Exposed skin, including torso, extremities, and face, and intertriginous areas and buttocks are the primary affected sites in children. In adults, most cases are sexually transmitted and lesions are seen on the thighs, genital region, and lower abdomen. Not typically seen on palms or soles.	Any site but most frequently involves fingers, dorsal hands, elbows, and knees.
Etiology	Infection by molluscum contagiosum virus, a double-stranded DNA virus of the Poxviridae family, through direct contact with infected skin or fomites. Autoinoculation is common, especially in children. The incubation period is between 2 and 6 w. The virus infects the epidermal keratinocytes and causes proliferation.	Infection by subtypes of human papillomavirus (HPV) by direct contact to infected skin or fomites. Incubation period is between 2 and 6 mo. HPV infects epidermal keratinocytes and causes proliferation.
Presentation	Grouped, firm, round, pink or skin-colored, 2-5 mm, papules with shiny, umbilicated surface. Lesions may be generalized in patients with atopic dermatitis or immunocompromised state. In individuals with HIV, large lesions ("giant molluscum"), greater than 1 cm in diameter, may be present.	Firm, keratotic, skin-colored papules with a rough, verrucous surface. Atopic dermatitis and immunosuppression increase risk of infection. Lesions may be associated with pain, pruritus, or functional impairment.
Histology	1. Epidermal hyperplasia forming an umbilicated papule with a central core of keratin *(Fig. 7.14.1)*. 2. Keratinocytes have a deep purple cytoplasm *(Fig. 7.14.2)*. 3. Superficial keratinocytes have large, eosinophilic, cytoplasmic inclusion bodies ("molluscum bodies" or "Henderson-Patterson bodies") *(Fig. 7.14.3)*. The inclusions are often present in the keratin core *(Fig. 7.14.4)*. 4. A variable amount of inflammation ranging from a minimal to dense mixed infiltrate.	1. Hyperkeratosis with discrete tiers of parakeratosis ("church spires") overlying epidermal papillomatous peaks *(Figs. 7.14.5 and 7.14.6)*. 2. Collections of blood in parakeratosis corresponding to black dots present clinically *(Fig. 7.14.5)*. 3. Coarse hypergranulosis in dells. The keratohyalin granules are smaller than molluscum bodies and are not present in the overlying stratum corneum *(Fig. 7.14.7)*. 4. Koilocytes may be present *(Figs. 7.14.5 and 7.14.7)*. 5. Dilated capillaries within elongate papillae *(Fig. 7.14.8)*. 6. Myrmecial form of palmoplantar wart has large, coarse eosinophilic cytoplasmic inclusions that resemble molluscum bodies *(Figs. 7.14.9 and 7.14.10)*. Acral location and papillomatous architecture of epidermis help to distinguish it from molluscum contagiosum.

7.14 Molluscum Contagiosum vs Verruca Vulgaris

	Molluscum Contagiosum	**Verruca Vulgaris**
Special studies	None.	None. PCR may be used to identify the HPV subtype.
Treatment	No treatment is necessary given that it is a self-limited condition. If treatment is desired, mechanical, chemical, immunomodulatory, and antiviral modalities are available. These include cryotherapy, curettage, shave excision, cantharidin, podophyllotoxin, and imiquimod. The antiviral agent, cidofovir, may be used in immunocompromised individuals with generalized or refractory lesions.	Treatment is not required unless necessitated by symptoms, concern for cosmesis, or in the setting of immunosuppression. Topical salicylic acid and cryotherapy are first-line therapies. Other modalities include cantharone, surgical excision or ablation, and topical immunogens. Bleomycin and 5-fluorouracil have been for recalcitrant lesions in adults.
Prognosis	A benign, self-limited infection with spontaneous resolution of lesions generally within 6-9 months.	A benign condition, not associated with malignancy. Spontaneous resolution typically occurs within 1 to 2 y in children. This may be longer in adults and immunocompromised individuals. Recurrences are frequently seen.

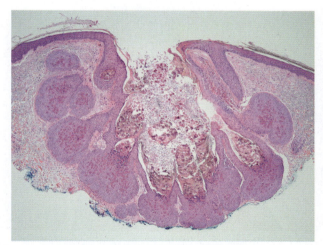

Figure 7.14.1 Molluscum contagiosum. Umbilicated papule with lobulated, endophytic epidermal hyperplasia and central keratin core.

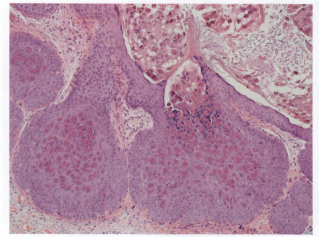

Figure 7.14.2 Molluscum contagiosum. Keratinocytes have deep purple cytoplasm and intracytoplasmic eosinophilic inclusions.

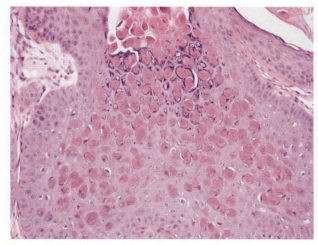

Figure 7.14.3 Molluscum contagiosum. Large, eosinophilic, cytoplasmic inclusions called "molluscum bodies" or "Henderson-Patterson bodies."

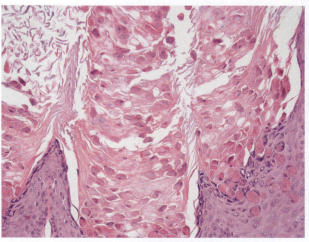

Figure 7.14.4 Molluscum contagiosum. Inclusions present within keratin core.

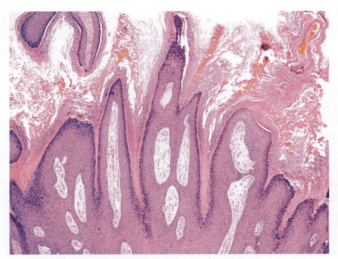

Figure 7.14.5 Verruca vulgaris. Papillomatous epidermal hyperplasia with hyperkeratosis and tiers of parakeratosis overlying papillomatous projections. Collections of blood present in stratum corneum.

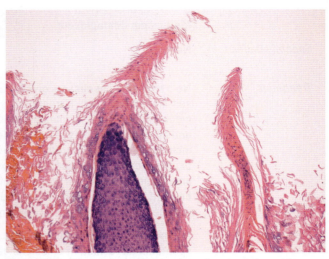

Figure 7.14.6 Verruca vulgaris. Discrete column of parakeratosis overlying papillomatous projection ("church spire").

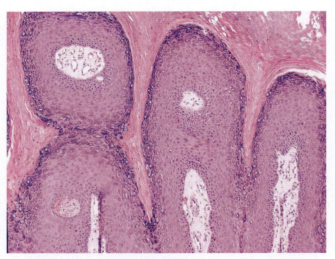

Figure 7.14.7 Verruca vulgaris. Coarse keratohyalin granules within dells between papillomatous projections and koilocytes in superficial epidermis.

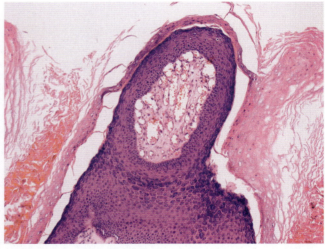

Figure 7.14.8 Verruca vulgaris. Dilated capillaries within elongated papillae.

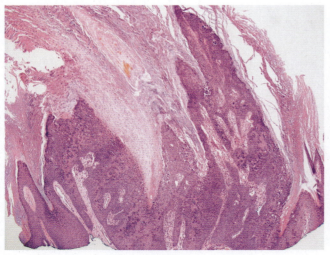

Figure 7.14.9 Verruca vulgaris. A myrmecial variant with papillomatous architecture and a thick stratum corneum of acral skin. Large, coarse, eosinophilic inclusions present in cytoplasm.

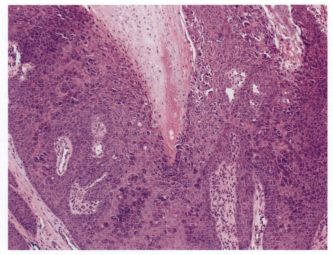

Figure 7.14.10 Verruca vulgaris. A myrmecial variant with large, coarse, eosinophilic inclusions in the cytoplasm that resemble those of molluscum contagiosum.

7.15 CONDYLOMA ACUMINATUM VS EPIDERMOLYTIC ACANTHOMA

	Condyloma Acuminatum	**Epidermolytic Acanthoma**
Age	Most commonly seen in teens and young adults.	All ages but predominately adults.
Location	Genital skin of the vulva, perineum, perianal region, penis, mons pubis, and groin.	Trunk, extremities, scrotum, and vulva.
Etiology	Virally mediated epithelial overgrowth caused by HPV. HPV subtypes 6 and 11 are most frequently detected, although there may be coinfection with high-risk subtypes, such as 16 and 18, among others. The virus is transmitted by contact with infected skin through genital, oral, or anal sex.	The etiology of the acanthoma is unknown, although trauma has been suggested. Epidermolytic hyperkeratosis is a histologic pattern due to aberrant epidermal maturation with diminution of keratin 1 and keratin 10 in the epidermis.
Presentation	Soft, smooth, sessile, skin-colored to brown lobulated papules and plaques with a cerebriform surface. May be solitary or multiple grouped lesions. Risk factors include immunosuppression, sexual activity at an early age, and multiple sexual partners.	Discrete, keratotic, skin-colored papule. May be solitary or multiple.
Histology	1. Epidermal hyperplasia with rounded papillomatosis (Figs. 7.15.1 and 7.15.2). 2. Hyperkeratosis with foci of immature parakeratosis with dark pyknotic nuclei (Fig. 7.15.3). 3. Epidermal keratinocytes show koilocytosis with perinuclear vacuoles, irregular hyperchromatic nuclei, and binucleation (Fig. 7.15.4). 4. Keratinocytes show orderly maturation with infection with low-risk subtypes (Fig. 7.15.3). 5. Variable dermal inflammation.	1. Orthohyperkeratosis and epidermal acanthosis with papillomatosis (Fig. 7.15.5). 2. Epidermolytic hyperkeratosis characterized by an intact basal layer and cytoplasmic vacuolization of the stratum spinosum with finely speckled to coarse keratohyalin granules in upper levels of the epidermis (Figs. 7.15.5 and 7.15.6). 3. Keratinocytes have indistinct cell borders (Fig. 7.15.7). 4. Cytoplasmic vacuolization may be mistaken for koilocytosis but the character of the keratohyalin granules, indistinct cell borders, and lack of nuclear atypia aid in distinction.
Special studies	Negative or patchy p16 staining (rather than block-like staining) of epidermal keratinocytes. PCR and in situ hybridization may also be utilized to detect HPV.	None.
Treatment	Destructive modalities include cryotherapy, trichloroacetic acid, podophyllotoxin, laser ablation, and surgical removal. Immunomodulating therapies, such as imiquimod and sinecatechins, may also be used. HPV vaccines, targeted for individuals between 9 and 25 y, are effective for prevention of the disease.	No treatment is necessary but typically removed to exclude other entities. May utilize liquid nitrogen or topical imiquimod or calcipotriol if treatment is desired.

(continued)

	Condyloma Acuminatum	**Epidermolytic Acanthoma**
Prognosis	A variable clinical course. Many cases resolve spontaneously within 2 y. Others may persist, increase in number, and grow in size. Recurrences may occur since the virus can persist after lesions regress. Coinfection with high-risk subtypes may be associated with development of malignancy.	Excellent. A benign lesion with no risk for malignancy.

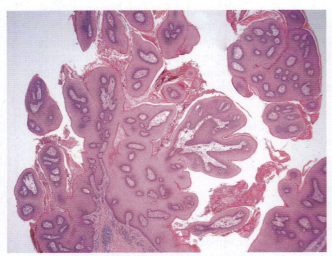

Figure 7.15.1 Condyloma acuminatum. Exophytic papule formed by epidermal hyperplasia with rounded papillomatosis.

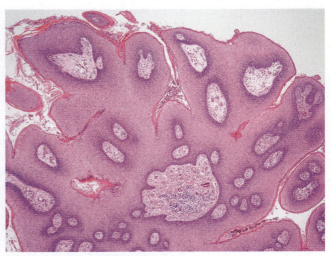

Figure 7.15.2 Condyloma acuminatum. Hyperkeratosis and parakeratosis overlying complex papillomatous epidermal hyperplasia.

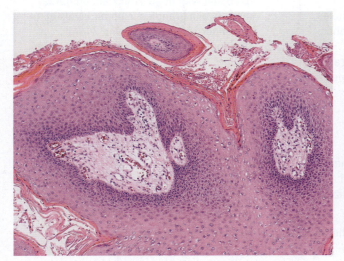

Figure 7.15.3 Condyloma acuminatum. Immature parakeratosis with dark, pyknotic nuclei.

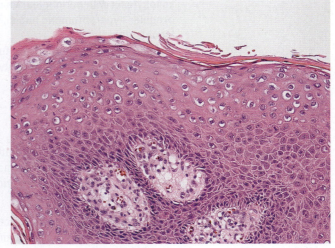

Figure 7.15.4 Condyloma acuminatum. Koilocytes in superficial epidermis characterized by perinuclear vacuolization, hyperchromasia, irregular nuclear contours, and binucleation.

7.15 Condyloma Acuminatum vs Epidermolytic Acanthoma

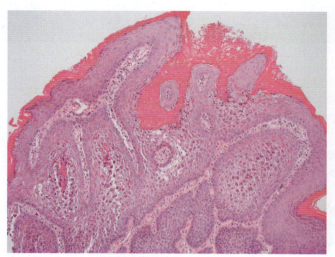

Figure 7.15.5 Epidermolytic acanthoma. Papillomatous epidermal hyperplasia with compact orthohyperkeratosis.

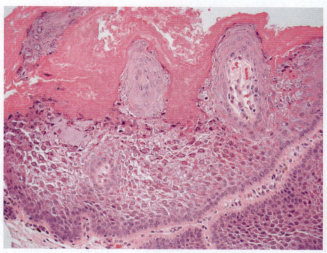

Figure 7.15.6 Epidermolytic acanthoma. Papillomatous epidermal hyperplasia with epidermolytic hyperkeratosis.

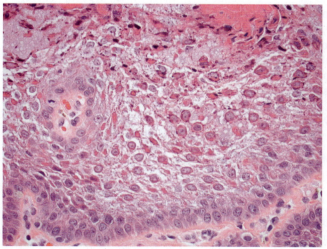

Figure 7.15.7 Epidermolytic acanthoma. Epidermolytic hyperkeratosis characterized by intact basal layer and cytoplasmic vacuolization with finely speckled to coarse keratohyalin granules in the superficial epidermis. The cell borders are indistinct.

7.16 LEPROSY VS SARCOIDOSIS

	Leprosy	**Sarcoidosis**
Age	All ages with bimodal peaks at 10-15 y and 30-60 y of age.	Any age. Typically presents in third to fourth decades.
Location	Preference for colder areas of the body including distal extremities, nose, ears, and mucous membranes.	Central face, extremities, and areas of trauma.
Etiology	Infection by *Mycobacterium leprae* and *Mycobacterium lepromatosis*, acid-fast, obligate intracellular bacilli. Humans are primary carriers of the organism, and transmission is through respiratory droplets.	Unknown. Pathogenesis postulated to involve dysregulation of the Th1 immune response to extrinsic antigens.
Presentation	Presentation is variable and dependent upon an individual's immunologic response to the infection. Categories include tuberculoid, borderline tuberculoid, mid-borderline, borderline lepromatous, and lepromatous. Most common presentation consists of single or grouped, well-delineated, hypopigmented or erythematous, hypoesthetic or anesthetic, macules or low plaques. Often, tender, enlarged peripheral nerves are also present.	Smooth macules or papules that may be violaceous, hyperpigmented, hypopigmented, or skin-colored.
Histology	1. A relatively normal epidermis and stratum corneum with exocytosis of rare lymphocytes along the basal zone *(Fig. 7.16.1)*. 2. Loose aggregates of epithelioid histiocytes forming granulomas within the reticular dermis. Granulomas assume a linear pattern following the neurovascular plexus and are associated with a variable infiltrate of lymphocytes *(Figs. 7.16.1 and 7.16.2)*. 3. Few histiocytes, lymphocytes, and plasma cells surround portion of nerve in reticular dermis *(Fig. 7.16.3)*. 4. AFB stain reveals acid-fast bacilli within histiocytes *(Fig. 7.16.4)*. Quantity of organisms dependent upon form of disease with few seen in tuberculoid form and many in lepromatous form.	1. A normal epidermis. 2. Granulomas present in the superficial dermis. May coalesce within the interstitium but are not perifollicular or preferentially surrounding nerves *(Fig. 7.16.5)*. 3. Granulomas are surrounded by a minimal to mild lymphocytic infiltrate ("naked granulomas") *(Figs. 7.16.5 and 7.16.6)*. 4. Granulomas composed of epithelioid histiocytes and multinucleate giant cells *(Fig. 7.16.7)*. 5. No mycobacteria on AFB stain.
Special studies	AFB or Fite stain to detect organisms. PCR may be used to confirm diagnosis.	Polarization to detect foreign material. Histochemical stains to exclude microorganisms (PAS or GMS stain for the fungus and AFB stain for mycobacteria).

7.16 Leprosy vs Sarcoidosis

	Leprosy	**Sarcoidosis**
Treatment	Treatment involves multiple-drug therapy in order to prevent resistance. First-line medications used include rifampin, dapsone, and clofazimine.	Based upon the extent and severity of disease. Topical and intralesional corticosteroids for limited disease. Systemic therapy for extensive disease or localized disease not responsive to therapy. Systemic therapies include antimalarial drugs, methotrexate, and tetracyclines.
Prognosis	Appropriate therapy generally leads to slow resolution of skin lesions but nerve damage is permanent. Disease progression or relapse is typically due to lack of compliance to treatment or high organism load. Immunological reactions may occur abruptly during or after initiation of therapy and have severe complications. Untreated infection can cause progressive and permanent damage with disfigurement.	A chronic disorder; prognosis depends upon the extent of cutaneous disease and involvement of other organ systems. Systemic involvement seen in approximately two-thirds of cases of cutaneous sarcoidosis. Involvement of the central face by erythematous plaques (lupus pernio variant) is associated with a high risk of concomitant pulmonary disease.

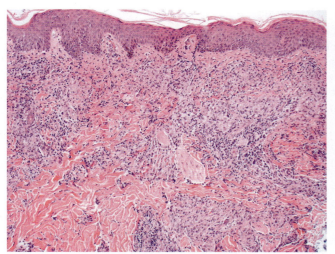

Figure 7.16.1 Leprosy. A normal epidermis with exocytosis of lymphocytes along basal zone and superficial band of histiocytes forming loose granulomas following the neurovascular plexus.

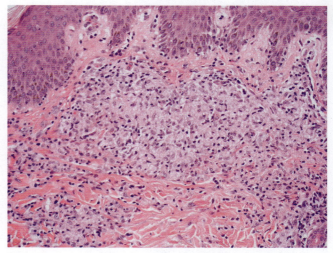

Figure 7.16.2 Leprosy. Epithelioid histiocytes forming noncaseating granulomas associated with lymphocytic infiltrate.

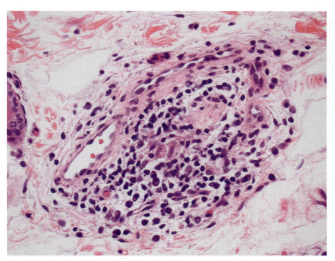

Figure 7.16.3 Leprosy. Few histiocytes, lymphocytes, and plasma cells surround portion of nerve in reticular dermis.

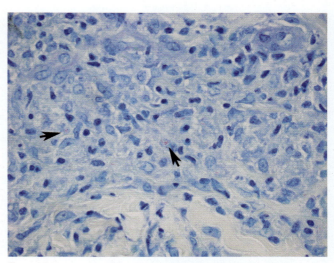

Figure 7.16.4 Leprosy. AFB stain reveals short acid-fast bacilli within histiocytes (arrows).

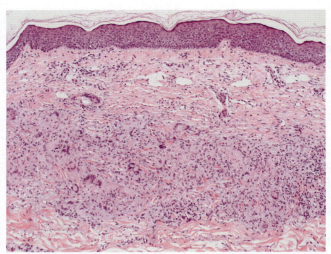

Figure 7.16.5 Sarcoidosis. A normal epidermis with underlying coalescing granulomatous inflammation. The granulomas are similar to those seen in leprosy but do not preferentially surround nerves.

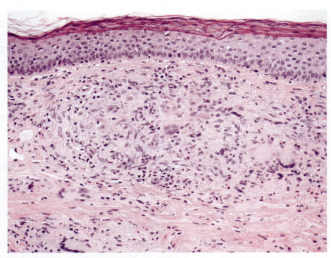

Figure 7.16.6 Sarcoidosis. Granulomas are composed of epithelioid histiocytes with sparse surrounding lymphocytic infiltrate.

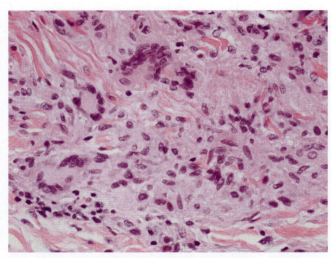

Figure 7.16.7 Sarcoidosis. Epithelioid histiocytes and multinucleate giant cells.

7.17 ATYPICAL MYCOBACTERIUM VS ERYTHEMA NODOSUM

	Atypical Mycobacterium	**Erythema Nodosum**
Age	All ages but primarily adults in the United States.	Any age; most commonly between 25 and 40 y of age; women more often than men.
Location	Dependent upon organism and mode of acquisition of infection. Direct inoculation typically occurs on extremities but other sites of trauma, surgery, and compromised skin barrier may be involved.	Extensor surfaces of legs and knees; less commonly on thighs, arms, calves, and face.
Etiology	Infection by nontuberculous mycobacterium that include the rapidly growing organisms (*Mycobacterium abscessus*, *Mycobacterium fortuitum*, and *Mycobacterium chelonae*) and slowly growing organisms (*Mycobacterium marinum*, *Mycobacterium ulcerans*, *Mycobacterium haemophilum*). Cutaneous involvement is the result of hematogenous dissemination, local spread from deep infection, or direct inoculation of the skin. Organisms are present in the environment, including water and soil sources.	Delayed-type hypersensitivity due to exposure to a variety of antigens. Underlying causes include infection, medications, malignancy, inflammatory bowel disease, and other inflammatory processes. Between 30% and 50% of cases are idiopathic.
Presentation	A wide variety of presentations including papules, plaques, nodules, pustules, abscesses, cellulitis, necrotic ulcers, and draining sinuses. May have solitary lesions but typically multiple with a sporotrichoid pattern of spread.	Abrupt onset of tender, erythematous, nonulcerated, fixed nodules on bilateral shins. May have a prodrome of fever, fatigue, and arthralgias.
Histology	1. A deep-seated inflammatory infiltrate involving septal and lobular components of subcutaneous tissue *(Fig. 7.17.1)*. 2. Septal fibrosis associated with dense mixed inflammation *(Fig. 7.17.2)* 3. Loose granulomas and neutrophilic abscesses with areas of fibrinoid degeneration *(Figs. 7.17.3 and 7.17.4)*. Miescher granulomas are not present. 4. Short bacilli present on AFB stain *(Fig. 7.17.5)*.	1. Septal panniculitis with widening of the subcutaneous septae by fibrosis and inflammation *(Fig. 7.17.6)*. Minimal extension into fat lobules. No necrosis or fibrinoid degeneration. 2. Inflammation includes lymphocytes, histocytes, neutrophils, and eosinophils, especially in early lesions *(Figs. 7.17.7 and 7.17.8)*. 3. Noncaseating granulomas including Miescher radial granulomas characterized by macrophages surrounding cleft-like spaces with or without clusters of neutrophils *(Fig. 7.17.9)*.
Special studies	AFB and/or Fite stains to detect organisms. Culture and PCR for confirmation.	PAS or GMS and AFB stains to exclude fungal and mycobacterial infection.

(continued)

	Atypical Mycobacterium	Erythema Nodosum
Treatment	Dependent upon the causative organism, the patient's immunological status, and the extent of disease. Medications typically used include clarithromycin, azithromycin, rifampin/ethambutol, and minocycline. Solitary or limited lesions may be amenable to surgical excision.	Treatment is not generally necessary but nonsteroidal anti-inflammatory agents and potassium iodide may be used for symptomatic relief. Intralesional or systemic glucocorticoids are alternative therapies for nonresponsive cases.
Prognosis	Infections can generally be successfully treated with appropriate therapy. Elderly and immunocompromised individuals are at higher risk for complications. Without treatment, infections can become more widespread and lead to severe disfigurement and disability.	Nodules spontaneously resolve within 2 mo but may have postinflammatory hyperpigmentation.

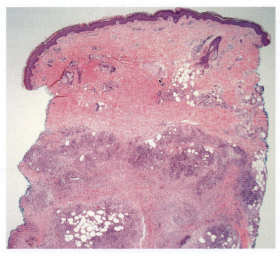

Figure 7.17.1 Atypical mycobacterium. Deep, dense inflammation that involves both septal and lobular components of subcutaneous tissue.

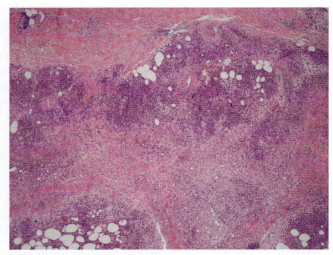

Figure 7.17.2 Atypical mycobacterium. Septal fibrosis with dense mixed inflammation.

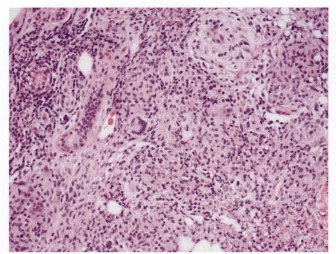

Figure 7.17.3 Atypical mycobacterium. Epithelioid histiocytes and multinucleate giant cells forming granulomas associated with lymphocytes, plasma cells, and neutrophils.

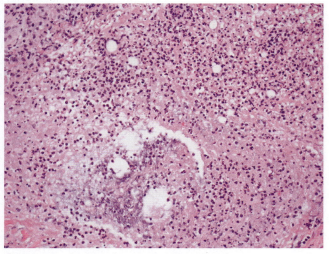

Figure 7.17.4 Atypical mycobacterium. Neutrophilic microabscess formation with fibrinoid degeneration.

7.17 Atypical Mycobacterium vs Erythema Nodosum

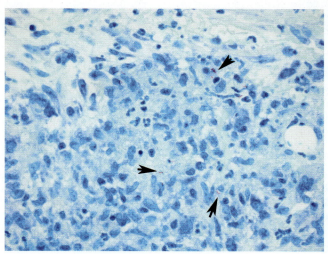

Figure 7.17.5 Atypical mycobacterium. AFB stain reveals acid-fast bacilli (arrows).

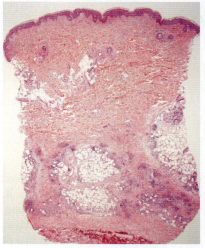

Figure 7.17.6 Erythema nodosum. Septal panniculitis with widening of the septae by fibrosis and inflammation. Fat lobules are encroached upon but not significantly involved by inflammation.

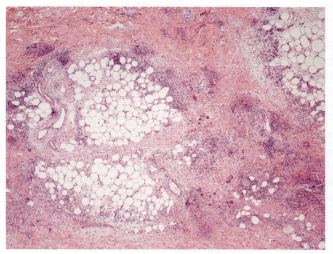

Figure 7.17.7 Erythema nodosum. Mixed inflammation within septae that are widened by edema and fibrosis. No necrosis or fibrinoid degeneration.

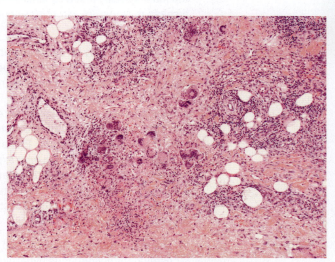

Figure 7.17.8 Erythema nodosum. Mixed inflammation includes neutrophils, eosinophil, lymphocytes, and histiocytes, forming loose granulomas.

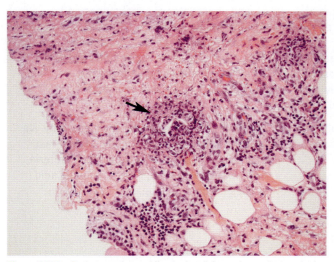

Figure 7.17.9 Erythema nodosum. Miescher's radial granulomas characterized by macrophages surrounding cleft-like spaces with clusters of neutrophils (arrow).

7.18 NOCARDIOSIS VS ACTINOMYCOSIS

	Nocardiosis	**Actinomycosis**
Age	Primary affects adults.	Any age with peak incidence between 40 and 50 y of age.
Location	Any site may be involved.	Head and neck including mandibular region, cheek, jaw, and chin.
Etiology	Infection by gram-positive aerobic bacilli of the *Nocardia* genus. It is acquired by direct inoculation presenting as a localized process or secondarily involves the skin when disseminated from a primary pulmonary infection. The majority of primary infections are caused by *Nocardia brasiliensis* and the main species involved in disseminated disease is *Nocardia asteroides* complex.	Infection caused by anaerobic, filamentous, gram-positive bacteria of the genus *Actinomyces*. Pathogenic species include *A. israelii*, *Actinomyces naeslundii*, *Actinomyces viscosus*, and *Actinomyces odontolyticus*. The organisms are commensal in the oropharynx, gastrointestinal tract, and female genital tract. Infection is initiated with disruption of the mucosal barrier and alteration of the resident microbiologic flora.
Presentation	Primary lesions may be acute and present as a superficial infection forming nodules or pustules that may progress in a sporotrichoid (lymphocutaneous) fashion. Other manifestations include cellulitis, ulceration, and abscess formation. Chronic primary lesions present as mycetoma. Primary lesions are due to direct inoculation with exposure to plants and soil. Disseminated infection is typically seen in immunocompromised individuals with development of pustules, nodules, and abscesses.	An indurated nodule that progresses into abscesses and sinus tracts. Sinus tracts discharge yellow, thick, sulfur granules. Fistula formation may also be present.
Histology	1. The epidermis may be ulcerated or show pseudoepitheliomatous hyperplasia *(Fig. 7.18.1)*. 2. The dermis has granulation tissue with dense mixed inflammation composed of lymphocytes, histiocytes, and aggregates of neutrophils *(Fig. 7.18.2)*. 3. Filamentous, thin bacilli with hyphae-like branching that are weakly gram-positive with a beaded appearance, partially acid-fast, and GMS-positive *(Figs. 7.18.3-7.18.5)*.	1. Epidermal ulceration with dense inflammation *(Fig. 7.18.6)*. 2. A dense mixed inflammatory infiltrate with sheets of foamy histiocytes and aggregates of lymphocytes and neutrophils *(Fig. 7.18.7)*. 3. Neutrophilic abscess formation *(Fig. 7.18.8)*. 4. A mass of filamentous bacteria forming sulfur granule and demonstrating Splendore-Hoeppli phenomenon *(Fig. 7.18.9)*.
Special studies	Tissue Gram, Fite, and GMS stains. Culture or PCR analysis for confirmation and speciation.	Tissue Gram stain showing gram positivity. No staining with acid-fast or modified acid-fast stains helps distinguish it from mycobacteria and *Nocardia*. Culture, PCR, and nuclei acid probes for confirmation.

	Nocardiosis	**Actinomycosis**
Treatment	An isolated cutaneous infection is treated with oral trimethoprim-sulfamethoxazole. Severe or disseminated infection is often treated with combination therapy consisting of two intravenous antibiotics. Susceptibility studies guide the choice of antibiotics.	Long-term, high-dose penicillin is first-line therapy. Doxycycline, amoxicillin, clindamycin, and minocycline are alternate antibiotics that have shown efficacy. Surgical debridement may be needed in complicated cases involving critical spaces.
Prognosis	Primary lesions typically resolve within few weeks of the start of treatment. Relapses are not uncommon, despite appropriate therapy.	Generally good response to appropriate antibiotic therapy with clearing of infection.

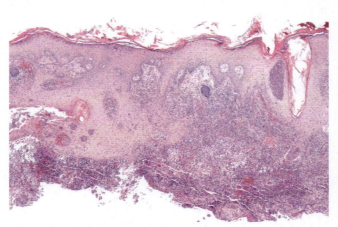

Figure 7.18.1 Nocardiosis. Pseudoepitheliomatous epidermal hyperplasia with dense mixed inflammation and microabscess formation.

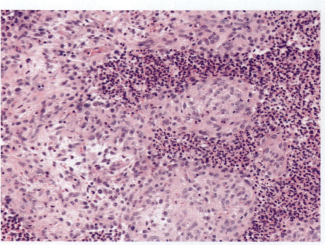

Figure 7.18.2 Nocardiosis. Dense neutrophil-rich inflammation with aggregates of histiocytes and reactive vessels.

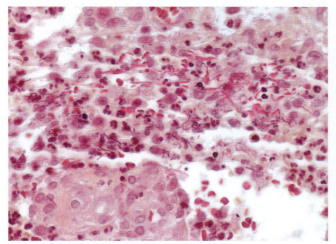

Figure 7.18.3 Nocardiosis. Tissue Gram stain showing thin, filamentous, weakly gram-positive bacilli that have a branched and somewhat beaded appearance.

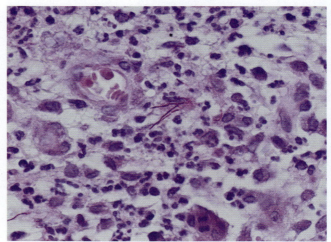

Figure 7.18.4 Nocardiosis. Filamentous bacilli on Fite stain.

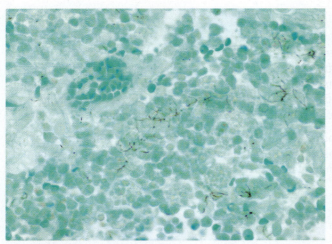

Figure 7.18.5 Nocardiosis. Thin, filamentous, branching bacilli on GMS stain.

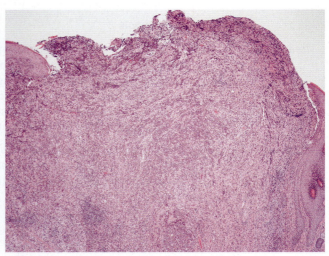

Figure 7.18.6 Actinomycosis. Epidermal ulceration with dense mixed inflammation within dermis.

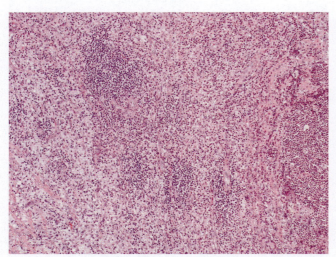

Figure 7.18.7 Actinomycosis. Sheets of foamy histiocytes and lymphocytes with aggregates of neutrophils.

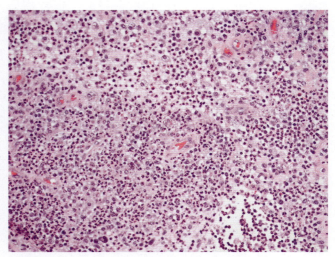

Figure 7.18.8 Actinomycosis. Neutrophilic microabscess formation.

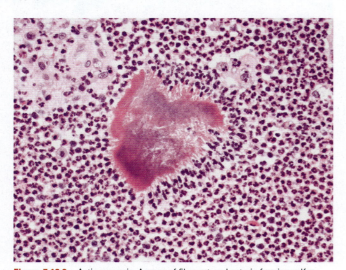

Figure 7.18.9 Actinomycosis. A mass of filamentous bacteria forming sulfur granule and demonstrating Splendore-Hoeppli phenomenon.

7.19 SECONDARY SYPHILIS VS LUPUS ERYTHEMATOSUS

	Secondary Syphilis	**Lupus Erythematosus**
Age	Adults, primarily young and middle-aged.	Fourth to fifth decades; women more frequently than men.
Location	Trunk and extremities. Involvement of palms and soles characteristic.	Sun-exposed areas favored. Localized forms most commonly on head and neck, especially scalp and ears. Generalized forms also involving extensor forearms and hands. Palms and soles spared.
Etiology	Infection by spirochete *Treponema pallidum*. Develops 3-10 w after primary chancre. Most infections are sexually acquired.	Autoimmune disease with contributions from genetic (HLA) and environmental (UV exposure and smoking) factors.
Presentation	Symmetric scaly, copper-colored or reddish-brown macules, papules, and plaques. Often accompanied by fever, fatigue, myalgias, and lymphadenopathy.	Well-demarcated, erythematous macules or papules with scale. Late-stage lesions with peripheral hyperpigmentation surrounding central hypopigmentation and atrophy.
Histology	1. Mild irregular epidermal acanthosis with reactive changes (Fig. 7.19.1). 2. Basal zone vacuolization with lymphocytes in each vacuole (Fig. 7.19.1). 3. Perivascular and interstitial inflammatory infiltrate of plasma cells and lymphocytes (Fig. 7.19.2). 4. Endothelial swelling with obliterative endarteritis (Fig. 7.19.3). 5. Spirochetes identified in the dermis with silver stain (Steiner or Warthin-Starry) (Fig. 7.19.4) or immunohistochemistry for *T. pallidum*.	1. A superficial and deep perivascular and periadnexal lymphocytic infiltrate (Fig. 7.19.5). 2. Epidermal interface vacuolar change with exocytosis of a small number of lymphocytes (Fig. 7.19.6). Note that the infiltrate is composed primarily of lymphocytes and plasma cells are not prominent. No obliterative endarteritis. 3. Mucin deposition within the reticular dermis with colloidal iron or Alcian Blue stain (Fig. 7.19.7).
Special studies	Silver stain (Steiner or Warthin-Starry) or immunohistochemistry for *T. pallidum* to detect spirochetes. Serologic testing with rapid plasma reagin (RPR) and/or Venereal Disease Research Laboratory (VDRL) tests to aid in confirmation.	Colloid iron or Alcian Blue stain to detect extracellular mucin. Direct immunofluorescence (lesional lupus band test) sometimes utilized in unclear cases to detect granular deposits of IgG, IgM, and sometimes IgA at dermal-epidermal junction.
Treatment	Intramuscular penicillin G benzathine is preferred treatment. Doxycycline or ceftriaxone may be substituted if unable to take penicillin. Clinical and serologic monitoring is recommended to assess response to therapy.	Strict sun avoidance and protection. Localized disease treated with topical corticosteroids or calcineurin inhibitors. Widespread or scarring disease treated with antimalarials drugs or other systemic immunosuppressants if refractory to antimalarials.

(continued)

	Secondary Syphilis	**Lupus Erythematosus**
Prognosis	Resolution of symptoms with appropriate therapy is generally seen in individuals with syphilis without underlying immunocompromise, neurosyphilis, or cardiovascular infection. If untreated, can progress to disseminated and tertiary disease with significant morbidity including neurologic and cardiovascular complications.	An unpredictable course with exacerbations and remissions. May cause considerable morbidity even when limited to the skin. Approximately 10%-20% may progress to systemic lupus erythematosus.

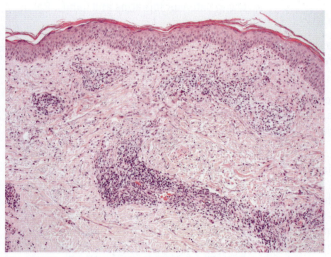

Figure 7.19.1 Secondary syphilis. Mild irregular epidermal hyperplasia with exocytosis of lymphocytes along the basal zone.

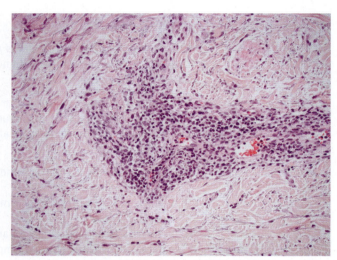

Figure 7.19.2 Secondary syphilis. A moderately dense perivascular infiltrate composed of lymphocytes and aggregates of plasma cells.

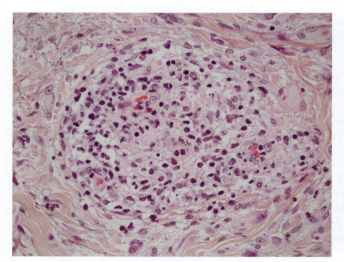

Figure 7.19.3 Secondary syphilis. Endothelial cell swelling with obliterative endarteritis.

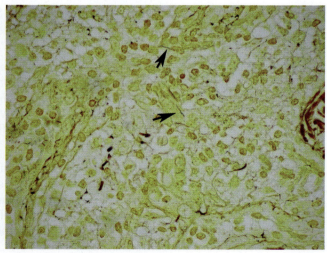

Figure 7.19.4 Secondary syphilis. Silver stain demonstrates spirochetes around dermal vessels (arrows).

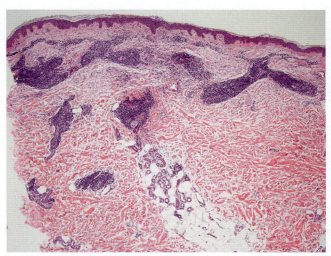

Figure 7.19.5 Lupus erythematosus. A moderately dense superficial and deep perivascular and periadnexal lymphocytic infiltrate.

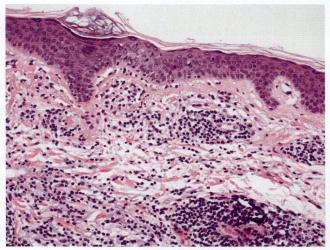

Figure 7.19.6 Lupus erythematosus. Interface vacuolar change with exocytosis of a small number of lymphocytes.

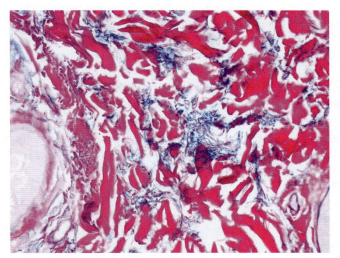

Figure 7.19.7 Lupus erythematosus. Copious mucin deposition in reticular dermis on colloidal iron stain.

7.20 SECONDARY SYPHILIS (CONDYLOMA LATA) VS PSORIASIS

	Secondary Syphilis (Condyloma Lata)	**Psoriasis**
Age	Adults, primarily young to middle age.	Any age, peak onset in young adulthood.
Location	Anogenital region, primarily, although other sites, including medial thighs, inframammary folds, and axillae, have been reported. Areas of heat, moisture, and friction preferentially involved.	Bilateral and symmetric; elbows, knees, buttock, scalp. May involve genital region as "inverse psoriasis."
Etiology	Infection by spirochete *T. pallidum*. Manifestation of secondary syphilis that develops 3-10 w after primary chancre. Most infections are sexually acquired.	Complex, multifactorial disease resulting from a combination of genetic, environmental, and immunologic factors. There is a genetic predisposition associated with certain HLA alleles, with HLA-Cw6 being most strongly associated. Environmental triggers are many and include infection, trauma, alcohol ingestion, medications, and cold weather. The triggers evoke excess T-cell activity that causes stimulation of epidermal keratinocytes with an increase in keratinocyte turnover rate.
Presentation	Smooth, moist, flat-topped, gray-pink, papules and plaques. Lesions are typically nontender but may be malodorous.	Monomorphic, sharply demarcated erythematous plaques covered by silvery scale.
Histology	1. Parakeratosis with entrapped serum and neutrophils *(Figs. 7.20.1* and *7.20.2).* 2. Psoriasiform epidermal hyperplasia with intercellular edema and exocytosis of lymphocytes and neutrophils *(Figs. 7.20.2* and *7.20.3).* 3. A dense perivascular infiltrate of lymphocytes and numerous plasma cells *(Fig. 7.20.4).* 4. Endothelial swelling *(Fig. 7.20.5).* 5. Numerous spirochetes identified with silver stain *(Fig. 7.20.6)* and immunohistochemical stain for *T. pallidum (Fig. 7.20.7).*	1. Hyperkeratosis and parakeratosis overlying psoriasiform epidermal hyperplasia with thinning of the suprapapillary plate *(Fig. 7.20.8).* 2. Foci of parakeratosis with entrapped neutrophils *(Figs. 7.20.8* and *7.20.9).* 3. Neutrophilic microabscesses in superficial epidermis and stratum corneum *(Figs. 7.20.10).* A dermal infiltrate of lymphocytes but no appreciable plasma cell component. 4. Dilated, tortuous thin-walled vessels in papillae *(Figs. 7.20.10).*
Special studies	Silver stain (Steiner or Warthin-Starry) or immunohistochemistry for *T. pallidum* to detect spirochetes. Serologic testing with RPR and/or VDRL tests to aid in confirmation.	PAS to exclude a superficial fungal infection.
Treatment	Intramuscular penicillin G benzathine is preferred treatment. Doxycycline or ceftriaxone may be substituted if unable to take penicillin. Clinical and serologic monitoring is recommended to assess response to therapy.	Treatment is based upon the extent and severity of disease along with comorbidities. Limited disease is treated with topical corticosteroids and emollients. Phototherapy may be added for moderate to severe disease. Alternatively, systemic agents including retinoids, methotrexate, cyclosporine, and a variety of biologic immune modifying agents, may be used.

7.20 Secondary Syphilis (Condyloma Lata) vs Psoriasis

	Secondary Syphilis (Condyloma Lata)	**Psoriasis**
Prognosis	Resolution of symptoms with appropriate therapy is generally seen in individuals with syphilis without underlying immunocompromise, neurosyphilis, or cardiovascular infection. If untreated, can progress to a disseminated and tertiary disease with significant morbidity including neurologic and cardiovascular complications.	A chronic disease characterized by exacerbations and remissions. Individuals with cutaneous psoriasis are at risk for development of psoriatic arthritis.

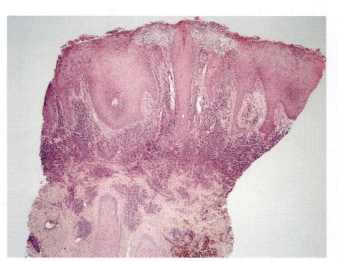

Figure 7.20.1 Secondary syphilis (condyloma lata). Irregular psoriasiform epidermal hyperplasia with dense band of inflammation in superficial dermis.

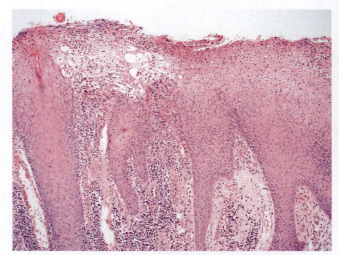

Figure 7.20.2 Secondary syphilis (condyloma lata). Ragged parakeratosis overlying irregular epidermal hyperplasia with focally prominent intercellular edema and inflammatory cell exocytosis.

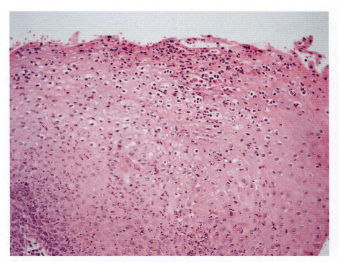

Figure 7.20.3 Secondary syphilis (condyloma lata). Diffuse neutrophilic exocytosis within epidermis.

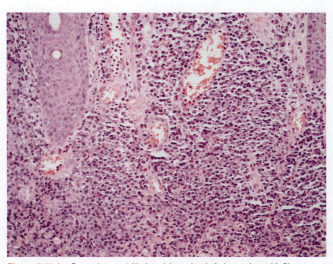

Figure 7.20.4 Secondary syphilis (condyloma lata). A dense dermal infiltrate consisting of numerous plasma cells.

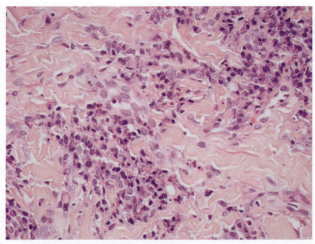

Figure 7.20.5 Secondary syphilis (condyloma lata). A plasma cell infiltrate and reactive vessels with endothelial cell swelling.

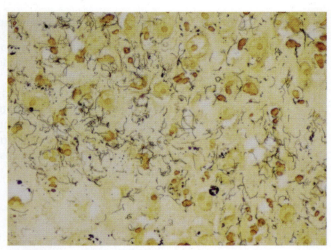

Figure 7.20.6 Secondary syphilis (condyloma lata). Numerous spirochetes identified within epidermis with silver stain.

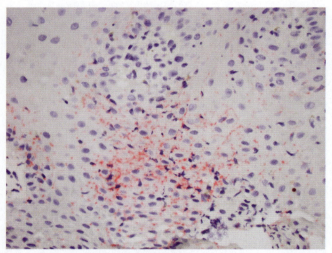

Figure 7.20.7 Secondary syphilis (condyloma lata). Spirochetes identified on immunohistochemical stain for *T. pallidum*.

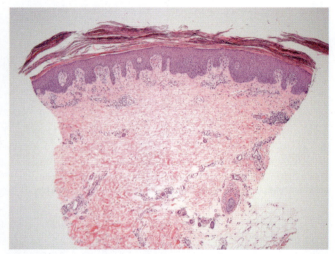

Figure 7.20.8 Psoriasis. Hyperkeratosis and parakeratosis overlying psoriasiform epidermal hyperplasia.

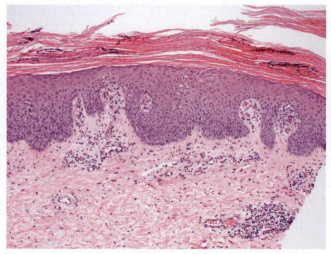

Figure 7.20.9 Psoriasis. Foci of parakeratosis alternating with orthokeratosis. Neutrophils are entrapped within the parakeratosis. Neutrophilic exocytosis in an area of hypogranulosis.

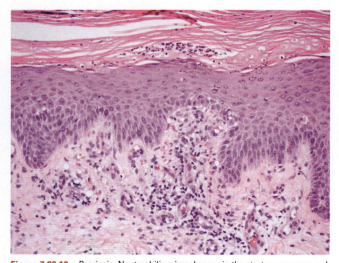

Figure 7.20.10 Psoriasis. Neutrophilic microabscess in the stratum corneum and tortuous, dilated capillaries in papillae.

7.21 SCABIES VS DEMODICOSIS

	Scabies	**Demodicosis**
Age	All ages may be affected.	Adults, primarily after the age of 40 y, with predilection for elderly.
Location	Predilection for finger webspaces, wrists, axillae, umbilicus, areolae, buttocks, lower abdomen, and genital region.	Primary form occurs mainly on the face (perioral, periorbital, and periauricular regions) and neck. Secondary form may involve trunk as well as face.
Etiology	Infestation by the female mite of *Sarcoptes scabiei* that burrows into the stratum corneum and deposits eggs. Transmission is by close personal contact or through contaminated clothing or linens.	Human mites *Demodex follicularis* and *Demodex brevis* are normal inhabitants of hair follicles and sebaceous glands. Mites may cause pathology that is classified as primary and secondary forms of demodicosis.
Presentation	Intensely pruritic papules or burrows, consisting of slightly elevated tortuous lines, which are often excoriated. Some cases may have a nodular component. Crusted scabies occurs in immunocompromised or debilitated individuals and consists of lichenified plaques with thick scale and crusting.	The primary form can present in several ways that include discrete, white spicules involving sebaceous hair follicles without significant erythema (spiculate demodicosis); erythematous papulopustules (papulopustular demodicosis); madarosis and scaling of eyelids with dry eye and chalazion formation (ocular demodicosis); and scaling of external ear canal (auricular demodicosis). Secondary demodicosis is more extensive and usually associated with immunosuppression.
Histology	1. The stratum corneum is thickened by hyperkeratosis and parakeratosis with crust formation *(Fig. 7.21.1)*. 2. A dense dermal inflammatory infiltrate with numerous eosinophils *(Fig. 7.21.2)*. 3. Formation of burrow (space between stratum corneum and epidermis) within which intact mites, ova, and scybala (feces) are found *(Figs. 7.21.3-7.21.5)*. Mites are within the interfollicular areas, not specifically in follicular lumens, like demodex. 4. Fragments of chitinous exoskeleton form curled scrolls and remnants of eggshells form pink "pigtails" *(Fig. 7.21.6)*.	1. Follicular dilatation and hyperkeratosis *(Figs. 7.21.7* and *7.21.8)*. 2. Follicular infundibula are distended by numerous demodex mites *(Figs. 7.21.9* and *7.21.10)*. 3. Mites have a chitinous exoskeleton and eight legs *(Figs. 7.21.10)*. 4. Variable density and composition of perifollicular inflammation dependent upon type of presentation.
Special studies	None. Skin scrapings with mineral oil can also be performed for diagnosis.	None. May perform mineral oil skin scraping to detect and quantitate mites.
Treatment	Topical permethrin is first-line treatment, especially in children. Oral ivermectin may also be used and is preferred for outbreaks in living facilities or cases of crusted scabies. Antihistamines may be needed to control pruritus.	Treatment and preventative strategies include cleansing face, hair, and eyelashes. Treatment with acaricides, including ivermectin cream, topical permethrin, benzyl benzoate solution, and metronidazole gel. Oral ivermectin may be used for heavy infestation or in the setting of HIV infection.

(continued)

	Scabies	Demodicosis
Prognosis	Resolution of the infestation generally occurs with adequate treatment. Retreatment may be necessary in cases of persistent infestation or reinfestation. Complications include secondary bacterial infection and prurigo nodularis due to rubbing and scratching.	Generally responds to therapy and has a good prognosis, although immunocompromised individuals may have a more prolonged and severe course. Recurrence is more common when associated with other follicular inflammatory disorders such as rosacea and acne.

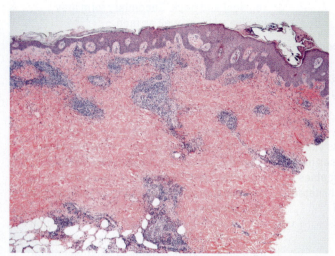

Figure 7.21.1 Scabies. Superficial and deep dermal inflammation with overlying epidermal hyperplasia, focal parakeratosis, and crust formation.

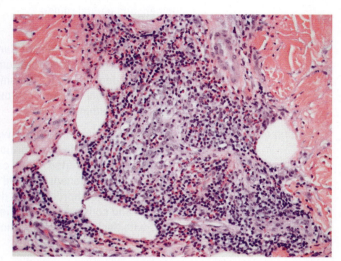

Figure 7.21.2 Scabies. Dermal inflammation including numerous eosinophils.

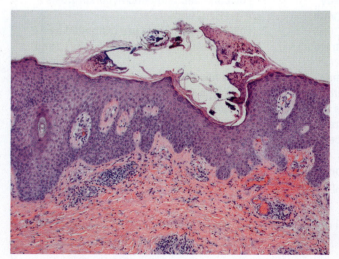

Figure 7.21.3 Scabies. Formation of a burrow between the stratum corneum and the epidermis with an overlying crust. Scabies mite is evident within the burrow.

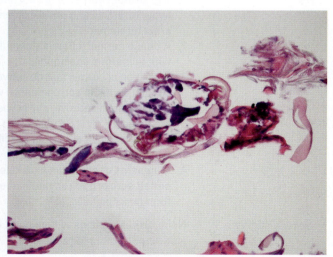

Figure 7.21.4 Scabies. Higher magnification of scabies mite.

7.21 Scabies vs Demodicosis

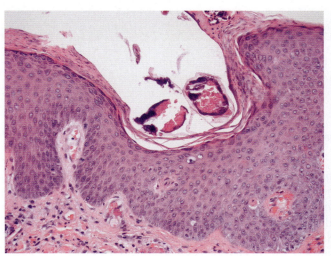

Figure 7.21.5 Scabies. Ova and scybala within burrow.

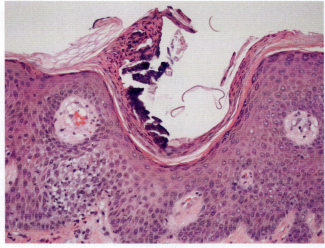

Figure 7.21.6 Scabies. Remnants of eggshells form curled "pigtails."

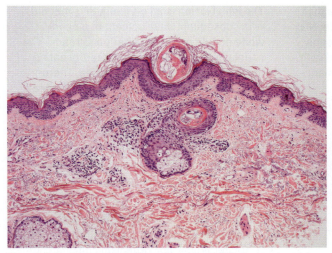

Figure 7.21.7 Demodicosis. Follicular dilatation with follicular hyperkeratosis and perifollicular chronic inflammation.

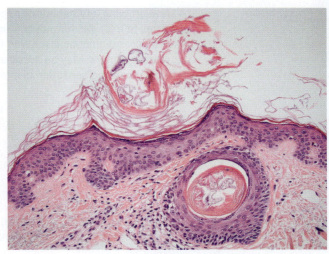

Figure 7.21.8 Demodicosis. Follicular dilatation with follicular hyperkeratosis and perifollicular chronic inflammation. Note demodex in hyperkeratosis and within follicular lumen.

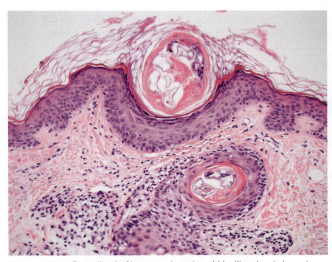

Figure 7.21.9 Demodicosis. Numerous demodex within dilated and plugged follicle. Mild perifollicular lymphocytic infiltrate.

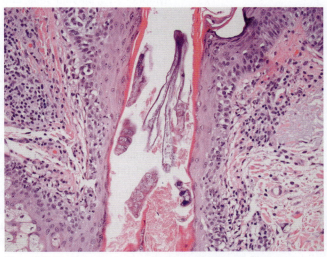

Figure 7.21.10 Demodicosis. *Demodex* mites within distended follicular lumen.

7.22 MYIASIS VS TUNGIASIS

	Myiasis	**Tungiasis**
Age	Any age.	Any age.
Location	Exposed skin at any site, typically face, upper extremities, and trunk.	Typically feet but any body site may be involved.
Etiology	Infestation with dipterous larvae (maggots) from *Dermatobia hominis* (botfly) found in Central and South America, *Cordylobia anthropophaga* (tumba, blowfly) found in Africa, and *Cochliomyia hominivorax* (screwworm fly) found in tropical locals in Old and New World. Fly eggs are transferred to human host by mosquito or fly vector.	Penetration of the skin by female members of *Tunga penetrans*, a sand flea found in tropical and subtropical regions of the world. This is followed by significant hypertrophy of the abdominal segments and ultimate shedding of eggs.
Presentation	A slow-growing, erythematous papule that enlarges to a tender, furuncular nodule. May have a serosanguinous discharge through a central punctum. May be associated with pruritus, pain, and sensation of movement.	The initial lesion is an erythematous macule with subsequent development of a pearly white nodule one to 2 d after penetration. The nodule has a central black dot representing the anal-genital opening of the flea. There is often progressive erythema with possible ulceration and desquamation of the skin. Three to 5 w after penetration, there is involution after death of the parasite with scar formation. Infestation by multiple sand fleas is not uncommon and produces a tumorous growth. There may be pain, pruritus, and sensation of a foreign body.
Histology	1. Reactive epidermal hyperplasia, hyperkeratosis, and parakeratosis *(Fig. 7.22.1)*. 2. Expansion of the dermis by a dense, diffuse, mixed inflammatory infiltrate of lymphocytes, plasma cells, and numerous eosinophils *(Fig. 7.22.2)*. 3. Detached portions of larva in subcutis including undulating eosinophilic exoskeleton, pigmented spicule, and internal organs *(Figs. 7.22.3-7.22.5)*.	1. Reactive epidermal hyperplasia with mixed dermal inflammation *(Fig. 7.22.6)*. 2. An intraepidermal organism composed of an outer thick eosinophilic cuticle and a central cavity containing elements of the digestive tract, trachea, and developing eggs *(Figs. 7.22.7-7.22.9)*. Striated muscle runs from the head to terminal orifice.
Special studies	None. Microbiologic species identification based upon morphology of larvae.	None.
Treatment	Surgical extraction or suffocation of larvae by occlusion of the punctum by petroleum jelly, pork fat, or mineral oil has been utilized.	Surgical extraction of the flea.
Prognosis	Larvae mature in 8-12 w and exit the skin on their own. Surgical extraction is curative if removal is desired before full maturation. Secondary bacterial infections may occur.	Although self-limited, individuals may experience severe pain, difficulty walking, and secondary infections from fissures and ulceration. Preventative measures include wearing of closed-toe shoes and daily inspection of feet.

7.22 Myiasis vs Tungiasis

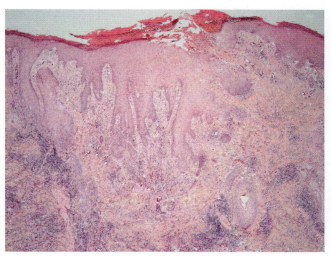

Figure 7.22.1 Myiasis. Reactive epidermal hyperplasia with hyperkeratosis and parakeratosis.

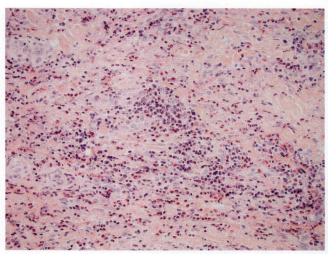

Figure 7.22.2 Myiasis. A dense dermal inflammatory infiltrate with numerous eosinophils.

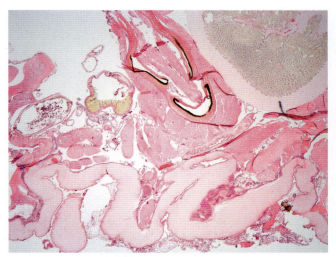

Figure 7.22.3 Myiasis. Portions of larva with undulating eosinophilic exoskeleton and internal organs.

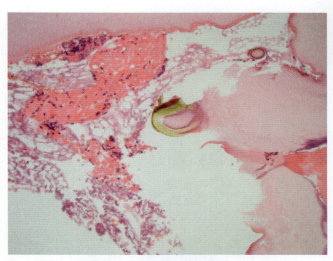

Figure 7.22.4 Myiasis. Pigmented spicule aids in diagnosis.

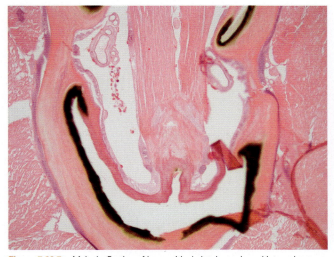

Figure 7.22.5 Myiasis. Portion of larva with skeletal muscle and internal organs.

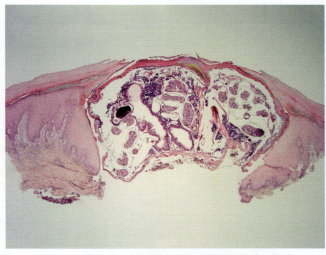

Figure 7.22.6 Tungiasis. Reactive epidermal hyperplasia associated with intraepidermal organism and mixed inflammatory infiltrate.

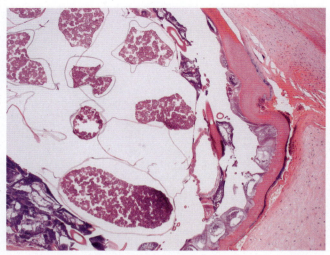

Figure 7.22.7 Tungiasis. Intraepidermal organism with eosinophilic exoskeleton and internal organs.

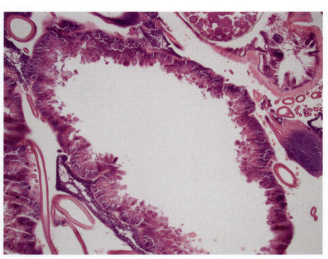

Figure 7.22.8 Tungiasis. Internal organs including portions of reproductive and digestive tracts.

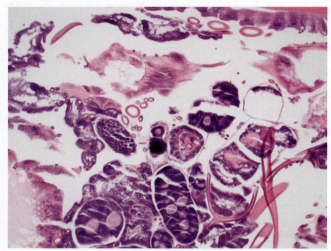

Figure 7.22.9 Tungiasis. Internal organs including portions of reproductive and digestive tracts.

SUGGESTED READINGS

Chapter 7.1

Brazel M, Desai A, Are A, Motaparthi K. Staphylococcal scalded skin syndrome and bullous impetigo. *Medicina*. 2021;57(11):1157.

Campois TG, Zucoloto AZ, de Almeida Araujo EJ, et al. Immunological and histopathological characterization of cutaneous candidiasis. *J Med Microbiol*. 2015;64(8):810-817.

Chapters 7.2-7.5

Darmstadt GL, Lane AT. Impetigo: an overview. *Pediatr Dermatol*. 1994;11(4):293-303.

Day T, Borbolla Foster A, Phillips S, et al. Can routine histopathology distinguish between vulvar cutaneous candidosis and dermatophytosis? *J Low Genit Tract Dis*. 2016;20(3):267-271.

Drolshagen H, Zoumberos N, Shalin S. Bullous tinea. *Arch Pathol Lab Med*. Published online 2023.

Groves JB, Nassereddin A, Freeman AM. Erythrasma. In: *StatPearls*. StatPearls Publishing; 2022.

Hartman-Adams H, Banvard C, Juckett G. Impetigo: diagnosis and treatment. *Am Fam Physician*. 2014;90(4):229-235.

Hudson A, Sturgeon A, Peiris A. Tinea versicolor. *JAMA*. 2018;320(13):1396.

Johnston GA. Treatment of bullous impetigo and the staphylococcal scalded skin syndrome in infants. *Expert Rev Anti Infect Ther*. 2004;2(3):439-446.

Kelly BP. Superficial fungal infections. *Pediatr Rev*. 2012;33:e22-e37.

Leung AK, Barankin B, Lam JM, Leong KF, Hon KL. Tinea versicolor: an updated review. *Drugs Context*. 2022;11. 2022-9-2.

Mendez-Tovar LJ. Pathogenesis of dermatophytosis and tinea versicolor. *Clin Dermatol*. 2010;28(2):185-189.

Meymandi S, Silver SG, Crawford RI. Intraepidermal neutrophils: a clue to dermatophytosis? *J Cutan Pathol*. 2003;30(4):253-255.

Nardi NM, Schaefer TJ. Impetigo. In: *StatPearls*. StatPearls Publishing; 2022.

Riquelme IL, Moyano EG. Axillary and inguinal erythrasma. *CMAJ*. 2021;193(39):E1535.

Ross A, Shoff HW. Staphylococcal scalded skin syndrome. In: *StatPearls*. StatPearls Publishing; 2021.

Chapters 7.6-7.7

Caldito EG, Antia C, Petronic-Rosic V. Cutaneous blastomycosis. *JAMA Dermatol*. 2022;158(9):1064.

Carrasco-Zuber JE, Navarrete-Dechent C, Bonifaz A, Fich F, Vial-Letelier V, Berroeta-Mauriziano D. Cutaneous involvement in the deep mycoses: A review. Part II -systemic mycoses. *Actas Dermosifiliogr*. 2016;107(10):816-822.

DiCaudo DJ. Coccidioidomycosis: a review and update. *J Am Acad Dermatol*. 2006;55(6):929-942; quiz 943-945.

Fernandez-Flores A, Saeb-Lima M, Arenas-Guzman R. Morphological findings of deep cutaneous fungal infections. *Am J Dermatopathol*. 2014;36(7):531-553; quiz 554-556.

Garcia Garcia SC, Salas Alanis JC, Flores MG, Gonzalez Gonzalez SE, Vera Cabrera L, Ocampo Candiani J. Coccidioidomycosis and the skin: a comprehensive review. *An Bras Dermatol*. 2015;90(5):610-619.

Hernandez AD. Cutaneous cryptococcosis. *Dermatol Clin*. 1989;7(2):269-274.

Noguchi H, Matsumoto T, Kimura U, Hiruma M, Kusuhara M, Ihn H. Cutaneous cryptococcosis. *Med Mycol J*. 2019;60(4):101-107.

Saccente M, Woods GL. Clinical and laboratory update on blastomycosis. *Clin Microbiol Rev*. 2010;23(2):367-381.

Chapter 7.8

Bhattacharjee R, Narang T, Chatterjee D. Cutaneous chromoblastomycosis: a prototypal case. *J Cutan Med Surg*. 2019;23(1):98.

Carrasco-Zuber JE, Navarrete-Dechent C, Bonifaz A, Fich F, Vial-Letelier V, Berroeta-Mauriziano D. Cutaneous involvement in the deep mycoses: a literature review. part i-subcutaneous mycoses. *Actas Dermosifiliogr*. 2016;107(10):806-815.

Caviedes MP, Torre AC, Eliceche ML, Valdivia Monteros DC, Volonteri VI, Galimberti RL. Cutaneous phaeohyphomycosis. *Int J Dermatol*. 2017;56(4):415-420.

Kundu R, Handa U, Punia RS, Singla N, Chander J, Attri AK. Phaeohyphomycosis: cytomorphologic evaluation in eleven cases. *Acta Cytol*. 2020;64(5):406-412.

Queiroz-Telles F, de Hoog S, Santos DWCL, et al. Chromoblastomycosis. *Clin Microbiol Rev*. 2017;30(1):233-276.

Revankar SG. Phaeohyphomycosis. *Infect Dis Clin North Am*. 2006;20(3):609-620.

Chapter 7.9

Bernardeschi C, Foulet F, Ingen-Housz-Oro S, et al. Cutaneous invasive aspergillosis: retrospective multicenter study of the french invasive-aspergillosis registry and literature review. *Medicine (Baltimore)*. 2015;94(26):e1018.

Chang H, Wang PN, Huang Y. Cutaneous mucormycosis. *Infection*. 2018;46(6):901-902.

Isaac M. Cutaneous aspergillosis. *Dermatol Clin*. 1996;14(1):137-140.

Manesh A, Rupali P, Sullivan MO, et al. Mucormycosis-A clinico-epidemiological review of cases over 10 years. *Mycoses*. 2019;62(4):391-398.

Nakashima K, Yamada N, Yoshida Y, Yamamoto O. Primary cutaneous aspergillosis. *Acta Derm Venereol*. 2010;90(5):519-520.

Shields BE, Rosenbach M, Brown-Joel Z, Berger AP, Ford B A, Wanat KA. Angioinvasive fungal infections impacting the skin: background, epidemiology, and clinical presentation. *J Am Acad Dermatol*. 2019;80(4):869-880.e5.

Chapter 7.10

Ahuja A, Bhardwaj M, Agarwal P. Cutaneous histoplasmosis in HIV seronegative patients: a clinicopathological analysis. *Dermatology*. 2021;237(6):934-939.

de Vries HJC, Schallig HD. Cutaneous leishmaniasis: a 2022 updated narrative review into diagnosis and management developments. *Am J Clin Dermatol.* 2022;23(6):823-840.

Gurel MS, Tekin B, Uzun S. Cutaneous leishmaniasis: a great imitator. *Clin Dermatol.* 2020;38(2):140-151.

Handler MZ, Patel PA, Kapila R, Al-Qubati Y, Schwartz RA. Cutaneous and mucocutaneous leishmaniasis: differential diagnosis, diagnosis, histopathology, and management. *J Am Acad Dermatol.* 2015;73(6):911-926; 927-928.

Lin MJ, Mazzoni D, Gin D. Disseminated cutaneous-only histoplasmosis in a patient with AIDS. *Australas J Dermatol.* 2019;60(4):e330-e332.

Raggio B. Primary cutaneous histoplasmosis. *Ear Nose Throat J.* 2018;97(10-11):346-348.

Chapter 7.11

Bäck O, Faergemann J, Hörnqvist R. Pityrosporum folliculitis: a common disease of the young and middle-aged. *J Am Acad Dermatol.* 1985;12(1 pt 1):56-61.

Bressan AL, Silva RSd, Fonseca JCM, Alves MdFGS. Majocchi's granuloma. *An Bras Dermatol.* 2011;86(4):797-798.

Castellanos J, Guillén-Flórez A, Valencia-Herrera A, et al. Unusual inflammatory tinea infections: Majocchi's granuloma and deep/systemic dermatophytosis. *J Fungi (Basel).* 2021;7(11):929.

Chou WY, Hsu CJ. A case report of Majocchi's granuloma associated with combined therapy of topical steroids and adalimumab. *Medicine (Baltimore).* 2016;95(2):e2245.

Ilkit M, Durdu M, Karakaş M. Majocchi's granuloma: a symptom complex caused by fungal pathogens. *Med Mycol.* 2012;50(5):449-457.

Peres FLX, Bonamigo RR, Bottega GB, Staub FL, Cartell AS, Bakos RM. Pityrosporum folliculitis in critically ill COVID-19 patients. *J Eur Acad Dermatol Venereol.* 2022;36(3):e186-e188.

Chapters 7.12-7.13

Bader MS. Herpes zoster: diagnostic, therapeutic, and preventive approaches. *Postgrad Med.* 2013;125(5):78-91.

Engin B, Kutlubay Z, Çelik U, Serdaroğlu S, Tüzün Y. Hailey-Hailey disease: a fold (intertriginous) dermatosis. *Clin Dermatol.* 2015;33(4):452-455.

Hoyt B, Bhawan J. Histological spectrum of cutaneous herpes infections. *Am J Dermatopathol.* 2014;36(8):609-619.

Leinweber B, Kerl H, Cerroni L. Histopathologic features of cutaneous herpes virus infections (herpes simplex, herpes varicella/zoster): a broad spectrum of presentations with common pseudolymphomatous aspects. *Am J Surg Pathol.* 2006;30(1):50-58.

Schmidt E, Kasperkiewicz M, Joly P. Pemphigus. *Lancet.* 2019;394(10201):882-894.

Whitley RJ, Roizman B. Herpes simplex virus infections. *Lancet.* 2001;357(9267):1513-1518.

Wick MR. Bullous, pseudobullous, & pustular dermatoses. *Semin Diagn Pathol.* 2017;34(3):250-260.

Chapter 7.14

Aboud AMA, Nigam PK. Wart. In: *StatPearls.* StatPearls Publishing; 2022.

Chen X, Anstey AV, Bugert JJ. Molluscum contagiosum virus infection. *Lancet Infect Dis.* 2013;13(10):877-888.

Forbat E, Al-Niaimi F, Ali FR. Molluscum contagiosum: review and update on management. *Pediatr Dermatol.* 2017;34(5):504-515.

Meza-Romero R, Navarrete-Dechent C, Downey C. Molluscum contagiosum: an update and review of new perspectives in etiology, diagnosis, and treatment. *Clin Cosmet Investig Dermatol.* 2019;12:373-381.

Stulberg DL, Hutchinson AG. Molluscum contagiosum and warts. *Am Fam Physician.* 2003;67(6):1233-1240.

Chapter 7.15

Abbas O, Wieland CN, Goldberg LJ. Solitary epidermolytic acanthoma: a clinical and histopathological study. *J Eur Acad Dermatol Venereol.* 2011;25(2):175-180.

Chan MP. Verruciform and condyloma-like squamous proliferations in the anogenital region. *Arch Pathol Lab Med.* 2019;143(7):821-831.

Diţescu D, Istrate-Ofiţeru AM, Roşu GC, et al. Clinical and pathological aspects of condyloma acuminatum: review of literature and case presentation. *Rom J Morphol Embryol.* 2021;62(2):369-383.

Ginsberg AS, Rajagopalan A, Terlizzi JP. Epidermolytic acanthoma: a case report. *World J Clin Cases.* 2020;8(18):4094-4099.

Hijazi MM, Succaria F, Ghosn S. Multiple localized epidermolytic acanthomas of the vulva associated with vulvar pruritus: a case report. *Am J Dermatopathol.* 2015;37(4):e49-e52.

Nelson EL, Bogliatto F, Stockdale CK. Vulvar Intraepithelial Neoplasia (VIN) and condylomata. *Clin Obstet Gynecol.* 2015;58(3):512-525.

Pennycook KB, McCready TA. Condyloma Acuminata. In: *StatPearls.* StatPearls Publishing; 2022.

Chapter 7.16

Maymone MBC, Laughter M, Venkatesh S, et al. Leprosy: clinical aspects and diagnostic techniques. *J Am Acad Dermatol.* 2020;83:1-14.

Rai VM, Balachandran C, Mathew M. Cutaneous sarcoidosis masquerading as lepromatous leprosy. *Indian J Lepr.* 2006;78(4):365-369.

Reibel F, Cambau E, Aubry A. Update on the epidemiology, diagnosis, and treatment of leprosy. *Med Mal Infect.* 2015;45(9):383-393.

Rongioletti F, Gallo R, Cozzani E, Parodi A. Leprosy: a diagnostic trap for dermatopathologists in nonendemic area. *Am J Dermatopathol.* 2009;31(6):607-610.

Singh A, Ramesh V. Histopathological features in leprosy, post-kala-azar dermal leishmaniasis, and cutaneous leishmaniasis. *Indian J Dermatol Venereol Leprol.* 2013;79(3):360-366.

Zumla A, James GD. Sarcoidosis and leprosy: an epidemiological, clinical, pathological and immunological comparison. *Sarcoidosis*. 1989;6(2):88-96.

Chapter 7.17

Bartralot R, Pujol RM, García-Patos V, et al. Cutaneous infections due to nontuberculous mycobacteria: histopathological review of 28 cases comparative study between lesions observed in immunosuppressed patients and normal hosts. *J Cutan Pathol*. 2000;27(3):124-129.

Chowaniec M, Starba A, Wiland P. Erythema nodosum: review of the literature. *Reumatologia*. 2016;54(2):79-82.

Gonzalez-Santiago TM, Drage LA. Nontuberculous mycobacteria: skin and soft tissue infections. *Dermatol Clin*. 2015;33(3):563-577.

Lee WJ, Kang SM, Sung H, et al. Non-tuberculous mycobacterial infections of the skin: a retrospective study of 29 cases. *J Dermatol*. 2010;37(11):965-972.

Nogueira LB, Garcia CN, Costa MSCD, de Moraes MB, Kurizky PS, Gomes CM. Non-tuberculous cutaneous mycobacterioses. *An Bras Dermatol*. 2021;96(5):527-538.

Pérez-Garza DM, Chavez-Alvarez S, Ocampo-Candiani J, Gomez-Flores M. Erythema nodosum: a practical approach and diagnostic algorithm. *Am J Clin Dermatol*. 2021;22(3):367-378.

Chapter 7.18

Akhtar M, Zade MP, Shahane PL, Bangde AP, Soitkar SM. Scalp actinomycosis presenting as soft tissue tumour: a case report with literature review. *Int J Surg Case Rep*. 2015;16:99-101.

Bandeira ID, Guimarães-Silva P, Cedro-Filho RL, de Almeida VRP, Bittencourt AL, Brites C. Primär kutane nokardiose. *J Dtsch Dermatol Ges*. 2019;17(3):327-329.

Doyle C, Costa Blasco M, MacEneaney O, Ryan C, Ní Raghallaigh S. Disseminated cutaneous nocardia. *Int J Dermatol*. 2023;62(1):e29-e31.

Ngow HA, Wan Khairina WMN. Cutaneous actinomycosis: the great mimicker. *J Clin Pathol*. 2009;62(8):766.

Patil D, Siddaramappa B, Manjunathswamy BS, et al. Primary cutaneous actinomycosis. *Int J Dermatol*. 2008;47(12):1271-1273.

Ramos-E-Silva M, Lopes RS, Trope BM. Cutaneous nocardiosis: a great imitator. *Clin Dermatol*. 2020;38(2):152-159.

Chapters 7.19-7.20

Aung PP, Wimmer DB, Lester TR, Tetzlaff MT, Prieto VG. Perianal condylomata lata mimicking carcinoma. *J Cutan Pathol*. 2022;49(3):209-214.

Bhugra P, Maiti A. Secondary syphilis. *N Engl J Med*. 2020;383(14):1375.

Liu XK, Li J. Histologic features of secondary syphilis. *Dermatology*. 2020;236(2):145-150.

Murphy M, Kerr P, Grant-Kels JM. The histopathologic spectrum of psoriasis. *Clin Dermatol*. 2007;25(6):524-528.

Pourang A, Fung MA, Tartar D, Brassard A. Condyloma lata in secondary syphilis. *JAAD Case Rep*. 2021;10:18-21.

Seline AE, Swick BL. Secondary syphilis. *Cutis*. 2016;97:16;45;46.

Shatley MJ, Walker BL, McMurray RW. Lues and lupus: syphilis mimicking systemic lupus erythematosus (SLE). *Lupus*. 2001;10(4):299-303.

Walkty A, Shute L, Hamza S, Embil JM. Condyloma lata. *IDCases*. 2021;26:e01321.

Chapter 7.21

Chandler DJ, Fuller LC. A review of scabies: an infestation more than skin deep. *Dermatology*. 2019;235(2):79-90.

Chen W, Plewig G. Human demodicosis: revisit and a proposed classification. *Br J Dermatol*. 2014;170(6):1219-1225.

Elston DM. Demodex mites as a cause of human disease. *Cutis*. 2005;76(5):294-296.

Kito Y, Hashizume H, Tokura Y. Rosacea-like demodicosis mimicking cutaneous lymphoma. *Acta Derm Venereol*. 2012;92(2):169-170.

Richards RN. Scabies: diagnostic and therapeutic update. *J Cutan Med Surg*. 2021;25(1):95-101.

Thomas C, Coates SJ, Engelman D, Chosidow O, Chang AY. Ectoparasites: scabies. *J Am Acad Dermatol*. 2020;82(3):533-548.

Chapter 7.22

Cardoso AEC, Cardoso AEO, Talhari C, Santos M. Update on parasitic dermatoses. *An Bras Dermatol*. 2020;95:1-14.

Cestari TF, Pessato S, Ramos-e-Silva M. Tungiasis and myiasis. *Clin Dermatol*. 2007;25(2):158-164.

Coates SJ, Thomas C, Chosidow O, Engelman D, Chang AY. Ectoparasites: pediculosis and tungiasis. *J Am Acad Dermatol*. 2020;82(3):551-569.

Globerson J, Yee D, Olsen S, Bender B. Punked by the punctum: domestically acquired cutaneous myiasis. *Cutis*. 2022;110(2):E37-E39.

Maier H, Hönigsmann H. Furuncular myiasis caused by dermatobia hominis, the human botfly. *J Am Acad Dermatol*. 2004;50(2 suppl):S26-S30.

McGraw TA, Turiansky GW. Cutaneous myiasis. *J Am Acad Dermatol*. 2008;58(6):907-926; quiz 927-929.

Robbins K, Khachemoune A. Cutaneous myiasis: a review of the common types of myiasis. *Int J Dermatol*. 2010;49(10):1092-1098.

INDEX

Note: Page numbers followed by *f* indicate figures.

CHAPTER 1 (INFLAMMATORY DISEASES OF THE EPIDERMIS)

Acute generalized exanthematous pustulosis *vs.* psoriasis (pustular type), 29–30, 30*f*–31*f*
Allergic contact dermatitis *vs.* irritant contact dermatitis, 2, 3*f*
Atopic dermatitis (eczema) *vs.* mycosis fungoides, 8–9, 9*f*–10*f*

Dermatomyositis *vs.* lupus erythematosus (discoid), 70–71, 71*f*–72*f*
Dermatophytosis *vs.* nummular dermatitis, 15, 16*f*–17*f*
Dyshidrotic dermatitis *vs.* palmoplantar pustular psoriasis, 6, 7*f*

Erythema annulare centrifugum *vs.* pityriasis rosea, 11, 12*f*
Erythema multiforme
   vs. fixed drug eruption, 60, 61*f*
   vs. graft-versus-host disease, acute, 58, 59*f*
   vs. morbilliform drug eruption, 62, 63*f*
   vs. pityriasis lichenoides et varioliformis acuta, 56, 57*f*

Fixed drug eruption *vs.* erythema multiforme, 60, 61*f*

Graft-versus-host disease, acute *vs.* erythema multiforme, 58, 59*f*
Guttate psoriasis *vs.* pityriasis rosea, 13, 14*f*

Hypertrophic lichen planus *vs.* squamous cell carcinoma, 42–43, 43*f*–44*f*

Irritant contact dermatitis *vs.* allergic contact dermatitis, 2, 3*f*

Langerhans cell histiocytosis *vs.* lichen nitidus, 48, 49*f*–50*f*
Lichen nitidus *vs.* Langerhans cell histiocytosis, 48, 49*f*–50*f*
Lichen nitidus *vs.* lichen striatus, 45, 46*f*–47*f*
Lichenoid drug eruption *vs.* lichen planus, 37, 38*f*
Lichen planus
   vs. lichenoid drug, 37, 38*f*
   vs. lichen planus–like keratosis, 35, 36*f*
   vs. lichen sclerosus, 39–40, 40*f*–41*f*
   vs. lupus erythematosus, 32, 33*f*–34*f*
Lichen planus–like keratosis *vs.* lichen planus, 35, 36*f*
Lichen simplex chronicus *vs.* psoriasis, 26–27, 27*f*–28*f*
Lichen sclerosus
   vs. lichen planus, 39–40, 40*f*–41*f*
   vs. radiation dermatitis, chronic, 67–68, 68*f*–69*f*
Lichen striatus *vs.* lichen nitidus, 45, 46*f*–47*f*
Lupus erythematosus
   vs. dermatomyositis, 70–71, 71*f*–72*f*
   vs. lichen planus, 32, 33*f*–34*f*
   vs. polymorphous light eruption, 73, 74*f*–75*f*
Lymphomatoid papulosis *vs.* pityriasis lichenoides et varioliformis acuta, 53, 54*f*–55*f*

Morbilliform drug eruption *vs.* erythema multiforme, 62, 63*f*
Mycosis fungoides *vs.* atopic dermatitis (eczema), 8–9, 9*f*–10*f*

Nummular dermatitis
   vs. dermatophytosis, 15, 16*f*–17*f*
   vs. psoriasis (plaque type), 18–19, 19*f*–20*f*

Palmoplantar pustular psoriasis *vs.* dyshidrotic dermatitis, 6, 7*f*
Photoallergic dermatitis *vs.* phototoxic dermatitis, 4, 5*f*
Phototoxic dermatitis *vs.* photoallergic dermatitis, 4, 5*f*
Pityriasis lichenoides chronica *vs.* pityriasis lichenoides et varioliformis acuta, 51, 52*f*
Pityriasis lichenoides et varioliformis acuta
   vs. erythema multiforme, 56, 57*f*
   vs. lymphomatoid papulosis, 53, 54*f*–55*f*
   vs. pityriasis lichenoides chronica, 51, 52*f*
Pityriasis rosea
   vs. erythema annulare centrifugum, 11, 12*f*
   vs. guttate psoriasis, 13, 14*f*
Pityriasis rubra pilaris *vs.* psoriasis (plaque type), 23–24, 24*f*–25*f*
Polymorphous light eruption *vs.* lupus erythematosus (subacute cutaneous), 73, 74*f*–75*f*
Psoriasis
   vs. acute generalized exanthematous pustulosis, 29–30, 30*f*–31*f*
   vs. lichen simplex chronicus, 26–27, 27*f*–28*f*
   vs. nummular dermatitis, 18–19, 19*f*–20*f*
   vs. pityriasis rubra pilaris, 23–24, 24*f*–25*f*
   vs. seborrheic dermatitis, 21, 22*f*

Radiation dermatitis, chronic *vs.* lichen sclerosus, 67–68, 68*f*–69*f*

Seborrheic dermatitis *vs.* psoriasis (plaque type), 21, 22*f*
Squamous cell carcinoma *vs.* hypertrophic lichen planus, 42–43, 43*f*–44*f*
Staphylococcal scalded skin syndrome *vs.* toxic epidermal necrolysis, 64–65, 65*f*–66*f*

Toxic epidermal necrolysis *vs.* staphylococcal scalded skin syndrome, 64–65, 65*f*–66*f*

CHAPTER 2 (INFLAMMATORY DISEASES OF THE DERMIS)

Allergic contact dermatitis *vs.* arthropod assault reaction, 104, 105*f*–106*f*
Arthropod assault reaction
   vs. allergic contact dermatitis, 104, 105*f*–106*f*
   vs. urticaria, 107, 108*f*–109*f*

Behcet disease *vs.* Sweet syndrome, 139, 140*f*–141*f*

Cryoglobulinemic vasculitis *vs.* leukocytoclastic vasculitis, 118–119, 119*f*–120*f*

Eosinophilic granulomatosis with polyangiitis *vs.* granulomatosis with polyangiitis, 121, 122*f*–123*f*
Eruptive xanthoma *vs.* granuloma annulare, 92, 93*f*–94*f*
Erythema chronicum migrans *vs.* urticaria, 110, 111*f*
Erythema elevatum diutinum *vs.* granuloma faciale, 136, 137*f*–138*f*

Foreign body granuloma *vs.* sarcoidosis, 87, 88*f*

Granuloma annulare
   vs. eruptive xanthoma, 92, 93*f*–94*f*
   vs. necrobiosis lipoidica, 81, 82*f*–83*f*
Granuloma faciale
   vs. erythema elevatum diutinum, 136, 137*f*–138*f*
   vs. Sweet syndrome, 133, 134*f*–135*f*
Granulomatosis with polyangiitis *vs.* eosinophilic granulomatosis with polyangiitis, 121, 122*f*–123*f*
Granulomatous rosacea *vs.* sarcoidosis, 84, 85*f*–86*f*

IgA vasculitis *vs.* leukocytoclastic vasculitis, 115, 116*f*–117*f*
Interstitial granuloma annulare
   vs. interstitial granulomatous drug reaction, 95, 96*f*–97*f*
   vs. palisaded neutrophilic granulomamtous dermatitis, 98, 99*f*–100*f*
Interstitial granulomatous drug reaction *vs.* interstitial granuloma annulare, 95, 96*f*–97*f*

Leukocytoclastic vasculitis
   vs. cryoglobulinemic vasculitis, 118–119, 119*f*–120*f*
   vs. IgA vasculitis, 115, 116*f*–117*f*
   vs. pigmented purpuric dermatitis, 124, 125*f*–126*f*
Lichen sclerosus
   vs. morphea, 147, 148*f*–149*f*
   vs. plasma cell mucositis, 145, 146*f*

Morphea *vs.* lichen sclerosus, 147, 148*f*–149*f*

Necrobiosis lipoidica
   vs. granuloma annulare, 81, 82*f*–83*f*
   vs. necrobiotic xanthogranuloma, 89, 90*f*–91*f*
Necrobiotic xanthogranuloma *vs.* necrobiosis lipoidica, 89, 90*f*–91*f*

Palisaded neutrophilic granulomamtous dermatitis *vs.* interstitial granuloma annulare, 98, 99*f*–100*f*
Pernio *vs.* tumid lupus erythematosus, 142, 143*f*–144*f*
Pigmented purpuric dermatitis
   vs. leukocytoclastic vasculitis, 124, 125*f*–126*f*
   vs. stasis dermatitis, 127, 128*f*–129*f*
Plasma cell mucositis *vs.* lichen sclerosus, 145, 146*f*
Pyoderma gangrenosum *vs.* Sweet syndrome, 130, 131*f*–132*f*

Rheumatoid nodule *vs.* subcutaneous granuloma annulare, 101, 102*f*–103*f*

Sarcoidosis
- vs. foreign body granuloma, 87, 88f
- vs. granulomatous rosacea, 84, 85f–86f

Stasis dermatitis vs. pigmented purpuric dermatitis, 127, 128f–129f

Subcutaneous granuloma annulare vs. rheumatoid nodule, 101, 102f–103f

Sweet syndrome
- vs. Behcet disease, 139, 140f–141f
- vs. granuloma faciale, 133, 134f–135f
- vs. pyoderma gangrenosum, 130, 131f–132f

Tumid lupus erythematosus vs. pernio, 142, 143f–144f

Urticaria
- vs. arthropod assault reaction, 107, 108f–109f
- vs. erythema chronicum migrans, 110, 111f
- vs. urticarial vasculitis, 112, 113f–114f

Urticarial vasculitis vs. urticaria, 112, 113f–114f

CHAPTER 3 (VESICULOBULLOUS DISEASE)

Benign familial pemphigus (Hailey-Hailey disease)
- vs. Darier disease, 205–206, 206f–207f
- vs. pemphigus vulgaris, 200–201, 201f–202f
- vs. transient acantholytic dermatosis (Grover disease), 203, 204f

Bullous pemphigoid
- vs. dermatitis herpetiformis, 164–165, 165f–166f
- vs. epidermolysis bullosa acquisita, 158–159, 159f–160f
- vs. pemphigus vulgaris, 155–156, 156f–157f
- vs. porphyria cutanea tarda, 173–174, 174f–175f

Darier disease
- vs. benign familial pemphigus (Hailey-Hailey disease), 205–206, 206f–207f
- vs. pemphigus vulgaris, 185–186, 186f–187f
- vs. transient acantholytic dermatosis (Grover disease), 188–189, 189f–190f

Dermatitis herpetiformis
- vs. bullous pemphigoid, 164–165, 165f–166f
- vs. linear IgA dermatosis, 170, 171f–172f

Epidermolysis bullosa acquisita
- vs. bullous pemphigoid, 158–159, 159f–160f
- vs. porphyria cutanea tarda, 179–180, 180f–181f

Epidermolysis bullosa vs. porphyria cutanea tarda, 182–183, 183f–184f

Linear IgA dermatosis
- vs. bullous pemphigoid, 161–162, 162f–163f
- vs. dermatitis herpetiformis, 170, 171f–172f

Mucous membrane (cicatricial) pemphigoid vs. bullous pemphigoid, 176–177, 177f–178f

Pemphigoid (herpes) gestationis vs. polymorphic eruption of pregnancy, 167, 168f–169f

Pemphigus foliaceus
- vs. bullous impetigo, 194–195, 195f–196f
- vs. pemphigus vulgaris, 191–192, 192f–193f

Pemphigus vulgaris
- vs. benign familial pemphigus (Hailey-Hailey disease), 200–201, 201f–202f
- vs. bullous pemphigoid, 155–156, 156f–157f
- vs. Darier disease, 185–186, 186f–187f
- vs. pemphigus foliaceus, 191–192, 192f–193f
- vs. transient acantholytic dermatosis (Grover disease), 197–198, 198f–199f

Polymorphic eruption of pregnancy vs. pemphigoid (herpes) gestationis, 176–177, 177f–178f

Porphyria cutanea tarda
- vs. bullous pemphigoid, 173–174, 174f–175f
- vs. epidermolysis bullosa, 182–183, 183f–184f
- vs. epidermolysis bullosa acquisita, 179–180, 180f–181f

Transient acantholytic dermatosis (Grover disease)
- vs. benign familial pemphigus (Hailey-Hailey disease), 203, 204f
- vs. Darier disease, 188-189, 189f–190f
- vs. pemphigus vulgaris, 197–198, 198f–199f

CHAPTER 4 (DISORDERS OF THE ADNEXAE)

Acne keloidalis nuchae vs. hidradenitis suppurativa, 237–238, 238f–239f

Acne rosacea vs. acne vulgaris, 229, 230f–231f

Acne vulgaris
- vs. acne rosacea, 229, 230f–231f
- vs. Favre-Racouchot syndrome, 232, 233f

Alopecia areata
- vs. androgenetic alopecia, 211, 212f–213f
- vs. telogen effluvium, 217–218, 218f–219f
- vs. trichotillomania, 220–221, 221f–222f

Androgenetic alopecia
- vs. alopecia areata, 211, 212f–213f
- vs. telogen effluvium, 214, 215f–216f

Central centrifugal cicatricial alopecia vs. lichen planopilaris, 226–227, 227f–228f

Discoid lupus erythematosus alopecia vs. lichen planopilaris, 223–224, 224f–225f

Favre-Racouchot syndrome vs. acne vulgaris, 232, 233f

Follicular infundibular cyst vs. hidradenitis suppurativa, 234–235, 235f–236f

Hidradenitis suppurativa
- vs. acne keloidalis nuchae, 237–238, 238f–239f
- vs. follicular infundibular cyst, 234–235, 235f–236f

Infectious folliculitis vs. keratosis pilaris, 240, 241f

Keratosis pilaris vs. infectious folliculitis, 240, 241f

Lichen planopilaris
- vs. central centrifugal cicatricial alopecia, 226–227, 227f–228f
- vs. discoid lupus erythematosus alopecia, 223–224, 224f–225f

Telogen effluvium
- vs. alopecia areata, 217–218, 218f–219f
- vs. androgenetic alopecia, 214, 215f–216f

Trichotillomania vs. alopecia areata, 220–221, 221f–222f

CHAPTER 5 (DISORDERS OF THE SUBCUTIS)

Alpha-1 antitrypsin deficiency panniculitis vs. pancreatic panniculitis, 273–274, 274f–275f

Behcet disease vs. erythema nodosum, 248, 249f–250f

Calciphylaxis vs. Monckeberg medial calcific sclerosis, 276, 277f

Cold panniculitis vs. lupus panniculitis, 266–267, 267f–269f

Eosinophilic fasciitis vs. scleroderma, 259–260, 260f–261f

Erythema nodosum
- vs. Behcet disease, 248, 249f–250f
- vs. nodular vasculitis, 245, 246f–247f
- vs. traumatic panniculitis, 251, 252f

Infectious panniculitis vs. pancreatic panniculitis, 270, 271f–272f

Lipodermatosclerosis
- vs. morphea, 256–257, 257f–258f
- vs. traumatic panniculitis, 253, 254f–255f

Lupus panniculitis
- vs. cold panniculitis, 266–267, 267f–269f
- vs. subcutaneous panniculitis-like T-cell lymphoma, 262–263, 263f–265f

Monckeberg medial calcific sclerosis vs. calciphylaxis, 276, 277f

Morphea vs. lipodermatosclerosis, 256–257, 257f–258f

Nodular vasculitis
- vs. erythema nodosum, 245, 246f–247f
- vs. polyarteritis nodosa, 278–279, 279f–280f

Pancreatic panniculitis
- vs. alpha-1 antitrypsin deficiency panniculitis, 273–274, 274f–275f
- vs. infectious panniculitis, 270, 271f–272f

Polyarteritis nodosa vs. nodular vasculitis, 278–279, 279f–280f

Scleroderma vs. eosinophilic fasciitis, 259–260, 260f–261f

Subcutaneous panniculitis-like T-cell lymphoma vs. lupus panniculitis, 262–263, 263f–265f

Traumatic panniculitis
- vs. erythema nodosum, 251, 252f
- vs. lipodermatosclerosis, 253, 254f–255f

CHAPTER 6 (ALTERATIONS OF THE EPIDERMIS AND DERMIS)

Acanthosis nigricans
- vs. confluent and reticulated papillomatosis, 292, 293f
- vs. granular parakeratosis, 290, 291f

Adult colloid milium vs. nodular amyloidosis, 324, 325f–326f

Calcinosis cutis vs. gouty tophus, 318–319, 319f–320f

Chondrodermatitis nodularis helicis vs. prurigo nodularis, 287, 288f–289f

Confluent and reticulated papillomatosis vs. acanthosis nigricans, 292, 293f

Cutaneous myxoma vs. focal cutaneous mucinosis, 312, 313f–314f

Digital mucous cyst vs. focal cutaneous mucinosis, 315, 316f–317f

Exogenous ochronosis vs. minocycline-induced hyperpigmentation, 338–339, 339f–340f

Focal cutaneous mucinosis
- vs. cutaneous myxoma, 312, 313f–314f
- vs. digital mucous cyst, 315, 316f–317f

Gouty tophus
- vs. calcinosis cutis, 318–319, 319f–320f
- vs. nodular amyloidosis, 321, 322f–323f

Granular parakeratosis vs. acanthosis nigricans, 290, 291f

Hypertrophic scar vs. keloid, 333, 334f

Ichthyosis vulgaris vs. X-linked ichthyosis, 297–298, 298f–299f

Keloid vs. hypertrophic scar, 333, 334f

Lichen planus–like keratosis vs. porokeratosis, 294, 295f–296f

Mid-dermal elastolysis vs. pseudoxanthoma elasticum, 330–331, 331f–332f

Minocycline-induced hyperpigmentation vs. exogenous ochronosis, 338–339, 339f–340f

Nephrogenic systemic fibrosis vs. scleroderma, 306–307, 307f–308f
Nodular amyloidosis
   vs. adult colloid milium, 324, 325f–326f
   vs. gouty tophus, 321, 322f–323f

Porokeratosis vs. lichen planus–like keratosis, 294, 295f–296f
Postinflammatory hypomelanosis vs. vitiligo, 284–285, 285f–286f
Pretibial myxedema
   vs. scleredema, 300, 301f–302f
   vs. scleromyxedema, 309–310, 310f–311f
Prurigo nodularis vs. chondrodermatitis nodularis helicis, 287, 288f–289f
Pseudoxanthoma elasticum
   vs. mid-dermal elastolysis, 330–331, 331f–332f
   vs. solar elastosis, 327–328, 328f–329f

Scleredema
   vs. pretibial myxedema, 300, 301f–302f
   vs. scleroderma, 303–304, 304f–305f
Scleroderma
   vs. nephrogenic systemic fibrosis, 306–307, 307f–308f
   vs. scleredema, 303–304, 304f–305f
Scleromyxedema vs. pretibial myxedema, 309–310, 310f–311f
Solar elastosis vs. pseudoxanthoma elasticum, 327–328, 328f–329f

Tattoo vs. tumoral melanosis, 335, 336f–337f
Tumoral melanosis vs. tattoo, 335, 336f–337f

Vitiligo vs. postinflammatory hypomelanosis, 284–285, 285f–286f

X-linked ichthyosis vs. ichthyosis vulgaris, 297–298, 298f–299f

CHAPTER 7 (INFECTIOUS DISEASES AND INFESTATIONS OF THE SKIN)

Actinomycosis vs. nocardiosis, 398–399, 399f–400f
Aspergillosis vs. mucormycosis, 370–371, 371f–372f
Atypical mycobacterium vs. erythema nodosum, 395–396, 396f–397f

Benign familial pemphigus vs. varicella-zoster virus (VZV) infection, 383–384, 384f–385f
Blastomycosis
   vs. coccidioidomycosis, 364–365, 365f–366f
   vs. cryptococcosis, 360–361, 361f–363f
Bullous dermatophytosis vs. dyshidrotic dermatitis, 351, 352f–353f
Bullous impetigo vs. staphylococcal scalded skin syndrome, 345–346, 346f–347f

Chromomycosis vs. phaeohyphomycosis, 367–368, 368f–369f
Coccidioidomycosis vs. blastomycosis, 364–365, 365f–366f
Condyloma acuminatum vs. epidermolytic acanthoma, 389–390, 390f–391f
Condyloma lata (secondary syphilis) vs. psoriasis, 404–405, 405f–406f
Cryptococcosis vs. blastomycosis, 360–361, 361f–363f
Cutaneous candidiasis vs. dermatophytosis, 357–358, 358f–359f

Demodicosis vs. scabies, 407–408, 408f–409f
Dermatophytosis
   vs. cutaneous candidiasis, 357–358, 358f–359f
   vs. erythrasma, 348–349, 349f–350f
   vs. tinea versicolor, 354–355, 355f–356f
Dyshidrotic dermatitis vs. bullous dermatophytosis, 351, 352f–353f

Epidermolytic acanthoma vs. condyloma acuminatum, 389–390, 390f–391f
Erythema nodosum vs. Atypical mycobacterium, 395–396, 396f–397f
Erythrasma vs. dermatophytosis, 348–349, 349f–350f

Herpes simplex infection vs. pemphigus vulgaris, 380–381, 381f–382f
Histoplasmosis vs. leishmaniasis, 373–374, 374f–376f

Leishmaniasis vs. histoplasmosis, 373–374, 374f–376f
Leprosy vs. sarcoidosis, 392–393, 393f–394f
Lupus erythematosus vs. secondary syphilis, 401–402, 402f–403f

Majocchi granuloma vs. pityrosporum folliculitis, 377–378, 378f–379f
Molluscum contagiosum vs. verruca vulgaris, 386–387, 387f–388f
Mucormycosis vs. aspergillosis, 370–371, 371f–372f
Myiasis vs. tungiasis, 410, 411f–412f

Nocardiosis vs. actinomycosis, 398–399, 399f–400f

Pemphigus vulgaris vs. herpes simplex infection, 380–381, 381f–382f
Phaeohyphomycosis vs. chromomycosis, 367–368, 368f–369f
Pityrosporum folliculitis vs. Majocchi granuloma, 377–378, 378f–379f
Psoriasis vs. secondary syphilis (condyloma lata), 404–405, 405f–406f

Sarcoidosis vs. leprosy, 392–393, 393f–394f
Scabies vs. demodicosis, 407–408, 408f–409f
Secondary syphilis
   lupus erythematosus vs., 401–402, 402f–403f
   psoriasis vs., 404–405, 405f–406f
Staphylococcal scalded skin syndrome vs. bullous impetigo, 345–346, 346f–347f

Tinea versicolor vs. dermatophytosis, 354–355, 355f–356f
Tungiasis vs. myiasis, 410, 411f–412f

Varicella-zoster virus (VZV) infection vs. benign familial pemphigus (Hailey-Hailey disease), 383–384, 384f–385f
Verruca vulgaris vs. molluscum contagiosum, 386–387, 387f–388f